CARDIAC PACEMAKERS

Publication Number 680

AMERICAN LECTURE SERIES®

A Monograph in

The BANNERSTONE DIVISION *of*
AMERICAN LECTURES IN LIVING CHEMISTRY

Edited by

I. NEWTON KUGELMASS, M.D., Ph.D., Sc.D.

Consultant to the Departments of Health and Hospitals
New York, New York

CARDIAC PACEMAKERS

By

HAROLD SIDDONS, M.Ch., F.R.C.S.

Senior Thoracic Surgeon
St. George's Hospital
London, England

and

EDGAR SOWTON, M.D., M.R.C.P.

Assistant Director
Institute of Cardiology, University of London
Honorary Physician, National Heart Hospital
London, England

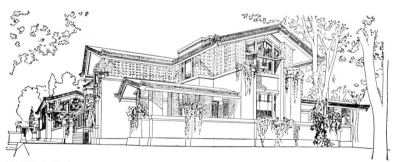

CHARLES C THOMAS · PUBLISHER
Springfield · Illinois · U.S.A.

Published and Distributed Throughout the World by
CHARLES C THOMAS • PUBLISHER
BANNERSTONE HOUSE
301-327 East Lawrence Avenue, Springfield, Illinois, U.S.A.
NATCHEZ PLANTATION HOUSE
735 North Atlantic Boulevard, Fort Lauderdale, Florida, U.S.A.

© 1967, by CHARLES C THOMAS • PUBLISHER
Library of Congress Catalog Card Number: 67-12042

With THOMAS BOOKS *careful attention is given to all details of
manufacturing and design. It is the Publisher's desire to present books
that are satisfactory as to their physical qualities and artistic possibilities
and appropriate for their particular use.* THOMAS BOOKS *will be true
to those laws of quality that assure a good name and good will.*

To our wives

FOREWORD

Oᴜʀ Lɪᴠɪɴɢ Cʜᴇᴍɪsᴛʀʏ Sᴇʀɪᴇs was conceived by Editor and Publisher to advance the newer knowledge of chemical medicine in the cause of clinical practice. The interdependence of chemistry and medicine is so great that physicians are turning to chemistry and chemists to medicine in order to understand the underlying basis of life processes in health and disease. Once chemical truths, proofs and convictions become sound foundations for clinical phenomena, key hybrid investigators clarify the bewildering panorama of biochemical progress for application in everyday practice, stimulation of experimental research and extension of postgraduate instruction. Each of our monographs thus unravels the chemical mechanisms and clinical management of many diseases that have remained relatively static in the minds of medical men for three thousand years. Our new Series is charged with *nisus élan* of chemical wisdom, supreme in choice of international authors, optimal in standards of chemical scholarship, provocative in imagination for experimental research, comprehensive in discussions of scientific medicine and authoritative in chemical perspective of human disorders.

Dr. Siddons and Dr. Sowton of London present the medical, chemical and electronic basis of artificial pacing of the heart to overcome heart block, which produces a very slow natural rate as a result of complete or partial dissociation between atria and ventricle electrical excitation and contraction. If dissociation is complete, contraction of the ventricle has to depend on rhythmic activity of tissue in the A-V node or peripheral to it, which is slow and unreliable. If dissociation is partial between atrium and ventricle, it may be inefficient but leads to complete dissociation with all its consequences. The etiology of chronic disease of the conducting tissue remains obscure without coronary or myocardial disease; hence the need for chemical therapy and cardiac pacing. The most serious clinical manifestations of atrioventricular conduction block are recurrent Stokes-Adams attacks. Episodes of cerebral ischemia resulting from intervals of cardiac arrest are due to a conduction defect in the bundle of His which prevents transmission of impulses from the pacemaker to the ventricles now under the control of an ectopic ventricular pacemaker. It beats regularly but unreliably at 20 to 40 beats per minute and may stop, causing loss of consciousness from cardiac standstill.

The pacemaker of the heart is the trigger that simulates the pump to compress and relax once about every 1.3 seconds, 24 hours a day for life with self-contained oscillators, revealed by recordings from microelectrodes inserted into the pacemaker cells. Animal electricity was known to the ancients from the hundred species of fish that generate currents in warm waters far in excess of domestic requirement—up to 600 v in the electric eel, enough to kill man or beast with its discharge. Their muscle cells are connected in series like a layer-built battery for communication, navigation and defense. Man could not study the behavior of electrical currents until he found some way of producing and controlling them. It is no wonder, therefore, that we have not developed an electrical common sense like the mechanical common sense which has almost become instinctive. There is really nothing more mysterious about electrical forces than about the forces which lift weights or pull trains; in fact, it is the latter which are more complicated. Galvani (1791) stirred scientists by restoring life to dead animals electrically and founded electrophysiology and neurology, while Volta refuted the thesis by generating electricity from metallic sheets and created electrical engineering. The eighteenth century medical world was startled when electricity applied to the heart revived a child who fell from a window and was taken up without signs of life. Stimulation produced no effect until the shocks directed through the chest elicited pulsations and lead to complete recovery within a week. Physicians were already familiar with effects of discharges from Leyden jars upon the lifeless muscles of executed criminals. Burns (1809) passed electric shocks through the chest when vital signs ceased; Walshe (1862), faradic stimulation of cardiac sympathetic nerves; Duchenne (1870), stimulation of the pericardium of an arrested heart in diphtheria; Gould (1920), a needle electrode directly into an infant's myocardium; Zoll (1952) resuscitated a heart in proven ventricular standstill by external electrical stimulation; Chardack (1960), a completely implanted pacemaker.

Cardiac arrest has long been recognized as the initial event in death from functional inability of the heart to maintain effective circulation by its pumping mechanism. The cardiac output can be rendered inefficient and the heart in asystole or in arrhythmia. Diagnosis is presumptive, but made when a conscious patient suddenly becomes unconscious with peripheral pulses absent and the heart beat inaudible. Circulation and respiration exchange must be restored within three minutes before the brain and heart have suffered irreversible damage. Asystole responds to the external cardiac pacemaker applied across the intact chest wall. The shock initiates a ventricular contraction with impulses delivered at a physiological rate of 60 to 80 beats per minute up to 200 v. Persisting Stokes-Adams attacks respond to endocardial pacing with an electric needle inserted directly into the myocardium through the anterior chest wall. The pacemaker is adjusted to deliver 65 to 75 impulses per minute to enable the stroke volume of the heart to increase with the demands of activity. Long-term pacing involves: epicardial electrodes with a buried abdominal pacemaker; endocardial-jugular pacing with an external pacemaker; or endocardial jugular pacing with an implanted pacemaker. The cardiac pacemakers studied by the authors have provided not only an effective therapeutic tool but the means of controlling heart rate, the confirmation of a supernormal phase of A-V conduction and repolarization of ventricular muscle, the elucidation of the nature of arrhythmias, the enhancement of postextrasystolic potentiation and other advances in understanding the circulation of man. Electronic technology is restoring normal cardiac dynamics, reestablishing equilibrial homeostasis and reviving meaningful lives. Why should a man die who has a pacemaker in his chest? *Medicus curat, Nature sanat morbus.*

*New occasions teach new duties
Time makes ancient good uncouth,
He must onward still and upward
Who would keep abreast of truth.*

I. NEWTON KUGELMASS, M.D., PH.D., SC.D., *Editor*

PREFACE

ARTIFICIAL PACING OF THE HEART provides one of the earliest examples of the extension of the use of electronic apparatus beyond
its usual role in clinical medicine. Instead of being used only for
investigation, recording and measurement, electronic equipment
is being used directly for long-term treatment in patients living
relatively normal lives outside hospital. Such patients must rely
for help and advice, not only on their doctors, but also on electronic engineers, metallurgists and physicists; they suffer the ills
of the body and also the failures of their equipment. They are
prone to the faulty transistor or the leaking capacitor, as well as
to heart failure or cardiac infarction. This association between
surgical, medical and technological skills has led to a dynamic
increase in the field of pacing over the past eight years, and in
this monograph we have attempted to collect the information
available at the present time. Our own experience covers some
200 patients, and we have had the opportunity of using pacemakers manufactured in the USA, in England and in various
countries in Europe; we have been able to employ all the main
methods of pacing, using external and internal pacemakers, with
electrodes placed in the myocardium at operation or trans-
venously, with rechargeable or mercury batteries, with induction
or radio frequency power supplies, with fixed-rate or variable
rate, and atrial-triggered units. Much of this clinical experience
was obtained at St. George's Hospital, London, but one of us
(E.S.) was also associated for some time with work in this field
in Stockholm and is now at the National Heart Hospital, London.
In addition to presenting much new material of our own we have
been very fortunate in that many colleagues in other countries
have provided us with hitherto unpublished information. It is

against this background that we have attempted to review the literature.

Our interest in artificial pacing has brought us patients from a wide area and we are grateful to all the doctors who have referred patients. Many patients were sent to Dr. Aubrey Leatham, Cardiologist to both St. George's and the National Heart Hospitals, and he has been kind enough to allow us to share in the responsibility of their care; we are much indebted to him. It is a pleasure to thank Mr. J. G. Davies, on whom the technical aspects of our work so often depend. He designed and made many of the pacemakers we have used.

The provision of 24-hour emergency services and the organization of "pacemaker clinics" at both St. George's and National Heart Hospitals has involved a large number of people and although for clarity we have referred to the patients treated at these hospitals as our own series we are very well aware of the great contributions made by others. Our experience could not have been gained without the assistance and long hours of work of doctors, nurses, x-ray staff and technicians at both centers.

The Appendix contains details of more than 25 pacemakers manufactured in seven countries and includes every unit of which we have knowledge in the world. In most instances, the data was provided by the manufacturers, who have often allowed us access to previously unavailable information, including the basic circuits of this equipment, and we are most grateful to them.

HAROLD SIDDONS
EDGAR SOWTON

CONTENTS

CARDIAC PACEMAKERS

Chapter 1

HISTORICAL REVIEW

STOKES-ADAMS DISEASE

THE ASSOCIATION OF A VERY SLOW PULSE with syncopal attacks has been known for many years and is usually referred to as Stokes-Adams disease or, in Continental Europe, as Morgagni-Adams-Stokes disease. The classical paper of Morgagni, Venice (1761),[529] describes two elderly men, one a grave and worthy priest, the other a merchant from Padua, whose pulses were exceptionally slow and who suffered from epileptic seizures; but even at that date Morgagni was able to refer to a previous report of similar patients written by Marcus Gerbezius, Nuremberg (1719).[267] Morgagni however, was the first to observe that the attacks were preceded by a total absence of the pulse.

Eight further detailed reports—Spens (1793),[722] Burnett (1927),[87] Mayo (1838),[504] Gibson (1838),[269] Law (1840),[421] Holberton (1841),[333] Worthing (1841),[819] including that of Adams (1827),[10] recorded the association of a very slow pulse with syncope or epileptiform seizures, before Stokes in 1846 [737] was able to summarize some of these earlier papers and add two new cases himself. Of the seven cases of which Stokes had knowledge, five had had aortic valve disease. The first evidence of associated coronary disease was in the autopsy report on one of Worthington's two patients, whose coronary arteries "had turned to bone." In 1899, Huchard [344] suggested the name "Stokes-Adams Disease." The condition was described in horses as early as 1837.[23, 597] The history of the condition including subsequent papers, has been surveyed by Lewis in 1958.[443]

THE CONDUCTION SYSTEM

Pioneer work on the conduction system of the heart was done in 1883 by Gaskell [262] who, after working on tortoise hearts, was able to stipulate that there must be a bridge of something other than fibrous tissue between the atria and ventricles, a theory quite contrary to anatomical teaching up to that time. His[322] in Germany and Kent[394] in England described the conducting bundle bridging the gap, both papers appearing in 1893, though the men had been working independently.

In 1906, Tawara[756] of Jena described in greater detail the conducting tissue, named the atrioventricular node, and put forward the view that the fibers already named after Purkinje in 1839[565] were part of the conducting system. In 1907, Keith[390] in England described and named the sino-atrial node, the specialized tissue having the most highly developed property of rhythmicity. This is the *natural pacemaker*, the normal site of initiation of the electrical stimulus to the heart.

ELECTRICAL STIMULATION OF THE HEART

As early as 1819, Aldini[15] had attempted electrical stimulation of the heart in decapitated criminals, and had recommended galvanism for syncope. In 1858, Lister[467] did some experimental work on rabbits which led Walshe, in 1862,[785] in his book *Diseases of the Heart*, to recommend galvanic stimulation for cardiac arrest. Galvanism was used by Duchenne in 1870.[199] He claimed success in treating a diphtheritic patient with a slow pulse, and in 1929, Gould in Sydney, Australia, demonstrated an electrical apparatus with which he had resuscitated a baby.[352]

The first report of attempts to restart the heart of an intact animal was by Hyman in 1932.[352] Bigelow and Callaghan in 1950[44] and in 1951[93] repeated this and showed that rapid electrical stimulation could take over the rate when in normal rhythm.

Cardiac arrest at operation was successfully treated by mechanical stimulation of the sino-atrial node by Sweet in 1947,[745] and Zoll in 1952[825] restarted the arrested human heart with electrical stimulation through the chest wall. In 1957, Allen and Lillehei[17] described the pacing of patients who developed heart block at operation by means of electrodes placed on the heart. Various techniques have been described by which a conducting needle or wire can be pushed through the intact chest wall to contact the ventricle as an electrode, Thevenet in 1958 [757] being the first to use this approach.

Pacing by means of an insulated wire passed along a vein to within the atrium was achieved in the experimental animal in 1954 by Hopps [342] and applied clinically by Leatham in 1959.[165] In 1958, Furman [257] had shown that much lower voltage was sufficient with the electrode in the ventricle, and in 1959 [258] he used this technique on a patient, so introducing the present method of endocardial pacing.

Senning in 1958,[208, 681, 682] was the first to implant an electrical pacemaker, this particular unit being powered from inside but charged electrically from outside the body. The patient survives and is still being paced eight years later.[408] In 1959, Greatbatch [288] patented a pacemaker, and success with this embedded unit powered by mercury cells was reported by Chardack in 1960.[135] In 1961, Zoll [828] reported similar success with another unit. Electrodes were placed on the ventricle at thoracotomy, and this technique proved the most popular for long-term pacing over the ensuing years.

Techniques by which an apparatus outside the body transmits power through the intact skin to an implanted receiver is based on previous work by Loucks in 1933 [479] and Chaffee and Light in 1934 [119] who used electromagnetic induction as an experimental technique to stimulate the nervous system. The scientific basis and early clinical applications of this technique have been reviewed by Mauro (1964).[503] These methods were applied clinically for radio frequency stimulation of the heart in block by Glenn in 1959 in the USA [279] and by Abrams working independently, using simple induction in England in 1960.[8] To eliminate the risk of fracture of wire within the body, Cammilli in 1961 [97] and Schuder in 1962 [663] designed receiver units actually placed on the heart, thus avoiding any implanted wires.

The endocardial venous electrode (electrode catheter) with an external pacemaker, although it avoided a thoracotomy, was not generally adopted as a means of prolonged pacing owing to the risk of septicemia from organisms from outside entering the blood stream along the track of the wire. However, in 1962, Lagergren and Johansson [409] modified this technique by using a long subcutaneous track for the wire before it entered the vein, and thereby reduced the risk of septicemia. In 1963, Lagergren,[409] Siddons [692] and Zucker [840] reported the use of the venous electrode in association with an implanted unit. Abrams [7] and Glenn [855] have combined the induction methods with endocardial electrodes.

Most implanted pacemakers containing their own power source are preset at a fixed rate, though various techniques for altering this rate temporarily have been developed and will be referred to below (see page 92). Butterworth and Poindexter in 1942 [89, 90] experimented in cats and dogs with apparatus which picked up the P wave from the atrium and amplified it before transmitting it to the ventricle. Folkman and Watkins in 1957 [234] used such an apparatus to pace the ventricle of dogs in which an atrioventricular dissociation had been created; they thus achieved physiological changes in rate and gained the benefit of the atrial contraction filling the ventricle immediately prior to its contraction. In 1963, Nathan [548] introduced for clinical use a completely implantable pacemaker of this type.

Up to this time, all pacing had been done to cover periods of failure of ventricular contraction or to speed up the heart from the very slow rate so often seen in complete block. In 1964 a new technique of slowing the heart from an abnormally rapid rate and of increasing contractibility was introduced both by Chardack [131] and by Braunwald *et al.*,[67, 69] as a result of experimental work initiated by Lopez, Edelist and Katz.[476] This technique, using paired stimuli, will be discussed in Chapter 11.

Chapter 2

ETIOLOGY OF STOKES-ADAMS DISEASE

CONGENITAL HEART BLOCK

CONGENITAL COMPLETE heart block has been recognized for many years and is suggested by the history of a slow pulse or syncopal attacks in early childhood, particularly in the absence of infections.[821] The group of patients usually considered together as having "congenital A-V block" probably includes those with several different etiological factors. Some have an absence or malformation of the conduction system,[437, 511] while an intrauterine myocarditis has also been suggested as a cause.[413, 460] Over half the cases occur in association with other congenital cardiac abnormalities,[541] which have been reviewed by Lev [437] and by Hudson.[345]

Unless complete heart block is diagnosed before birth there must be some doubt whether it is truly congenital or whether neonatal complications were the cause; in his series of 178 cases reported from 14 different centers, Michaëlsson [511] found that of the cases without additional congenital heart disease over 40 per cent had complications during delivery, and in 14 per cent cesarean section had been performed. Complete heart block has been diagnosed *in utero*,[353, 541] and Gochberg [280] was able to review 25 cases diagnosed antenatally. The usual cause in these patients is fibrosis below the level of the A-V node before its division into right and left main branches.

Uncomplicated congenital complete heart block is relatively rare, and Gochberg [280] found only three examples in 67,000 deliveries at the Boston Lying-in Hospital between 1936 and 1962; this is equivalent to one case in every 22,000 live births. Michaëlsson [511] estimated the incidence at one in 10,000 to 20,000 liveborn infants and found that in the absence of complicating congenital heart disease, complete block was more common in girls.

There is probably a familial association since the condition has been noted among siblings [511] and may be present in several successive generations.[263, 389] In Nadas' series of 61 children with complete heart block, there was a history of another member of the family having some degree of block in 10 per cent.[541]

Complete heart block occurred in 60 per cent of cases of corrected transposition reviewed by Rotem and Hultgren,[638] who comment that the presence of complete A-V block in a child or young adult should raise the possibility of corrected transposition. This diagnosis accounted for five of the 61 young patients with heart block described by Nakamura and Nadas.[541] The heart block in corrected transposition may first appear during adult life, and Schaefer and Rudolf [654] have described a man who developed congestive heart failure following sudden onset of complete heart block at the age of 36.

Complete heart block is also found in association with ostium primum defects [784, 822] when it is probably due to interruption of the bundle by fibrous tissue. Somerville [711] found the incidence of heart block in this condition to be 5 per cent; she notes that this incidence is increased to 30 per cent in a group of patients with severe disability and points out that the incidence rises with increasing age.

In the absence of complicating cardiac lesions, the prognosis is good,[102, 189] and survival to the age of 57 has been recorded.[85] There is usually a decrease in the ventricular rate with increase in age,[541] but constant ventricular rates up until the age of 15 or an increase in rate with age have also been reported.[511] On exercise there is a considerable increase in the ventricular rate and cardiac output, and the capacity for physical exercise is often near normal.[338, 354, 373, 511]

Stokes-Adams attacks occur, but are rare in patients with congenital complete A-V block,[239, 263, 366, 389, 583] and the risk for an individual patient has been estimated at about 10 per cent.[511] The first attack may occur at any time and has been recorded at the age of 44.[278] Stokes-Adams attacks in this group, as with the acquired disease, may prove fatal and may be precipitated by exercise.[872] Over 5 per cent of Michaëlsson's patients died during a syncopal attack. Artificial pacing has been utilized in a few

patients with congenital heart block and may prove lifesav-
ing.[278, 512, 541, 751] This form of therapy should probably be applied earlier rather than later since the prognosis of congenital
heart block is considerably worse under the age of one year.[413]

POSTSURGICAL HEART BLOCK

Heart block is a well-recognized complication of cardiac operations involving procedures in the region of the conducting
tissues when it is due to actual damage, edema or an inflammatory reaction involving the A-V node, the bundle or their blood
supply. The rhythm change usually occurs during the course of
the operation, but occasionally may develop in the postoperative
period.[455, 458] In 1963, Lillehei reported that approximately 10
per cent of the patients undergoing open heart surgery for VSD,
tetralogy of Fallot or atrioventricularis communis developed
transient or permanent complete heart block;[455] it may also be
produced as a result of operations for aortic stenosis.[679] The block
may be only temporary, and of patients who survive the immediate postoperative interval approximately 75 per cent revert to
sinus rhythm in the first four weeks.[455, 653] It has been estimated
that permanent heart block complicates about 1 per cent of operations for ventricular septal defects and endocardial cushion
defects.[268, 486]

The prognosis of persisting surgically induced heart block is
very bad without pacing,[454, 485, 486] about three-quarters of the
patients who were still in heart block four weeks after the operation dying later in Stokes-Adams attacks.[454] The prognosis is said
to be better when the rhythm change occurs in the postoperative
period rather than during the operation itself.[458]

Drug treatment of this group of patients is unsatisfactory, and
it is now the usual practice for myocardial electrodes to be placed
during operation in any patient with evidence of delayed A-V
conduction. The ventricles can then be paced if necessary during
the operation and in the postoperative phase; this technique has
led to a great reduction in the immediate mortality of postsurgical heart block.[796] The mortality without pacing is considerably
lower (12.5%) in patients who show intermittent complete heart
block in the postsurgical phase as compared to those patients

with persistent complete heart block (80%),[455] and most authors are in agreement that long-term pacing must be instituted in all patients in whom postsurgical complete heart block persists beyond four weeks.[455] The late recurrence of a transitory postsurgical block may necessitate artificial pacing.[596, 805]

ISCHEMIC HEART DISEASE

Complete heart block complicates about 5 per cent of acute myocardial infarction and is a grave prognostic feature; [142, 145, 186, 413, 516, 607] it accompanies posterior infarction more commonly than anterior.[245, 389] In 90 per cent of survivors heart block is transient and sinus rhythm returns within two weeks,[186, 245, 658] and the long-term mortality among patients returning to sinus rhythm is the same as for those who did not develop complete heart block.[142] It is apparent that myocardial infarction will only rarely result in persistent complete heart block,[430] although 9 of 100 cases of complete heart block reported by Kay [389] were associated with recent cardiac infarction. In Papp's series [568] of 150 cases of acute myocardial infarction, the only four patients with complete heart block gave no history of chest pain, and it is possible that patients of this type do not seek medical advice at the time of development of heart block. Occasionally, heart block and Stokes-Adams attacks occur only in association with angina.[845, 865] The management of complete heart block developing during acute myocardial infarction is discussed in Chapter 11.

Coronary artery disease has been widely accepted in the past as the predominant cause of complete heart block, but the evidence for this diagnosis is often unconvincing. Penton [589] quotes 43 per cent of a series of 251 patients, and other authors have quoted figures of 69 per cent,[820] 73 per cent,[640] 52 per cent,[389] 48 per cent [245] and 42 per cent [888] as being due to disease of coronary arteries. The diagnosis in these patients rests on clinical and electrocardiographic evidence, and the difficulties of diagnosing ischemic heart disease in patients with complete heart block are considerable, while the presence of ischemic heart disease is to be expected in a proportion of patients with heart block and need have no etiological connection. A history of chest pain does not necessarily indicate infarction or angina; [306, 713] it may be produced by a change in rhythm, particularly as effort has been shown to precipitate heart block in certain patients.[240] The electrocardiograph is often difficult to interpret because left ventricular hypertrophy accompanies long-standing bradycardia,[583] while in addition, 60 per cent of patients with complete heart block have QRS complexes of the bundle branch block pattern (see p. 30).

Patients referred for artificial pacing form a selected group, and the incidence of coronary artery disease in this group is probably unduly low. Nearly all of these patients have experienced at least one Stokes-Adams attack and many have had multiple attacks over several years; it seems likely that these episodes, during which coronary perfusion is absent, represent severe biological stress. Patients with severe ischemic heart disease would be unlikely to survive repeated stresses of this type, and so a series of paced patients is probably heavily biased in favor of those who have unusually clear coronary arteries for their age and have successfully undergone a prolonged period of self-selection.[713] This theory is favored by the results of postmortem coronary angiography performed on 19 of our patients; [306] fifteen of these patients had normal coronary vessels and only two had slight coronary arterial disease. Also the study of serial histological sections of the conducting tissue of 40 of our patients revealed evidence of ischemia as the probable cause of the complete heart block in 5.[887] This suggestion that patients with heart block caused by ischemic heart disease often die during their first Stokes-Adams attack is supported by reports that the prognosis differs between patients with and without Stokes-Adams attacks. Those who have attacks survive statistically twice as long as those without,[589, 640] and both Johansson [366] and Gilchrist [273] reported that the prognosis was quite good if patients survived the first few months.

PRIMARY HEART BLOCK

There is now a considerable amount of evidence that a large proportion of patients, probably nearly 50 per cent, with acquired heart block have only minor cardiac lesions and typically show small areas of fibrosis involving the conducting system either alone or in association with scattered areas of fibrosis in the myocardium. These multiple localized sclerotic lesions frequently involve both right and left conducting branches rather than the main bundle of His and correlate well with the ECG changes.[434, 437, 483] In most patients the process is probably related only to advancing age,[437] but it is impossible to exclude old myocarditis or minor ischemic changes [662] as etiological factors. The end results are the same in that the lesions are small and hardly affect myocardial function at all unless A-V block is produced. It seems likely that patients of this type have been reported under different headings by different authors. In an analysis of 50 cases of complete heart block, Zoob and Shirley Smith [839] found no clear etiology in 30 and suggested the term "primary heart block" for this group. Autopsy of two of their patients disclosed only focal disease of the conducting tissue. Lev [437] described the condition as "sclerosis of the left side of the cardiac skeleton" and ascribed it to wear and tear resulting from the repeated pull of the left ventricular musculature. He noted that it can first be detected at about the age of 40. Lenègre [433] found "sclerosing degenerative changes in the A-V conducting system" to be present in 21 of his 44 patients (48%) without fresh myocardial infarction, and fibrosis of the conducting system has also been reported by many other authors.[187, 366, 437, 490, 589, 598, 687, 814] In his report of 48 cases of complete heart block, Yater [823] found that 19 (40%) showed no evidence of any cause apart from extremely localized fibrosis, and in particular these 19 cases had no evidence of myocardial ischemia. Ellis [206] was unable to identify the etiology in 14 of his 37 patients (38%) treated by pacing.

A possible mechanism for the development of A-V block in patients with clear coronary arteries was put forward by Biss [48] as a result of his study of five patients dying from Stokes-Adams attacks. He suggested that mild aortic incompetence resulted from senile dilatation of the aortic ring and the resulting regurgitant stream caused a jet lesion on the intraventricular septum with involvement of the underlying bundle of His.

Of 483 patients with Stokes-Adams disease reported in seven series published since 1961,[158, 206, 245, 366, 434, 713, 839] the etiology was unknown in 152 (32%) and there was no evidence of coronary artery disease in 278 (58%).

In a review of 552 patients with 1st, 2nd and 3rd degree heart block Moreau [527] assessed the etiology as being due to coronary atherosclerosis in 134 (24.3%) and to be unknown in 150 (27.2%).

Whatever the exact etiology, this concept of the disease of the conducting tissues with good myocardial function is supported by coronary angiograms performed not only post mortem [157, 687] but also in patients with complete heart block, when arteries to the conducting tissue have been shown to be normal.[237] The absence of significant myocardial disease in patients with primary heart block makes them ideal candidates for treatment with artificial pacemakers. We have often noted that such patients appear much younger than their years and consider that this is possibly related to a generalized absence of atheroma in keeping with the clear coronary arteries often found in patients with Stokes-Adams attacks.

CARDIOMYOPATHY

Cardiomyopathies of various types may be associated with complete heart block. Rossi [636] reports block occurring in amyloidosis, and patients with familial cardiomyopathy have been treated by artificial pacing.[294] Several of our own patients were diagnosed on clinical grounds as having cardiomyopathy, and postmortem studies of the hearts of some of our patients have indicated that this etiology may be more common than is usually appreciated.[169]

HYPERTENSION

Many authors have noted the apparent association between systolic hypertension and complete heart block, and some have indicated that the high blood pressure was a cause of Stokes-Adams disease.[158, 245, 261, 332, 389, 430, 527, 589, 640] The systolic hypertension of patients with complete heart block is in many instances no more than a reflection of the large stroke volume, and when the ventricular rate is increased by artificial pacing the blood pressure returns to normal levels (see p. 182).[42, 450, 687] The mean changes in blood pressure with pacing in 50 of our patients [713]

TABLE I

MEAN BLOOD PRESSURE CHANGES ON PACING IN 50 PATIENTS

	Mean Change in Systolic Pressure	Mean Change in Diastolic Pressure
25 men	−51.2 mm Hg	+6.4 mm Hg
25 women	−49.4 mm Hg	+3.6 mm Hg

are shown in Table 1. The overall effect of pacing was a fall in the systolic pressure of about 50 mmHg with a rise in the diastolic of about 5 mmHg. An elevated diastolic pressure during complete heart block, as opposed to a high systolic level, is of significance, and we consider that a diastolic pressure above 100 mmHg before pacing indicates the presence of true hypertension. When these criteria are adopted, hypertension is rare amongst patients treated with artificial pacemakers [306] and probably has no etiological significance.

DIPHTHERIA

Diphtheria has been described as causing Stokes-Adams attacks,[401] and there are many reports of heart block associated with diphtheritic attacks.[210, 229, 361, 490, 499, 500, 552, 734] Diphtheria has also been described as a cause of heart block persisting or developing in later life,[88, 445, 589, 612,] and nearly 18 per cent of our own cases gave a history of diphtheria in childhood.[306] As diphtheria used to be a common disease of childhood, and as the figures in a control population who did not develop complete heart block are not available, we feel, like Perrotin,[591] that the evidence implicating it as a cause of Stokes-Adams disease is unconvincing.

SYPHILIS

Syphilis has been implicated as a cause by several authors,[332, 378, 389] and this aspect of the subject has been reviewed by Lev.[436] The mechanism of block in this condition was usually a gumma involving the conducting system but this is now an exceptionally rare cause of complete heart block.

DIABETES

Diabetes occurred in 14 of 36 patients (39%) with heart block reported by Gadboys,[261] but this figure is unusually high, and

Johansson [366] reports an incidence of 7 per cent. In our own series three of the first hundred patients (3%) had diabetes.

VALVULAR DISEASE

Rheumatic fever may cause heart block during the acute phase,[101, 156, 243, 270, 292, 297, 437, 647,] but it is more likely to be important in the etiology of heart block when valvular disease results.[589, 640] Mitral valve disease, presumably rheumatic, has been implicated by several authors.[282, 322] In our own series,[306] 4 per cent of the patients gave a history of rheumatic fever, and one patient had mitral valve disease with conducting tissue involved in the heavily calcified annulus.

Aortic valve disease, particularly calcified aortic stenosis, has long been recognized as a cause of heart block, and, of the seven cases reported by Stokes,[737] five had aortic valve disease. The development of A-V dissociation may be long delayed, and Gilchrist [273] reports two patients who developed block at the ages of 85 and 62. The usual mechanism is involvement of conducting tissue by calcification, but traumatic block can occur during aortic valve surgery. Calcific aortic stenosis accounted for eight (22%) of Ellis's [206] 37 patients with Stokes-Adams disease, for five (11%) of Lenègre's 44 cases [433] and for three (3%) of our first 100 paced cases. Heart block may disappear after surgical correction of aortic stenosis.[492] Calcification of the mitral annulus with involvement of the bundle of His, the so-called Rytand's syndrome,[644, 645] is a relatively uncommon cause of complete heart block, although it occurred in one of our patients. One patient with Rytand's syndrome, in whom block appeared only when the atrial rate increased, has been reported by Day and Viar.[171]

RHEUMATOID ARTHRITIS

Rheumatoid arthritis was also present in 4 per cent of our series and has been described as an etiological factor in the development of heart block; [77, 284, 564] the block may precede the joint manifestations.[331] Apart from our own cases, artificial pacing has been reported by Hoffman and Leight.[331] The association of rheumatoid (ankylosing) spondylitis and heart block has been discussed by Julkunen and Luomanmäki.[375]

OTHER INFECTIONS

Many other infections have been implicated, and in endemic areas Chagas' disease is a common cause.[416, 629] Coura,[149] working in the area around Rio de Janeiro, found that among patients with symptomatic Chagas' disease, the incidence of Stokes-Adams attacks was 5 per cent; in an electrocardiographic study of 100 patients he found 15 with complete heart block, 13 with partial block, 50 with right bundle branch block and 6 with left bundle branch block. Successful treatment by artificial pacing has been reported.[317] Heart block has also been recorded in the course of scarlet fever,[39, 584] pneumonia,[746] influenza,[162] tuberculosis,[508] typhoid fever,[162, 609] typhus fever,[473] mumps,[630] measles,[141] rubella,[473] malaria,[609] amebic hepatitis,[610] pertussis [428] and sarcoidosis.[58, 519, 574, 593]

MISCELLANEOUS CAUSES OF HEART BLOCK

Unusual causes of heart block include non-specific myocarditis,[437, 812] myxedema,[427] progressive muscular dystrophy,[359 431] hemochromatosis,[592] cardiac lymphangitis,[637] Paget's disease,[310, 815, 820] calcified ventricular aneurysm,[406] non-penetrating chest wounds [585, 748] and tumors which involve the A-V node or bundle. These may be primary or secondary [491, 615, 640, 753, 823] and may be amenable to surgical treatment [437] or radiotherapy.[242, 873]

Pacing has been necessary in the treatment of A-V block from several rarer causes. Reports include patients with dermatomyositis [698] and systemic lupus erythematosus,[657] a condition in which A-V block may be more common than usually realized.[362, 523]

DRUGS AS A CAUSE OF HEART BLOCK

Digitalis

Digitalis overdose may prolong the PR interval and lead to complete A-V block,[244, 670] or may induce ventricular fibrillation.[21, 671] Stokes-Adams attacks are said to be rare in digitalis-induced block.[589] A Stokes-Adams attack due to digitalis-induced ventricular asystole in a 67-year-old woman was reported by Leon-Sotomayer; [435] external stimulation at 150 volts was ineffective, but pacing via an electrode catheter in the right ventricle was successfully continued for 24 hours. Tamura [753] produced experimental heart block in dogs with digitalis and noted that pacing of the ventricle could still be effective even in the presence of a high concentration of calcium. We have seen ventricular arrest from digitalis overdose in three patients, and in each case external pacing with electrodes on the chest wall restarted the heart.[714] The role of potassium in digitalis-induced block is difficult to assess since hyperkalemia is itself a cause of block [327] and this effect is increased by digitalis.[226] The whole field of the use of digitalis in complete heart block has been reviewed by Schwartz and Schwartz.[670, 671]

Quinidine

Quinidine may cause syncopal attacks due to asystole or to a rapid ventricular arrhythmia in patients with or without A-V conduction.[45, 395, 619, 685] Two of our own cases developed ventricular asystole during attempted reversion of atrial fibrillation to sinus rhythm with quinidine; in both patients pacing with external electrodes was successful.

Stokes-Adams attacks have also been reported as complications of treatment with streptomycin,[235] Prostigmin®,[40] pilocarpine,[118] potassium antimony tartrate [686] and procaine amide.[318, 413] It seems possible that pacing may have a very limited part to play in keeping such patients alive long enough for the toxic effects of drugs to disappear.

NEUROGENIC STOKES-ADAMS DISEASE

The vagal distribution includes fibers to both S-A and A-V nodes as well as to the atrium and the upper part of the bundle of His.[705] Vagal over-activity may inhibit impulse formation and cause or enhance A-V block. The effect of vagal stimulation in dogs with complete heart block was studied by Brockman.[74] In over 400 experiments on 32 dogs he was unable to produce ventricular asystole and could not demonstrate any alteration in ventricular myocardial contractility although atrial arrest always occurred. There was a minimal fall in ventricular rate (about 3%) and in aortic systolic blood pressure (about 4%) unless the ventricles were paced artificially, in which case vagal stimulation had no effect whatsoever on the ventricle.

As expected from these results, the clinical effects of excess vagal activity are seen in patients with intermittent heart block where cardio-inhibitory reflexes are important factors in provoking syncopal attacks.[671] Complete A-V block may rarely be provoked by vagal reflexes during Cheyne-Stokes respiration, particularly in patients receiving digitalis.[501] A similar observation has been made by Schwartz and Schwartz,[671] who reported that in some patients deep breathing could cause ventricular standstill and syncope after digitalization, and that this "pulmonary stretch reflex" could be present in patients with normal sinus rhythm, 2:1 or complete heart block.

Carotid sinus stimulation in dogs with complete heart block results in ventricular bradycardia or asystole and a profound negative inotropic effect on the ventricular muscles due to reflex diminution in cardiac sympathetic tone.[74] Spontaneous Stokes-Adams attacks due to a hypersensitive carotid sinus reflex or to excess vagal activity [224, 417, 588, 730, 770, 798] are very rare, but syncopal attacks are more likely to occur if the patient is digitalized [671] or if a carotid sinus tumor is present.[671, 798] Johansson has reported neurogenic Stokes-Adams attacks in two patients, one with a bronchial carcinoma [365] and one with gallbladder disease.[364] Excess vagal activity has also been implicated in patients with Stokes-Adams attacks due to sino-atrial block; such cases have been successfully treated by pacing with electrodes attached either to the ventricle [858] or to the atrium.[107]

INCIDENCE OF STOKES-ADAMS DISEASE

Estimates of the incidence with which complete heart block or Stokes-Adams disease occurs in the general population must necessarily be based on inadequate information, but several lines of approach may be used to obtain an approximate estimate. The incidence of complete heart block among members of hospital populations can be assumed to be higher than that among members of the general population and so calculations based on these figures are known to be too high. An analysis of 49,000 patients attending the University of Texas hospitals over a 25-year period was made by Wright,[820] who found that complete heart block occurred in 90 subjects (0.2%); complete heart block was found by Rowe and White [640] in 350 of 160,000 electrocardiograms taken between 1925 and 1955 at the Massachusetts General Hospital. If these figures were applicable to the general population of the United States they would represent an incidence of about 11,000 new cases of complete heart block every year, and it follows, therefore, that the actual incidence must be less than this.

Michaëlsson [511] has estimated that there is one case of *congenital* heart block in every 10,000 to 20,000 live births and that between one-third and one-half of these subjects will have additional congenital heart disease. The relative frequency of *congenital* and *acquired* heart block can be very approximately obtained from the literature; uncomplicated congenital heart block accounted for 5 per cent of the 140 patients in Gilchrist's series,[273] 6 per cent of Rowe and White's series [640] and 7 per cent of Wright's series.[820] A combination of these figures with those provided by Michaëlsson, together with the official figures for the birth rate in the United States, leads to an estimate of about 5,000 new cases of complete heart block arising each year in the United States.

More direct estimates of the incidence of heart block in the normal population are extremely scarce. Kantrowitz [381] has sug-

TABLE II

Method of Calculation	Incidence of New Cases of Heart Block/Million Population/Year	Comment
American hospital population	57	Higher than in general population
Extrapolated from incidence of congenital block	26	Method inaccurate but based on general population
Figures given by Kantrowitz	160–200	Considerably too high—based on highly selected series
Figures given by Johansson	63	Based on general population

gested that there may be 25,000 to 30,000 new cases each year
in the United States (about 160-200 per million population), but
as he based this figure on the number of patients seen personally
at a pacing center it is certainly too high. The best estimate at
present available is probably that of Johansson,[888] who, over a
15 year period (1951-1964), collected 193 new cases of complete
heart block from the fairly closed community of Malmö, Sweden.
This he calculated as 63 cases per million population per year.

TABLE III

Country	Approximate Estimate of New Cases of Complete Heart Block Each Year
Australia	550
Austria	365
Britain	2,500
Canada	965
Denmark	235
Finland	215
France	2,335
Germany	2,915
Holland	600
Israel	125
Italy	2,500
Japan	4,665
New Zealand	125
Norway	185
Sweden	375
Switzerland	290
United States of America	9,585

A comparison between these various methods of calculation
is shown in Table II, where the probable incidence of new cases
of complete heart block arising each year per million population
is given. The errors implicit in estimates based on such scanty
information and unsatisfactory methods of deduction are self-
evident, but a consideration of all the above figures leads us to
suggest that the likely incidence of complete heart block is, very
approximately, 50 new cases per million population per year.
Using population figures supplied by the London embassies of
various countries this incidence can be converted into the number of new cases of complete heart block which may be expected
each year in the countries concerned, and these results are shown
in Table III.

SUMMARY AND CONCLUSIONS

Congenital heart block occurs in one of 10,000 to 20,000 live births and is particularly associated with corrected transposition, ostium primum septal defects and complicated congenital heart disease. About half the cases are uncomplicated, and the survivors of this group account for about 6 per cent of all new cases of complete heart block.

Heart block developing during cardiac surgery is usually associated with operations on septal defects or the aortic valve. It is often temporary, but if it persists beyond four weeks postoperatively the prognosis is very bad unless long term pacing is undertaken.

About 5 per cent of patients with cardiac infarction develop acute heart block, which is more common with posterior lesions than anterior. In survivors the block usually remits within two weeks, but patients with persisting block account for about 10 per cent of all cases with chronic heart block.

Coronary atherosclerosis is not the major cause of chronic block; one-third to one-half of the patients with complete heart block have degenerative changes affecting mainly the conduction tissue ("primary heart block"), and patients with a history of many Stokes-Adams attacks may have unusually clear coronary arteries. Complete heart block is more common than is usually realized in collagen disorders and in cardiomyopathy.

The approximate incidence of complete heart block is estimated at 50 new cases per million population per year. Figures are given converting this incidence into the number of new cases to be expected each year in various countries.

Chapter 3

CLINICAL PRESENTATION

FREQUENCY OF STOKES-ADAM'S ATTACKS AMONG PATIENTS WITH COMPLETE HEART BLOCK

THE INCIDENCE HAS been variously quoted as being between 35 per cent [221] up to the more common figure of 67 per cent; [286, 589] it is sometimes stated that Stokes-Adam's attacks are rare in children and that the incidence increases directly with increasing age,[684] but we have been unable to find confirmation of this, and in our experience the age-related incidence of syncope has not been striking. In his series of 178 cases of congenital heart block collected from 14 centers in Finland and Sweden, Michaëlsson [511] reported that Stokes-Adams' attacks may occur at any time, and that 23 of his patients had died from this cause.

SYNCOPAL ATTACKS

A short period of extreme bradycardia or ventricular tachycardia will result in loss of cardiac output for a few seconds, and unconsciousness usually follows unless cerebral blood flow is restored within 5 to 10 seconds. A Stokes-Adams attack may be so short that unconsciousness is not lost and the patient merely staggers, but the more usual clinical picture is that the patient suddenly becomes completely unconscious. An experienced patient recognizes that an attack is imminent and so is often able to sit down before unconsciousness occurs. During the latent period there is extreme facial pallor which persists during the period of unconsciousness and may possibly develop into cyanosis. During an attack the pulse is absent or extremely slow, while heart sounds and blood pressure are absent. Dilatation of the pupils usually occurs, and if unconsciousness persists for long enough, there are frequently small muscular twitchings which may progress to convulsions or even focal neurologic phenomena which may leave permanent sequelae.[366] Increases in the depth and frequency of breathing during attacks have been described,[285] but respiration is usually gasping or stertorous and may cease if the attack is prolonged. The termination of a Stokes-Adams attack is usually as dramatic as the onset, and the subject recovers consciousness rapidly with the development of a red flush of the face and limbs. Attacks are usually of short duration and consciousness is recovered within one minute, but occasionally the patient does not really recover consciousness before a further attack develops.

Differentiation between attacks due to ventricular asystole and those due to rapid ventricular rhythms (tachyarrhythmia) may require electrocardiographic proof during a syncopal episode, but there are certain clinical features which are helpful in the differential diagnosis. If the pulse rate is normally slow, indicating complete heart block, but there are many ectopic beats and perhaps a history of short bursts of rapid irregular rhythm, then it is very likely that the syncopal attacks are due to ventricular tachyarrhythmia. The latent period before consciousness is lost is frequently greater when the attacks are due to ventricular tachycardia than when they are due to asystole, since the fall in cardiac output is less dramatic when the ventricle continues to beat; a history of consciousness being slowly lost over some 20 or 30 seconds is suggestive that the Stokes-Adams attack is due to a rapid ventricular rate. If the syncopal attacks occur at a time when the preceding pulse rate was normal, then it is unlikely that a rapid ventricular ryhthm is the cause, and asystole is much more likely; it is rare for syncopal attacks caused by asystole to occur without the preceding development of a short period of slow idioventricular rhythm. After a Stokes-Adams attack the pulse is often slow for a short period, even in patients who were previously in sinus rhythm, and this point may be helpful in the differential diagnosis, suggesting that the attack was due to ventricular asystole.

It is important to bear in mind that drug therapy may influence the cause of the attacks, and on several occasions we have noted that patients whose previous Stokes-Adams attacks were always due to ventricular asystole developed attacks due to rapid ventricular arrhythmias when taking sympathomimetic drugs.

DIFFERENTIATION OF STOKES-ADAMS ATTACKS
FROM EPILEPSY

Epilepsy is a common misdiagnosis in patients with Stokes-Adams attacks, particularly when sinus rhythm is present between syncopal episodes, and 5 per cent of the patients in our series had previously been diagnosed and treated for epilepsy. If the typical history of a slow pulse and a Stokes-Adams attack is available the differential diagnosis presents no difficulty, but the presence of any ECG abnormality in a patient with epilepsy should always raise the suspicion of Stokes-Adams disease. The suggestion of Portal [598] that "epilepsy plus right bundle branch block equals Stokes-Adams disease" will often be found to be correct. The main differentiating features favoring epilepsy are the characteristic aura followed by generalized tonic and clonic muscular constrictions, often associated with urinary incontinence and tongue biting, a sequence of events which does not occur normally during Stokes-Adams attacks. After the syncopal episode the epileptic patient commonly has a period of impaired consciousness with amnesia and perhaps temporary neurological deficit, while recovery from a Stokes-Adams attack is usually immediate, complete and may be associated with flushing. If a reliable witness of the attack is available, the most useful diagnostic point is that the pulse is absent during a Stokes-Adams attack but present during an epileptic attack; occasionally an electrocardiogram will be required for final differentiation. It should be noted that Stokes-Adams disease and epilepsy are not mutually exclusive diagnoses, and that the presence of one condition is no guarantee against the presence of the other also; in fact, epileptiform features may even be due to cerebral damage suffered during previous Stokes-Adams attacks. As Johansson [366] pointed out, a syncopal attack in a patient with heart block need not be a Stokes-Adams attack.

PRECIPITATING CAUSES OF STOKES-ADAMS ATTACKS

Attacks can occur in many circumstances, and we have witnessed attacks due to ventricular tachyarrhythmia and due to ventricular asystole even during sleep; such attacks may wake the patient. It is usually impossible to identify the precipitating

cause of syncopal attacks. Some patients are particularly liable
to attacks when changing posture.[666] Emotional factors have
been implicated in Stokes-Adams attacks of vagal origin,[790] but
Schwartz did not find emotional disturbances an important factor in precipitating attacks in patients in sinus rhythm.[666] It is
possible that the animal experiments reported by Citters [140] may
be relevant to human patients with complete heart block; in these
investigations, stimulation of a very localized area, less than
2 mm in depth, in the hypothalamus in dogs with complete heart
block provoked episodes of ventricular tachycardia with rates
of up to 280 beats per minute. An association between ventricular tachycardia and lesions in the central nervous system in
human subjects is suggested by electroencephalographic abnormalities associated with the ventricular arrhythmia,[791] and Nadas
has reported a case of a five-year-old girl in whom a fracture of
the base of the skull was followed by paroxysmal ventricular
arrhythmias which had not disappeared after a year.[539] It is
interesting to note that two of Johansson's [366] patients in whom
no etiology for syncopal attacks could be found had sustained
cerebral concussion earlier in their lives, one of the patients having a fractured skull.

Stokes-Adams attacks have been reported following severe
hemorrhage,[524] and reflexes from subdiaphragmatic organs have
frequently been implicated.[364, 799] The removal of an infected
gallbladder is said to be of therapeutic value occasionally.[364, 489]
Stokes-Adams attacks provoked by swallowing in a patient with
an esophageal diverticulum and bronchial carcinoma were reported by Johansson,[365] who reviewed the German literature
dealing with other patients whose syncopal attacks were provoked by stimulation of "trigger areas" in the neck. A very similar
situation has been described in a cow with Stokes-Adams attacks
provoked by massage of the neck in the region of the vagus
nerve; subsequently the heart was found to be normal, but the
vagus nerve had been punctured by a small piece of wire.[82]

Stokes-Adams attacks due to ventricular asystole are particularly likely to occur in patients with unstable heart block; [273, 413]
exercise may provoke alterations in the degree of heart block
or may result in the appearance of heart block in a patient who

has sinus rhythm when at rest, and this transient change in A-V
conduction may be associated with Stokes-Adams attacks.[240, 273]
Gilchrist states that in Type 2 partial block (see p. 29) there
is often a critical atrial rate of about 70 to 80 beats per minute;
if this rate is exceeded, 2:1 A-V block suddenly appears and the
degree of block increases as the atrial rate becomes faster. This
may be the mechanism involved in the development of heart
block during exercise and perhaps also explains the use of atropine as a provocative test.[273] It is interesting to note that the
PR interval in normal subjects progressively lengthens as the
atrial rate is increased by pacing with an artificial pacemaker,
leading to the eventual production of temporary complete heart
block (see p. 35).

PAIN

Patients with complete heart block frequently give a history
of chest pain which is often assumed to be anginal in type;[249]
it has been shown that coronary blood flow decreases with the
onset of heart block[727] and that it is lower at slow ventricular
rates than at normal or fast rates.[38, 429] A central chest pain occur-
ing in relation to the onset of complete heart block need not
indicate ischemic heart disease, and we have seen several patients who gave an excellent history of ischemic cardiac pain yet
at autopsy had clear coronary arteries with no evidence of ischemic changes in the myocardium.[306, 713] Possible alternative ex-
planations of the chest pain are distention of the left ventricle[240,
509] or of the aorta, and although Froment[249] considered the pain
to be due to myocardial ischemia, he reported three cases who
experienced pain associated with heart block but had no evidence of coronary artery disease; it seems likely that, whatever
the origin of the pain, it does not have the same significance as
true anginal pain experienced in sinus rhythm or when heart
block has been long established. In Fowler's[240] patients, pain
was repeatedly provoked by exercise but was associated with an
increase in the degree of block, being unrelieved by rest unless
the block remitted, and not occurring on effort unless the heart
block was also provoked.

LOW CARDIAC OUTPUT

Although a syncopal attack is the most dramatic presentation of patients with complete heart block, many patients suffered from additional symptoms related to a low cardiac output associated with bradycardia. The low output results in fatigue, clouding of the sensorium, slow cerebration,[161] poor exercise tolerance (particularly faintness on exertion) and sometimes heart failure and renal failure. Friedberg[246] reported that bradycardia alone does not produce congestive cardiac failure in human subjects, although it is a significant contributory cause; he claimed that coexistent myocardial or renal disease are needed for the development of impaired sodium excretion and heart failure. Many other miscellaneous complaints have also been made by the patients in our series; these complaints include abdominal pain, diarrhea, difficulty in hearing, dry mouth, inability to speak loudly, blurred vision, paresthesia of the limbs, nervousness, irritability and throbbing felt widely over the body. Some of these complaints are related to the low cardiac output or the wide pulse pressure of complete heart block, but the presentation is undoubtedly influenced by psychological factors.

Symptoms are particularly troublesome when heart block is of recent origin. Accommodation to the slow heart rate occurs over the next few weeks, with many patients improving considerably. Recovery from heart failure following surgical induction of heart block in dogs has been reported,[727] and we and others[413] have observed a similar clinical course in patients following the sudden onset of complete heart block. This adaptation to a slow ventricular rate occurs primarily by an increase in the maximum available stroke volume[338] (see p. 181), but an additional mechanism is a widening of the arterial-venous oxygen difference.

ELECTROCARDIOGRAPHIC FEATURES OF STOKES-ADAMS DISEASE

ECG During Syncopal Attacks

Stokes-Adams attacks are due to ventricular asystole or to very rapid ventricular activity; the distinction between short periods of asystole and a profound bradycardia [173, 571] is a matter of terminology only. A rapid ventricular arrhythmia may be a tachycardia or ventricular fibrillation, and the term "tachyarrhythmia" has been widely used in Europe.[413] Repeated syncopal attacks in the same subject are usually [182, 366, 714] but not invariably [413] related to the same arrhythmia. Parkinson [571] analyzed the electrocardiograms during Stokes-Adams attacks in eight patients of his own and 56 cases from the literature; he found ventricular asystole alone caused 55 per cent of the attacks and ventricular tachycardia with or without subsequent standstill in 45 per cent. In 100 of our own patients,[306] 77 per cent had attacks caused by ventricular asystole alone and 7 per cent caused by ventricular tachycardia alone; in the remaining 16 per cent the attacks were due to both asystole and ventricular tachycardia, so that in 83 per cent of the patients Stokes-Adams attacks were associated with at least short periods of ventricular standstill and could thus be terminated by pacing.

Atrial activity usually persists during Stokes-Adams attacks,[366, 413, 713] but there may be complete lack of atrial and ventricular activity.[770] Syncopal attacks which appear clinically to be identical with the Stokes-Adams syndrome have been reported in which the mechanism was a rapid ventricular response to atrial arrhythmias; [295] only one patient in our series experienced Stokes-Adams attacks due to supraventricular tachycardia without the preceding development of a ventricular bradycardia, and other authors have also noted that Stokes-Adams attacks due to rapid ventricular rhythms rarely arise from sinus rhythm.[413]

ECG apart from Syncopal Attacks

Heart block is usually classified under three headings—first, second and third degree block.

First degree block is present when the PR interval is longer than 0.20 seconds.

Second degree block is also referred to as "partial A-V block" or "incomplete heart block" and occurs in various forms; the common feature is that occasional atrial beats are not followed by ventricular contraction. Second degree block is usually subdivided into Type 1 and Type 2.[273, 520, 521] In Type 1, or "Wenckebach block," the PR interval becomes progressively longer until one ventricular beat is dropped and the cycle then repeats. This type of second degree block is usually transient and often associated with digitalis overdose. In Type 2 partial block the ventricle contracts in response to every second, third or fourth atrial contraction without alteration in the PR interval. The ratio of atrial to ventricular contractions is usually 2:1 or 3:1, with higher degrees occurring only rarely. Gilchrist [273] regards this type of second degree block as a frequent stage in the development of complete heart block and notes that if it apparently resolves, recurrence is so common that lasting recovery is very unlikely.

Third degree block, "complete heart block" or "A-V dissociation," occurs when all atrial impulses fail to reach the ventricle so that independent rhythms result. The atrial rate remains under the control of the sinus node, but the ventricular rate is governed by an idioventricular focus; when this focus is high in the ventricle, approaching the A-V node, the ventricular rate is usually faster than when the idioventricular focus is situated low in the body of the ventricles.

The electrocardiogram may be normal in the intervals between Stokes-Adams attacks, but this is rare: [146, 366, 668] established complete heart block is the rhythm most commonly found in association with Stokes-Adams attacks, the incidence being 80 per cent in our own series, 45 per cent in Burchell's series [85] and 38 per cent in Johansson's. [366]

There is often a prolonged PR interval or 2:1 block which may be intermittent and may be provoked by exertion. [85, 195, 240, 273] Ten per cent of our own patients were in 2:1 block before pacing. In Johansson's series, 19 of 42 patients (45%) had sinus rhythm between Stokes-Adams attacks; Burchell reported 24 per cent of his patients were in sinus rhythm before pacing; and in our own series the corresponding figure was 19 per cent. Such patients almost invariably reverted to periods of complete heart block, and other authors have also documented that complete A-V block was proven at some time in a very high proportion of their patients experiencing Stokes-Adams attacks. [206] Syncopal attacks may precede the onset of permanent heart block by a considerable period, [589] but are as common among patients with

2:1 block as those with established complete heart block [85] and may be particularly likely in patients with an unstable block.[273]

The QRS complexes are frequently abnormal and may differ from time to time in the same patient, particularly when intermittent A-V conduction occurs.[389] An analysis of 706 cases of Stokes-Adams disease taken from the literature (Table IV) shows

TABLE IV

Authors and Ref. Nos.	Year	Number of Cases	Cases with Widened QRS Complexes
Campbell [100]	1944	64	19
Graybiel and White [287]	1936	47	35
Johansson [366]	1961	42	20
Kay [389]	1948	100	47
Mouquin and Macrez [532]	1947	124	99
Penton [589]	1956	224	122
Sowton [713]	1963	61	55
Wright [820]	1956	44	19
Totals		706	416

that the QRS complexes were abnormally widened in 416, an incidence of 59 per cent.

The diagnostic significance of *bundle branch block* patterns in Stokes-Adams disease has been stressed by other authors.[59, 413, 738] Complete heart block occurs in approximately 5 per cent of cases with bundle branch block complexes.[241, 286]

The relative incidence of QRS complexes of right bundle branch block (RBBB) or left bundle branch block (LBBB) pattern varies considerably according to the selection of the patients in the series, and was approximately equal amongst Penton's cases.[589] Of our first 100 patients, 71 per cent had QRS complexes of RBBB type prior to pacing, and a high incidence of RBBB pattern complexes has also been noted by other authors.[389] The predominance of RBBB complexes is seen irrespective of the presence or absence of complete heart block [306] and may be related to the anatomical arrangement of the fibers of the conducting tissue. Conduction in the whole of the right bundle would be interrupted by a small lesion near the A-V node since the fibers are closely aligned, while the diffuse left bundle would not be wholly involved by such a lesion.

Atrial fibrillation occasionally occurs in conjunction with established or transient A-V block, and 10 per cent of Johansson's patients had this arrhythmia which was also noted by Burchell; it occurred in 7 per cent of our own patients. A QRS complex of supraventricular type is characteristic of congenital complete heart block,[389, 511] but occurred with a nodal rhythm in 7 per cent of Johansson's patients; 21 per cent of our own patients had QRS complexes of supraventricular type at some time prior to pacing.[306]

Liability to Stokes-Adams Attacks

Several authors have claimed that it may be possible to distinguish from the electrocardiogram patients who are especially liable to syncopal attacks. The features usually claimed to indicate a higher risk of syncopal attacks are: prolonged QRS duration; a rapid atrial rate; a slow ventricular rate; and a fixed PP interval which is not affected by the presence of a QRS complex.[332, 389] A marked shortening of the PP interval where the QRS complex is interposed (positive Erlanger-Blackman phenomenon),[287] a normal QRS duration, a slow atrial rate and a rapid idioventricular rate are claimed to indicate a relatively low risk of syncopal attacks.

Johansson's results tended to confirm this view although the numbers he reports are small.[366] The mean atrial rate in his patients with complete heart block and Stokes-Adams attacks was 97 beats per minute, while his patients without attacks had a mean atrial rate of 78 beats per minute. The Erlanger-Blackman phenomenon was negative in five patients with Stokes-Adams attacks and in only one patient without attacks; it was positive in two patients without attacks and in only one patient with Stokes-Adams attacks. These results could not be confirmed by Cosby,[147] who examined the atrial rate, ventricular rate, degree of variation of both rates, presence of changing A-V block and the width of the QRS complex in relation to the complications and prognosis of 100 patients with complete heart block. He found that none of these electrocardiographic criteria was significantly related to clinical state or prognosis.

ECG during Pacing

During stable ventricular pacing the typical electrocardiographic pattern shows a sharp initial deflection (due to the pacemaker stimulus) followed by a broadened QRS complex; the type of QRS complex depends upon the site of attachment of the electrodes. When pacing electrodes are attached to the left ventricle, this is activated first, and the spread of depolarization to the right ventricle is delayed so that the QRS complex has a right bundle branch block pattern. If the electrodes are on the right ventricle, the QRS pattern is that of left bundle branch block, and this distinction applies whether the electrodes are attached to the epicardial surface of the heart or whether a transvenous endocardial (catheter) electrode is used; to some extent the site of the electrode attachment can be predicted from the QRS pattern. It is worth noting that the auscultatory and phonocardiographic signs of right and left bundle branch block are also present in these circumstances and may be detected clinically, so that it is frequently possible to determine by auscultation the site of attachment of ventricular electrodes.[299, 715]

The amplitude of the deflection due to the pacemaker stimulus varies considerably between different leads of the electrocardiogram, but is normally considerably greater when unipolar stimulation is in use than when bipolar stimulation is used. The maximum amplitude of the stimulus deflection is naturally seen in the ECG lead orientated most nearly parallel to the vector of the stimulus, and this depends upon the relative placing in the tissues of the two pacemaker electrodes; it will usually be found that the maximum stimulus amplitude appears in one of the three standard leads. Since body position and respiration may cause alterations in the stimulus vector relative to the axes of the body, the height of the stimulus artifact may vary a little from time to time in any one patient, and frequently a respiratory variation can be detected. In electrocardiograms recorded at standard speed (25 mm/sec) there is usually no detectable delay between the stimulus deflection and the subsequent QRS complex, although when ECGs are recorded on a triggered oscilloscope for the investigation of possible pacing faults a delay can frequently be noted. Several aspects of the ECG during pacing are considered further in the sections relating to the investigation of pacing failure and cardiac threshold (pp. 122, 148).

When pacing occurs from a catheter electrode placed in the coronary sinus, the ECG pattern varies according to the position of the electrode within the sinus. If the catheter has been passed into the coronary sinus and along a coronary vein it may be stimulating the epicardial surface of the left ventricle with a resulting RBBB pattern QRS complex, while if the electrode is nearer the mouth of the coronary sinus, the right ventricle will be stimulated. There are no particular cardiographic features which distinguish coronary sinus pacing from endocardial pacing, although the rapid threshold rise characteristic of pacing from the coronary sinus leads to early pacing failure.

Pacing in the Presence of A-V Conduction

"Coronary sinus rhythm" has been produced experimentally in subjects without heart block by Lancaster,[411] who paced via an electrode catheter positioned at the os of the coronary sinus. The electrocardiogram showed a PR interval greater than 0.12 seconds with a P wave occurring before a normal QRS complex; the P wave was inverted in Leads 11, 111 and aVF. No complications occurred, and pacing of normal subjects by means of a bipolar electrode catheter placed against the atrial wall has also been reported by Braunwald [549, 631] without incident. We have also paced several patients in whom A-V conduction had returned with an atrial electrode catheter, but found that when the sinus rate exceeded the pacemaker rate atrial arrhythmias were commonly produced.[716] The usual arrhythmia was atrial flutter, and in no case did an arrhythmia persist for more than a minute or two after the cessation of atrial stimulation, which was carried out with an applied voltage of 2 v, an impulse duration of two milliseconds and a current of about 8 ma; presumably, this stimulus was powerful enough to induce the arrhythmia when it fell in the vulnerable period of the atrium.

When sinus rhythm is present, the S-A node competes with the artificial pacemaker for control of the heart rate, and the resulting rhythm depends upon the comparative rates of the two foci. When the pacemaker rate is considerably faster than the sinus rate, sinus rhythm is often suppressed and the atrium contracts after the start of ventricular systole due to retrograde conduction along the bundle of His. Retrograde and prograde conduction may occur intermittently and independently on different occasions either in sinus rhythm or in complete heart block, and the conduction time ("PR interval") is usually the same.[148, 465, 480, 713] Gerbaux [264] has also noted that in the presence of A-V conduction a retrograde P wave can be produced by artificial pacing and that the impulse then travels along the normal pathways in reverse.

When the sinus rate and the pacing rate are similar, cyclical interference between the two rhythms is often produced and the electrocardiogram then shows a regular pattern in which a few paced beats are succeeded by a few sinus beats before pacing reappears. As the sinus rate increases a larger proportion of the beats will be sinus in origin, and the approximate ratio of sinus beats to paced beats is given by the expression $\dfrac{P}{H-R} - 1$ where P is the pacemaker period in seconds (i.e., interval between two pacemaker stimuli), H is the sinus period in seconds, and R is the refractory period for sinus beats in seconds.[713] This type of cyclical interference has been noted by several authors and may occur whether the pacemaker rate is faster or slower than the sinus rate; the essential feature is that the two rates should be similar.

The more usual type of parasystole with the production of occasional paced beats and of fusion beats is frequently seen in patients with A-V conduction and an artificial pacemaker.[85, 563, 713, 828] From a study of the fusion beats produced by impulses from an artificial pacemaker and either the sinus node or a second artificial pacemaker, Linenthal and Zoll [462] were able to measure conduction times in the human heart. They concluded that conduction between the stimulation sites of the two electric pacemakers or retrograde conduction from an electrode site to the A-V node was via ordinary myocardium at a velocity of about 1 meter/sec; antegrade conduction in Purkinje tissue occurred at rates of 4.5-9 meters/sec. Burchell [85] reported a velocity of 0.5 meters/sec for transseptal conduction on the basis of similar measurements.

The interventricular conduction time has been studied in patients with two artificial pacemakers by Castellanos,[113] who concluded that the conduction time through muscle was the same whether the impulse travelled from left to right or from right to left.

Warner and Lewis [786] noted in normal subjects that the delay between the stimulus applied to the atrium and the appearance of a ventricular QRS complex lengthened as the pacing rate was increased, and this observation was confirmed by Carleton [107] and by Lister,[469] who showed that complete heart block was eventually produced by increasingly rapid pacing of the atrium. Lister noted that this was the opposite effect to that found normally when the heart rate was increased by exercise, since the PR interval then became shorter at faster rates. Linhart, Braunwald and Ross [466] also used a technique of pacing the atrium in unanesthetized subjects without heart block to investigate the A-V refractory period; extra impulses were inserted at various time intervals, and the shortest period in which the A-V system had recovered its ability to conduct was identified. The A-V refractory period averaged 350 milliseconds in the basal state but shortened by about ten milliseconds during exercise and during infusion of isoproterenol or atropine. Atrial tachycardia induced by pacing the atrium prolonged the A-V refractory period, and elevation of the arterial pressure by methoxamine also resulted in a considerable increase of the refractory period to about 600 milliseconds; this effect could be prevented by atropine and was presumably due to a vagal reflex.

The electrocardiographic findings associated with the "supernormal phase" are discussed on page 148.

SUMMARY AND CONCLUSIONS

Stokes-Adams attacks occur in about 60 per cent of patients with acquired complete heart block and in about 10 per cent of those with congenital block. A syncopal attack is probably due to ventricular asystole rather than tachycardia if the pulse rate is normal immediately before the episode; an attack is probably due to a rapid ventricular arrhythmia if consciousness is lost slowly over 20 to 30 seconds. Between half and three-quarters of all Stokes-Adams attacks are due to ventricular asystole alone; ventricular tachycardia alone accounts for 7 per cent of attacks, and both mechanisms occur in the remainder.

About 25 per cent of unpaced patients with Stokes-Adams attacks return to sinus rhythm at some time, but the ECG is rarely completely normal; widened QRS complexes are found in 60 per cent of cases, and partial block is often seen. The ECG is an unsatisfactory guide to prediction of which patients are liable to syncopal attacks.

During pacing the ECG reflects the position of the electrode on the ventricles; left bundle branch block complexes are found when the electrode is on the right ventricle and vice versa. When A-V conduction is present during pacing the resulting rhythm depends upon the rate of the artificial pacemaker. If the rate is fast, sinus rhythm may be suppressed, but if both paced and sinus rates are similar parasystole will be produced.

Measurements during pacing indicate that conduction through human myocardium occurs at 0.5-1.0 meters/second and about ten times faster through Purkinje tissue.

Chapter 4

DRUG TREATMENT

TREATMENT OF THE UNPACED PATIENT

Rational drug treatment of patients with heart block must be aimed at one or more of the four main objectives: (a) restoration of sinus rhythm; (b) increase in the rate of the idioventricular pacemaker; (c) the prevention of Stokes-Adams attacks; and (d) the treatment of heart failure.

If the patient has Stokes-Adams attacks, knowledge of the underlying mechanism is necessary before drug treatment can be fully satisfactory, since therapy is different when attacks are due to bradycardia or to tachycardia; if attacks are related to shifting heart block or if some precipitating mechanism can be identified, this also may influence the choice of therapy. The mechanisms and precipitating causes of Stokes-Adams attacks are discussed on page 24.

Sympathomimetic Drugs

Drugs of this type are indicated when the idioventricular rate is slow or when Stokes-Adams attacks are related to bradycardia or ventricular asystole. Although a large number of different sympathomimetic agents have been used in the past, the drugs in general use are epinephrine (Adrenalin®), isoproterenol (isoprenaline, isopropylnorepinephrine), either in the form of the hydrochloride (Aludrin®, Aleudrin®, Asdrin®, Isopro®, Isuprel®) or of the sulphate (Isonorin®, Norisodrine®), metaproterenol (orciprenaline, Alupent®) and ephedrine (see Fig. 1). It has been shown by Zoll[832] that even under similar experimental conditions, repeated trials of the same drug in the same patient may produce different results, but in general the results with different sympathomimetic amines differ only in degree. Weirich[797] found that the beneficial results of treatment with sympathomimetic amines

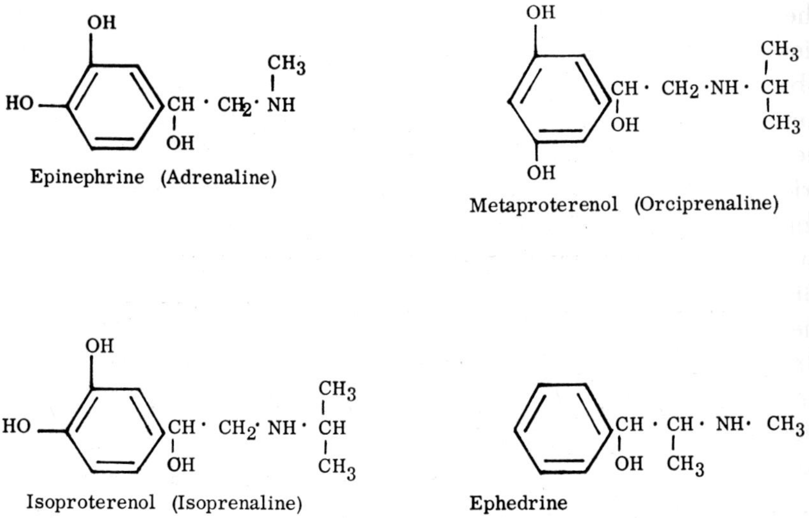

FIGURE 1. Structural formulae of epinephrine, metaproterenol, isoproterenol and ephedrine.

lasted for only about three weeks, but the experience of most workers is more encouraging, and we have maintained patients on these drugs for long periods.

Epinephrine (Adrenalin)

\The main action of epinephrine is to accelerate the idioventricular pacemaker,[355] and there is a direct relation between the degree of acceleration and the initial ventricular rate; the drug produces its greatest increase in ventricular rate when the initial rate is slow.\When the idioventricular rate is high, epinephrine has little effect. Sinus rhythm is only rarely restored, and larger doses than those providing relief do not result in greater acceleration of the idioventricular rate. The drug increases the atrial rate as well as the ventricular rate, but the atrial effect has no relation to the initial rate nor to the ventricular rates.\Epinephrine is contraindicated in patients with multiple ventricular ectopic beats or whose Stokes-Adams attacks are due to ventricular tachycardia; very small concentrations of epinephrine infused intravenously lower the threshold for ventricular fibrillation to the vicinity of the threshold for ventricular contraction,[77] but this effect is transient, lasting for approximately three minutes. Fatal ventricular fibrillation may be provoked by an intravenous injection of epinephrine in patients of this type. Several reports state that epinephrine is more likely than isoproterenol to produce rapid ventricular arrhythmias,[28, 551, 618] but this view was not supported by the findings of Zoll,[832] who could detect no difference in the tendency to provoke arrhythmias in 21 patients. Landergren and Biörck[413] recommend the use of intravenous epinephrine in patients with varying degrees of A-V block on the grounds that this drug stimulates the S-A pacemaker only moderately so that rapid ventricular rates do not occur during periods of 1:1 A-V conduction. It has also been used with success by Broustet,[78] who administered a total of 72 mg over 25 days to one of his patients.

The drug is given by injection. The usual dose for intramuscular or subcutaneous injection is 0.3 to 0.6 ml of 1:1,000 solution slowly injected over a period of several minutes, the rate of injection being governed according to the patient's response; a long-acting depot preparation in oil is also available. For intravenous use, a solution of 0.5 mg in 500 ml isotonic glucose has been recommended.[78] Our experience of the use of epinephrine in the management of patients with Stokes-Adams disease has been disappointing; we have found it troublesome and often ineffective in preventing recurrent syncopal attacks. Johansson[366] could detect no difference in animal experiments between epinephrine and norepinephrine in the production of ventricular ectopic beats.

Isoproterenol (Isoprenaline)

This is probably the most useful sympathomimetic drug in the treatment of Stokes-Adams disease. It stimulates impulse formation in both supraventricular and ventricular centers, produces increases in the atrial and idioventricular rates, improves A-V conduction and has a potent inotropic effect on the heart.[52, 243, 461, 594, 656, 709] It can be given intravenously in a drip containing 1 to 5 mg in 500 ml of 5 per cent dextrose, the drip rate being adjusted according to the rate response of the patient. This technique is preferred by Zoll to the use of an endocardial catheter for the short-term prevention of syncopal attacks.[829] If the drug is given by intramuscular or subcutaneous injection, its effects appear earlier and peak sooner than an injection of epinephrine.[12] The usual route of administration is sublingually, and most authors recommend doses of 10 to 30 mg taken frequently; it may be necessary to repeat the dose every 30 minutes.[413] Lillehei [450] reported that the rectal administration of isoproterenol was markedly superior to sublingual administration and claimed that it was often possible to prevent Stokes-Adams attacks by altering the route of administration from sublingual to rectal even when a lower total daily dose was used.

Isoproterenol may provoke ventricular ectopic beats or rapid ventricular arrhythmias and these may occur equally with large or small doses,[413] although it is claimed to be considerably less toxic than epinephrine in this respect.[239] It is advisable for the initial response to the drug to be assessed during hospital admission when an electrocardiogram can be monitored.[52]

If initial experience with short-acting isoproterenol preparations is satisfactory, maintenance therapy can be continued either with repeated sublingual tablets or with a delayed-release preparation (Saventrine®, Proternol®).[230, 557] These preparations are taken orally, and the dose varies from 30 mg every six hours up to 60 mg every two hours.[52] On several occasions we have noted that patients undergoing therapy with long-acting preparations have apparently responded with an increase in heart rate as judged from the apex or pulse, but that an electrocardiogram showed the increase to be due to multifocal ventricular ectopic beats. We have also seen dangerous ventricular tachycardias develop in patients taking large doses of sustained-action isoproterenol even when no preliminary abnormalities had been detected during the period of monitoring.

Differences in case selection and indications for pacemaker implantation make it impossible to compare the results to be expected from drug therapy between different centers, but it seems likely that nearly half the patients initially referred because of Stokes-Adams attacks may be treated successfully with long-term isoproterenol therapy.[52, 160] Karlson,[873] however, found the drug only prevented attacks in 10 per cent of his 47 patients.

Metaproterenol (Orciprenaline)

This sympathomimetic amine (Alupent ®) is widely employed in Continental Europe for the treatment of Stokes-Adams attacks. [179, 181, 315, 655] A usual route of administration is as an intravenous drip containing 5 mg in 200 ml of 5 per cent glucose and infused with a dose rate of 0.05 ml-0.125 ml a minute, the response being judged by the heart rate. Schaub [655] reported an increase in heart rate or a return to sinus rhythm with the use of this drug, and showed that in comparative studies carried out at rest and during exercise on a bicycle ergometer the heart rate, stroke volume and cardiac index could be increased progressively as the dose of orciprenaline was raised.

Ephedrine

This drug can be administered orally, the usual dose being 30 to 60 mg every four hours. Its action is to accelerate the idioventricular pacemaker, but we have found the drug usually inadequate in the treatment of Stokes-Adams attacks, while it also has the disadvantages of elevating the blood pressure, interfering with sleep and occasionally precipitating retention of urine.[355] It is contraindicated in the presence of multiple ventricular ectopic beats or transient rapid ventricular arrhythmias.

Comparison of Sympathomimetic Amines

Although these drugs all have similar actions on the heart rate and in the prevention of Stokes-Adams attacks, their other effects may differ considerably. Isoproterenol has little effect on the blood pressure but has greater positive chronotropic and inotropic actions than epinephrine.[414] This effect on myocardial contractility may result in an increase in stroke volume.[488, 725] Isoproterenol also improves A-V conductivity and stimulates impulse formation in supraventricular as well as in ventricular centers.[594] Epinephrine on the other hand causes considerable rise in blood pressure but has very little inotropic action, although it also normally improves A-V conductivity. There is little doubt that the sympathomimetic amine which is most widely used and which is the most satisfactory is isoproterenol, especially in its delayed release form.

Use of Sympathomimetic Amines in Ventricular Tachycardia

In our experience and in that of others,[413] rapid ventricular arrhythmias sufficient to cause Stokes-Adams attacks almost invariably arise from a slow heart rate and do not often occur directly from sinus rhythm. In such patients it may be possible to prevent any recurrence of attacks by treatment with sympathomimetic agents, and most authors are agreed that isoproterenol is the most satisfactory drug to use. For this application it is given by intravenous drip with the object of increasing the ventricular rate to a level at which arrhythmias arising from an ectopic focus do not occur; this "critical rate" may be produced by either a ventricular or a supraventricular focus, but provided the resultant ventricular rate is fast enough, alternative foci are suppressed and bursts of tachyarrhythmia are prevented. The essential feature in this mode of treatment is that the ventricular rate be maintained and that the site of origin of each contraction be identical; to achieve this frequent monitoring and alteration of the drip rate is essential. In effect, "titration" is carried out, the drip rate being increased whenever ventricular ectopic beats from a second focus appear. Good results have been reported by these means even when ventricular ectopic beats are common before treatment,[461, 618, 829, 832] and the method has been used by Matthews,[502] who employed very large doses in one case. In this patient, ventricular tachycardia invariably occurred whenever the ventricular rate fell below the critical level of 50 beats per minute, and isoproterenol hydrochloride had to be infused with increasing dosage to prevent the arrhythmia; the rate of infusion reached 154 mg/min with an average of 47 μg/min over 48 hours without evidence of cardiac or systemic toxicity. This patient was eventually successfully treated by implantation of an internal pacemaker. The critical ventricular rate of 50 beats per minute reported by Matthews is of the same order as that mentioned in most reports and agrees with our own experience also. Linenthal and Zoll [461] reported the use of intravenous isoproterenol in the prevention of ventricular tachycardia in eight patients; doses of 4 to 10 μg/min were needed to keep the idioventricular rate above the critical levels which varied from 40 to 65 beats per minute. We feel that this

IV drip technique [830] is satisfactory for short periods but is probably too dangerous for long-term use.[52]

Atropine

Vagal stimulation produces negligible effects on the ventricle of the dog in complete heart block,[74] and it is likely that a similar situation exists in patients, since atropine often has little effect on the ventricular rate in human subjects.[356] In some patients with complete heart block, however, there is an increase in ventricular rate following the intravenous injection of atropine,[272] and this is probably due to the vagal distribution to the conducting system at the level of the idioventricular pacemaker.

The effect of atropine on the atrial rate in complete heart block is variable and is unrelated to the ventricular response or to the initial atrial rate; in most instances there is an increase in atrial rate and this may result in an increase in the degree of partial A-V block.[273] The drug is theoretically indicated in the treatment of Stokes-Adams attacks or slow ventricular rates associated with increased vagal tone, and it has been used clinically by various authors,[720,799] sometimes in combination with other drugs such as ephedrine.[707] In our experience, patients with vagal-induced heart block are extremely rare, and since atropine only rarely abolishes even reflex block [356] we share the view of Landergren and Biörck [413] that this drug has no significant part to play in the therapy of complete heart block. The situation with regard to patients with established block can be summarized by stating that the drug is least helpful when it is most needed because at low ventricular rates the response to atropine is not appreciable.

Chlorothiazide

The use of this drug in the prevention of Stokes-Adams attacks was reported by Tobian,[761] who in 1964 [762] reported successful results on nine patients of whom eight were in incomplete block. The frequency of syncopal attacks decreased at the same time as the plasma potassium concentration fell. Landergren and Biörck [413] found that in their patients there was no consistent response to chlorothiazide and that when a beneficial effect was obtained it occasionally occurred several days before alterations in the plasma potassium level; they did however note that, in patients with permanent complete heart block and attacks due to asystole, chlorothiazide exerted a useful prophylactic effect.

Corticosteroids

Corticosteroids and ACTHs have been used in the treatment of Stokes-Adams attacks both in acute myocardial infarction [604] and in chronic cases,[247] and some benefit has been reported.[2, 3] Our experience, as well as that of others,[366, 413] is that steroids are indicated only in the presence of an acute inflammatory reaction relating to the heart block, when doses of up to 80 mg of prednisone a day may be tried; unless A-V conduction returns rapidly, therapy should be abandoned. Verel reported [777] that steroids are often effective in restoring sinus rhythm in patients with primary heart block,[839] but this effect is often only temporary, and heart block with Stokes-Adams attacks occurs despite maintenance therapy with corticosteroids.

The mechanism of action of corticosteroids is unknown. Lown [481] analyzed the PR interval in patients with Addison's disease and Cushing's disease, and showed that the mean conduction time was longer in patients with Addison's disease, suggesting that the steroids had a direct effect upon A-V conduction. The anti-inflammatory reaction of these drugs may be important in patients with acute heart block, and there are several other possible factors. Corticosteroids are known to increase catecholamine sensitivity of the cardiovascular system, at least in adrenalectomized dogs,[608] and the effects of steroids upon electrolyte balance, particularly upon potassium concentration, may be significant. The work of the Ann Arbor group,[535] demonstrating that the ventricular threshold for pacemaker stimuli is lowered by corticosteroids, may also be relevant in unpaced patients in whom a supraventricular impulse of subthreshold intensity might result in ventricular depolarization.

Molar Sodium Lactate

Bellet [27] reported that intravenous infusion of molar and half-molar sodium lactate solution produced an increase in ventricular rate and a diminution in frequency of syncopal attacks. The experience of other authors with the same technique has not been uniformly satisfactory,[192, 519, 832] and since many ventricular arrhythmias, including ventricular fibrillation, may be provoked,[537] this treatment should be confined to hospitalized patients; continuous monitoring of the ECG during treatment is recommended.[366, 413]

Other Drugs

Simple sedation has no specific effect upon Stokes-Adams attacks, but its use has been recommended [413] for patients who have rapid ventricular arrhythmias, and sedation has been shown to diminish the risk of ventricular fibrillation following acute coronary occlusions; [611] the observation reported by Citters [140] that dogs with complete heart block developed rapid ventricular tachycardias upon hypothalamic stimulation may be relevant in this respect.

Antiarrhythmic drugs, such as procaine amide or quinidine, are widely used in the suppression of ectopic foci, but, as they depress the velocity of conduction, the rate of intrinsic pacemakers and the myocardial contractility,[522] and may also precipitate rapid ventricular activity or ventricular fibrillation, they are usually considered to be contraindicated in the presence of complete heart block, particularly when it is associated with bursts of ventricular tachycardia.[170, 514, 619, 669] There are, however, several reports of successful use of this drug in the prevention of Stokes-Adams attacks due to rapid ventricular rhythms in patients without complete heart block.[188, 619, 739]

Digitalis has been suggested in the treatment of patients whose Stokes-Adams attacks are associated with a shifting A-V block, in the hope that complete heart block would be firmly established. This form of therapy, however, was felt to be impracticable by Schwartz and Schwartz,[670] who showed, by intravenous infusion of lanatoside C®, that it was impossible to establish fixed complete heart block without causing asystole of the ventricles at the same time. It is often considered that digitalis is contraindicated in the presence of complete heart block, but its beneficial action in cases of subclinical or even frank heart failure should outweigh all other considerations; occasionally,

Stokes-Adams attacks can be greatly reduced by maintenance therapy with digitalis, presumably because of its action in improving myocardial function and perhaps coronary flow.

Many other drugs have been recommended for the treatment of complete heart block, although the recommendations are often based on very small numbers of patients. Benzedrex® was reported as a very effective treatment in preventing exercise-induced block in one patient and was apparently equally satisfactory whether it was taken by inhalation or orally.[171] Nathanson [550] was able to prevent Stokes-Adams attacks for two months by oral treatment with hydroxyamphetamine, and the use of both methamphetamine [184] and of amphetamine itself [343] have been reported. Caffeine,[660] thyroxin [569] and barium chloride [143, 740] have been recommended in the past, and hypertonic glucose solution was also said to be effective.[697] Isosorbide dinitrate was used by Botti [845] in a patient with angina and transient block and proved more effective than nitroglycerin. One elderly patient apparently responded to a bradykinin antagonist, pyridinolcarbamate.[866] Treatment with most of these drugs has now been superseded by the use of more effective sympathomimetic amines or artificial pacemakers.

DRUG TREATMENT DURING ARTIFICIAL PACING

Heart failure is commonly present in patients with slow idioventricular rates from complete heart block, and improvement may occur when the ventricular rate is restored to normal levels by pacing. In many patients, however, the increase in ventricular rate does not by itself result in the maximum possible improvement. Many such patients will show further improvement when treated with an antifailure regime in addition to pacing, and the importance of digitalis in this respect has been emphasized by Kaiser.[379] Rowe and White [640] were unable to find any patient in their series of 350 cases with complete heart block in whom heart failure was precipitated or significantly aggravated by the development of block, and Friedberg [246] also claimed that bradycardia alone is not a cause of cardiac failure in human subjects. In our own series [713] we were unable to show any relationship between the development of cardiac failure and the idioventricular rate;

we have noted patients who did not develop failure despite a ventricular rate of less than 20 beats per minute, while others developed severe failure although the idioventricular rate never fell below 45 beats per minute. There seems little doubt that bradycardia can be a major contributory cause in the development of failure, but that severity of this complication depends upon the functional state of the myocardium itself. A critical evaluation of paced patients will often indicate the need for diuretic and digitalis therapy.

When the ventricular rate is controlled by an artificial pacemaker, toxic effects of drugs may be considerably modified, and drugs which are contraindicated for patients in complete heart block may be useful or even essential, while different indications may apply regarding drugs which are normally used in the treatment of heart block. Thus the vasopressor action of epinephrine or sympathomimetic amines has been utilized to maintain blood pressure during the immediate postoperative phase when pacemaker patients frequently experience a period of hypotension; [6, 277, 379] occasionally, sympathomimetic amines in this situation may actually contribute to arrhythmias during pacing.[379]

The acute effects of digitalization with lanatocide C in dogs with artificial pacemakers were studied by Grondin,[296] who found that doses of up to 0.04 mg/kg slowed the atrial and idioventricular rates but did not provoke significant arrhythmias; after two minutes anoxia, pacemaker-induced ventricular fibrillation developed in two animals. When larger doses of lanatocide C were given (0.16 mg/kg), ventricular arrhythmias were provoked, and ventricular fibrillation was frequently produced by stimuli falling in the vulnerable period (see p. 105). Acute digitalization was studied in six patients with fixed-rate pacemakers by Benchimol,[33] who showed that an injection of 1 mg of G-Strophanthin produced an inotropic action and so diminished the relative importance of the atrial transport mechanism for ventricular filling. Digitalization also caused a 20 per cent decrease in peripheral resistance which was not seen in patients during normal sinus rhythm, and it seems likely that the drug caused peripheral vasodilatation. Donoso[190] studied the effect of digitalis in paced patients and concluded that the drug was helpful only in patients in heart failure; and it is interesting that Borrie and Lichter [56] found they were unable to maintain life in sheep with surgically created complete heart block, despite artificial pacing, unless the sheep were digitalized. Sudden death occurred within 30 minutes of the creation of the block in all their non-digitalized experimental sheep, but two digitalized animals survived.

Isoproterenol was given to paced dogs by Grondin,[296] and caused an increase in the supraventricular rhythm by up to 125 beats per minute; the drug also produced increases in the ventricular rates of ten dogs with complete A-V block to as high as 250 beats per minute and resulted in the appearance of competing rhythms between the artificial pacemaker and the intrinsic ventricular focus. These workers concluded that during steady pacing the augmentation of the spontaneous rate by isoproterenol has no advantage, and the drug may even be dangerous because of its action in producing competition, leading to a situation in which pacemaker-induced ventricular fibrillation may occur. An alternative view was taken by Bellet,[303] who treated seven paced patients with intravenous or sublingual isoproterenol. He showed that an increase in cardiac output and stroke volume occurred both at rest and on exercise during the drug therapy and suggested that supplemental use of isoproterenol in paced patients would increase the cardiac output. Isoproterenol was also given intravenously to eight patients with fixed rate pacemakers by Benchimol,[32] who found that the drug produced changes similar to those of exercise; the cardiac index and left ventricular work increased by about 65 per cent, while the systemic blood pressure and peripheral resistance fell. A further action of isoproterenol in paced patients was reported by Haywood and Wyman,[314] who found that sublingual or intravenous administration of the drug would restore pacing in some patients who were no longer responding to the artificial stimulus; ephedrine did not restore pacing but merely increased the idioventricular rate.

Antiarrhythmic drugs have also been studied by several workers. Procaine amide was given to dogs with complete heart block by Grondin,[296] who found that, in moderate doses, its action in slowing the rate of the intrinsic rhythm was advantageous, since it abolished competing rhythms and so decreased the danger of ventricular fibrillation. When large doses were given, of the order of 125 mg/kg, the depressant action of the drug was overwhelming, and three dogs died in irreversible shock despite stable pacing. A further effect of moderate doses (50-75 mg/kg) was noted in that the electrical threshold for contraction increased by an average of 2 ma in four of eight experiments, while the supernormal phase of excitability also became less obvious in six of eight experiments and could not be located in the other two. This alteration in cardiac threshold by procaine amide has little consequence when applied to human subjects since pacemakers commercially available for clinical use provide stimuli well in excess of this small increase [139] (see p. 168). Procaine amide has also been recommended in the suppression of ectopic ventricular activity following the insertion of artificial pacemakers,[6, 125] and six of 34 patients reported by Kaiser [379] needed procaine hydrochloride or quinidine for this reason. A note of caution was introduced by Rothfeld, Zucker, Parsonnet and Lotti,[639] who produced competitive pacing in dogs with sinus rhythm by means of right ventricular bipolar catheters. No ill effects followed until quinidine was given intravenously (5-10 mg/kg), but in fourteen dogs ventricular fibrillation was then rapidly produced by the pacemaker stimulus (6 ma, 2 msec) falling in the vulnerable period; the authors conclude that quinidine should not be used in patients with competing rhythms. The use of beta-adrenergic blocking drugs such as pronethanol or propranalol is normally contraindicated in the presence of complete heart block because of their depressant action on the myocardium, but we have used pronethanol in one patient with intermittent heart block and supraventricular tachycardia in conjunction with an artificial pacemaker for a period of over a year,[719] and in other patients to suppress non-pacemade activity.[52] Investigations in our laboratory [50] have shown that the use of these drugs in paced patients results in a diminution of the cardiac output by up to 30 per cent both at rest and on exercise, and so very strong indications must be present before they are used.

The effects of drugs on the threshold for stimulation are discussed on page 168.

SUMMARY AND CONCLUSIONS

The relative merits of different drugs for the treatment of un-paced patients are discussed, together with side-effects, contra-indications and routes of administration. Isoproterenol is the most satisfactory sympathomimetic agent at present available and can be given orally, rectally or as an intravenous drip; delayed-release preparations are available for long-term use. Treatment should be started with small doses, and ECG monitoring carried out if pos-sible, because of the risk of provocation of rapid ventricular ar-rhythmias. About half of all patients with Stokes-Adams disease may be maintained successfully on isoproterenol therapy without pacing.

Paced patients often benefit from supplemental drug therapy with digitalis and diuretics, but sympathomimetic amines are usu-ally contraindicated because they tend to promote parasystole and at the same time lower the threshold for ventricular fibrillation. Antiarrhythmic drugs are frequently beneficial in small doses but dangerous in large doses.

Chapter 5

SHORT-TERM PACING

IMMEDIATE TREATMENT OF A STOKES-ADAMS ATTACK

IN THE EVENT OF cessation of circulation and its associated loss of consciousness in a Stokes-Adams attack, closed chest cardiac compression and artificial respiration are effective, as in cardiac arrest from other causes, but, if the apparatus for pacing is immediately at hand, it should be switched on, and this may obviate the necessity of cardiac compression. Pacing will be ineffective in persistent tachycardia or fibrillation, and these can only be diagnosed with an ECG, which should be attached to the patient at once. Ventricular tachyarrhythmias usually give way temporarily to brief periods of asystole, during which a pacemaker will take over and control the ventricle. In persistent fibrillation we have been able to maintain an adequate circulation on more than one occasion for more than an hour by closed chest cardiac compression together with artificial respiration, pending effective defibrillation.

INDICATIONS FOR SHORT-TERM PACING

1. As an emergency measure in a prolonged Stokes-Adams attack;
2. For rapidly recurring Stokes-Adams attacks, allowing assessment of drug treatment;
3. When an acute myocardial infarct is associated with multiple extrasystoles, or a slow rate from block;
4. As a preparation for setting up long-term pacing to improve the clinical state before implantation procedures;
5. To cover the risk of cardiac arrest during operations for implantation of pacemakers; [1, 693]
6. To cover anesthetics and operations on patients particularly susceptible to cardiac arrest, e.g., when there is a his-

51

tory of arrest in similar circumstances, and in all patients
with complete heart block; [774, 399]

7. As a trial to see whether pacing is beneficial, notably to
show whether cerebral or other symptoms are the result
of poor cardiac output correctable by pacing;

8. When block occurs during cardiac surgery;

9. To suppress ectopic ventricular activity (see p. 62).

METHODS

Artificial cardiac pacing can be instituted as an emergency by
three methods:

1. Using electrodes on the intact chest wall, when voltages
which cause painful convulsive muscular movements are
required;

2. Using a needle through the skin to make direct contact
with the ventricular muscle; and

3. Using a long wire (electrode "catheter") with its tip bare
of insulation passed along a vein to make contact with the
inside of the right ventricle.

1. Skin Electrode Pacing

The first recorded recovery following cardiac asystole treated
by electrical impulses pacing the heart was in 1952 by Zoll,[825] and
was achieved by transmitting an impulse through the intact chest
wall. The initial report was followed by a number of others [833,
834, 835, 836, 837, 838] recording his increasing experience, which
showed that, with suitable impulses, not only could asystole be
terminated, but also that continued pacing would prevent Stokes-
Adams attacks in those patients whose rhythm during attacks was
not asystole, but ventricular tachycardia, or included bouts of
fibrillation. As was to be expected from animal experiments,[257]
stimuli were not effective during established ventricular fibrillation. By 1955,[835] he was able to record resuscitation of 25 patients from Stokes-Adams attacks; in the same year, Douglas [191]
recorded successful pacing for one patient over a period of seven
days, and, in 1959, Jackson [358] recorded intermittent pacing up
to seven months; a limiting factor was the pain and skin burns
from repeated stimulation.[627]

As electrodes the plates usually used for ECG work are suitable, but in order to reduce the resistance of dry skin, electrode jelly or saline is essential. The plates, usually about 2 in. square, are applied to the front of the chest over the manubrium of the sternum and to the left axilla just lateral to the apex beat. Voltage of 50 to 200 is needed, and the impulse is usually of two milliseconds duration and should not exceed three milliseconds. We prefer to use apparatus with rate control (30-120), particularly in order to slow down gradually when weaning off pacing, and with voltage control, so that one can adjust to the minimum required.

When it is necessary to pace by this method after the return of consciousness, we have had to anesthetize patients for whom the pain from muscular contractions has proved intolerable, and although trouble from skin burns can be reduced by changing the electrode sites,[837] we use this technique only in emergency and for short periods. Electrodes can be fixed to the chest wall as a precautionary measure in special circumstances,[831] such as before anesthetizing a patient in heart block who is undergoing any form of surgery.

2. Percutaneous Myocardial Needle

With wires making direct contact with the myocardium, voltages of under 10 suffice. Thevenet [757] first described this technique, using a needle through the 4th or 5th left interspace. Lillehei [453, 454] recommends it, using a 20 gauge spinal needle, usually through the 6th space just to the left of the xiphoid, directing it towards the 2nd right costochondral junction at 30° to the chest wall. Once the heart beat is felt he advances a further 5 mm into the myocardium and then threads a size 0 braided surgical stainless steel uninsulated wire through the needle, advancing 1 cm into the myocardium. The needle is then withdrawn and the circuit completed with a subcutaneous needle as the other electrode. Other similar techniques have been described.[363, 441, 531, 599, 624, 625, 632] Roe [625] found, in one patient, that this percutaneous technique avoided repeated ventricular fibrillation apparently due to stimulating endocardially (method 3). Ross and Hoffman [635] designed a small portable pacemaker with two short electrodes which could be pushed through the skin to make contact with the myocardium.

There are other techniques with electrodes which do not reach the heart itself. Nicholson [554] and Lawrence [424] have recommended the insertion of needles through the chest wall as electrodes for monitoring the ECG so that, in the event of asystole, they can be used for pacing. Silverman,[700] when opening the chest by splitting the sternum in patients at risk, uses a subcutaneous needle near the apex and one in a similar position on the right side; the voltage required is half that needed with skin electrodes. Shafiroff and Linder [683] attempted pacing by means of electrodes in the esophagus. The threshold proved to be 30 to 50, at which level the tendency to muscle contractions and local tissue burning makes prolonged pacing impracticable.

3. Emergency Pacing with Endocardial Electrode (Electrode Catheter)

We consider this technique, which was developed at the Montefiore Hospital, New York,[258] the method of choice, provided suitable x-ray apparatus is available for positioning of the electrode. It requires very small currents which are painless and provoke no muscle twitching. The technique can be used safely for several days at a time, and with some minor modifications can be used as a long-term method of pacing (see p. 68).

Endocardial Electrodes

We have experience of the use of several different makes of endocardial catheters, including those made by the United States Catheter and Instrument Corp. (U.S.C.I.), by Medtronic, also of the USA, by Elema Schönander of Sweden, by Lucas of England and those designed at our own hospital. These electrodes are described in the appendix. Different makes vary in their flexibility, and rather different techniques are required to place them. Some are unipolar, in which case an "indifferent" electrode is placed subcutaneously conveniently near the site at which the wire traverses the skin. The relative advantages of unipolar and bipolar stimulation are discussed on pages 78 and 150.

The U.S.C.I. electrode wires are quite stiff at room temperature though they soften on warming after a few minutes in the body. The C50 electrode is unipolar; the C51 and C52 are bipolar, having their electrodes respectively 1 cm and 2 cm apart. They are made in various sizes, of which we prefer the No. 5 (French gauge), which is very considerably smaller than the Medtronic. No stiffener is required when passing the U.S.C.I. wires. When using a neck vein, if there is difficulty in getting into the superior vena cava [283] because of a tendency to pass out towards the axilla, it may be helpful temporarily to set the tip of the catheter into an acute bend. This can be carried out by immersing the terminal 5 cm in boiling water until it is extremely flexible, and then, while holding it in the required shape, quenching it in cold water for a few moments. This set will rapidly disappear after insertion into the blood stream, but it may persist long enough to enable an obstacle to be passed.

The Medtronic electrode "catheter," which is bipolar, is much more flexible and is passed with the aid of an internal stylet, which is pulled out when a satisfactory position has been achieved.

The Elema is also very flexible but has a relatively heavy tip; it was first used by Ekestrom.[205, 409] The most satisfactory method of placing it is probably that in use in Stockholm, in which the patient is positioned on a special table in such a way that the heavy electrode tip falls across the tricuspid valve and drops into the apex of the right ventricle, the movement of the electrode along the vein being aided by the operator feeding the wire in and by the streaming effect of the blood. For this technique to be satisfactorily employed it is essential that frequent minor movements of the patient can be performed easily and that the screening apparatus is capable of producing a good image with the patient in the lateral position. With this electrode it is sometimes impossible to pass the clavicular region from the external jugular vein and for prolonged pacing the internal jugular vein must be used. It may occasionally be helpful for a Cournand catheter (No. 10) to be passed over the soft Elema wire to aid in manipulation past the root of the neck.[682]

De Vos [183] in Holland has designed an electrode, the tip of which is positioned in the pulmonary artery, so that the electrode

placed 12 cm from the tip lies in the heart. With such an electrode, direct contact cannot be maintained permanently with
the ventricular wall, and thus the threshold required to maintain
stimulation must be high. Experience with this electrode has
been reported by Chaillet.[120]

Very fine insulated wires with small electrode tips have been
introduced recently as a method of endocardial stimulation.[308, 398] These are positioned by the blind technique described below
(p. 58).

Choice of a Vein

For emergency pacing it is essential that the electrode tip
be positioned in the right ventricle as speedily as possible, and
the U.S.C.I. electrode is usually chosen for this application. It
is passed from a jugular vein, from an arm vein [258, 598] or occasionally from the saphenous [710, 824] and may be inserted through
a thin-walled needle if the urgency of the situation requires extreme speed.[713, 840] The use of a leg vein limits the patient's mo-
bility and is only suitable for brief periods. The use of an arm
vein is suitable for periods of a few days, but carries with it the
risk of thrombophlebitis [258, 598] and of displacement of the electrode due to movements of the patient's arm. If possible, a
medial-going vein above the level of the elbow in the patient's
left arm should be chosen, since this introduces the minimum
disability to the patient from restriction of arm movement. For
emergency use we prefer to avoid the jugular vein, as we consider it the vein of choice for long-term pacing. A previous incision and wire coming through the skin in the neck would seri-
ously interfere with the sterility of the subsequent long-term
procedure. Details of technique for the use of jugular veins are
given in Chapter 6, p. 74.

Positioning the Electrode

The electrode wire is manipulated under x-ray control and,
because of its small size, is difficult to see unless an image in-
tensifier is available. The electrode is passed into the right ventricle in the usual way, and we recommend that it should be
passed through the pulmonary valve and be seen to reach into

the lung field, since this ensures that it has not entered the coronary sinus. It is then withdrawn into the body of the right ventricle and manipulated until the tip is positioned as nearly as possible in the apex of the ventricle. The electrode is cautiously advanced until the tip is lightly impacted among the trabeculae, and any redundant loops are then withdrawn so that the wire forms a smooth curve from the SVC into the apex of the ventricle. It is acceptable for a small indentation in the wire to appear at the level of the tricuspid valve, but if any redundant wire remains in the right atrium this will almost inevitably rotate and form a loop, with the result that the electrode tip becomes displaced and may even return to the right atrium. In our experience the position described is the only satisfactory one for pacing to be continued for more than a few hours, and most other authors are in agreement with this view,[134, 182, 283, 409, 413] although placing of the electrodes in the outflow tract of the right ventricle has been recommended.[575] Pacing with a bipolar system may be satisfactory when the electrodes are not touching the endocardium,[580] but we strongly recommend that both bipolar and unipolar electrodes be positioned so that the electrode wire runs under the right ventricular trabeculae, since we have found that stable pacing is far more likely to be achieved when this is done.

Throughout the procedure, care should be taken that the patient remains flat so that there is no possibility of air embolism. When a satisfactory position has been achieved it should be ascertained that the electrode is stable, and there should be no movement of the tip when the patient turns his body, sits up, shrugs his shoulders, coughs, strains or, when a jugular vein has been used, lifts his arms above his head. The opportunity may also be taken of checking that the pacing is satisfactory and that the threshold is very low (see Chapter 9). With a C50 or C51 electrode, stable pacing should be achieved with an applied voltage of about half a volt and a current of 1 to 1½ ma, the energy being of the order of 0.5 μj. With the Medtronic and Elema electrodes we find the corresponding values are 1 v, 1½ ma, and 3 μj.

It is wise that all patients should be carefully examined clinically when the endocardial electrode has been satisfactorily implanted, with particular attention being paid to the second heart sound. Since the stimulus is applied to the right ventricle, the pulmonary closure sound (P_2) will occur before the aortic closure sound (A_2), and the second heart sound will thus exhibit a reversed split with respiration,[299, 712] the situation being analogous to that found when a patient has a spontaneous left bundle branch block.[299] If the electrode has inadvertently been passed into the coronary sinus, the tip may have passed far enough along a coronary vein to be stimulating the left ventricle from its epicardial aspect, and in this case the reversed split of the second heart sound will not be present, A_2 and P_2 having their normal relationship with each other.[299]

As soon as practical after insertion of the endocardial electrode, the patient should have a chest x-ray taken erect with the standard technique, and an electrocardiogram recorded with a machine having a high-frequency response for comparison with future records (see Chapter 7).

Blind Positioning of Electrodes

In exceptional circumstances it may be necessary for an electrode to be placed in the right ventricle without fluoroscopic facilities being available. The most satisfactory procedure under these circumstances is probably the method recommended by Kimball [398] and by Harris,[308] in which a fine insulated wire terminating in a small electrode is introduced from a peripheral vein and advanced slowly at such a rate that the blood flow sweeps the tip through to the right ventricle. This procedure is essentially similar to that widely used for positioning of fine polythene catheters in the pulmonary artery, and it seems likely that in a high proportion of cases the insulated wire will also be swept along with the blood stream so that the tip passes the pulmonary valve. The final positioning of the tip within the right ventricle is carried out by monitoring an ECG cavity lead recorded along the wire, and the typical appearances to be expected when the recording electrode is in the SVC, right atrium, right ventricle, pulmonary artery and coronary sinus have been detailed by Watson.[788] If the electrocardiogram from an exploring electrode is displayed upon an oscilloscope, the atrial potentials can be easily recognized when the record is being obtained from the right atrium. As the tip of the exploring lead crosses the tricuspid valve into the ventricle in a patient with complete heart block there is a sudden dramatic alteration both in the amplitude and in the rate of potentials recorded, and it is immediately obvious that the right ventricle has been entered. It is possible for the U.S.C.I. electrodes (C50, etc.) to be positioned blind in the right ventricle by a very similar technique, and we have employed this method occasionally.[712]

An alternative method of blind positioning of a bipolar electrode (C51) has also been occasionally used clinically, particularly when the electrode has been displaced into the atrium in a patient already in hospital. The wire is connected to a pacemaker, which is then switched on and the wire manipulated until pacing occurs. We are aware of one patient to whom an attempt to pass a C51 electrode from an arm vein by this method caused considerable distress when the tip entered the jugular vein, but Hudson [346] has used this technique from the neck without difficulty.

We consider that the risks of blind positioning of all flexible wires are too high for the technique to be recommended, and the already-described alternative methods of emergency management of the patient, such as the use of an external pacemaker, percutaneous chest wall needle pacing or treatment with intravenous sympathomimetic amines should be used whenever possible.

Neufeld, working in Israel,[553] has described an ingenious experimental technique which does not require fluoroscopy, but depends on the electrode tip being magnetic and the use of a powerful magnet on the chest wall. The electrode is passed blindly via a vein to the ventricle. The magnet is then switched on to keep the electrode in contact with the ventricular wall.

Complications

The complications of this endocardial technique used for short-term pacing have not proved serious. Aseptic technique in passing the electrode wire is essential or a *bacteremia* will follow; [174] this is particularly to be avoided if there is valvular disease.[306] Should the electrode require repositioning in the ventricle, the risk is increased, due to the possibility of introducing organisms from the site of entry of the wire through the skin, for it is not easy to sterilize the wire and skin at the site of a partially healed incision.[673] We have had only two bacteremias from this method used for periods of up to four weeks in over 200 patients. We have only used antibiotic cover for the procedure when there appears to be a special risk, as after repositioning or in association with valvular disease. Zoll has never favored this technique; in 13 patients he had two septicemias among other complications.[827] This complication will also be discussed under long-term pacing on p. 70.

Another argument against this technique using the relatively stiff U.S.C.I. wire electrodes is the risk of *perforation* of the heart, which has been reported by many authors [64, 80, 134, 174, 238, 239, 306, 398, 544, 562, 582, 775, 824, 856] and may be even more common than is realized, though Furman [852] records 156 catheterizations with only two perforations; he stresses the lower incidence of this complication if an arm vein is avoided, and he used either a neck or a leg vein in his 156 cases. Serious ill effects are extremely rare, though death has been attributed to this cause.[239, 274] The risk may be greater in patients on anticoagulants.[674] In our experience of passing a wire electrode to the right ventricle for pacing on several hundred occasions, we are now aware that the tip certainly penetrated into the pericardium on seven occasions, and may have done so in others. It has always been an early complication, probably occurring while being positioned. With such penetration of the electrode the threshold required to pace may rise, resulting, if minimal currents are being used, in intermittent pacing; but we have never observed any rise in venous pressure or other untoward effects, though patients have occasionally complained of some precordial discomfort. Perforation can be diagnosed by the presence of a pericardial rub, by a rise in threshold required to pace, and occasionally by the diaphragm twitching with the impulses.[174] If the electrode in the pericardium makes contact with the left ventricle, the ECG pattern will change from left to right bundle branch pattern. Screening may reveal that the electrode tip is very close to the

edge of the cardiac silhouette, or there may be sufficient pericardial fluid to be diagnostic on x-ray. In one of our patients
perforation had not been diagnosed until the pericardium was
opened for the attachment of electrodes for long-term pacing,
and this has also been recorded by Brück [80] and Kimball.[398]
Chardack [134] has reported two perforations, one early and one
late; these occurred when he retained *in situ* the stylet of the
catheter of his design.[856] He subsequently recommended that the
stylet used to facilitate placing the electrode should be withdrawn, and with this variation of technique has had no perforations. Lagergren [407] has reported the use of the flexible Elema
endocardial electrode in 305 patients without perforation and
without wire fracture.

While perforation of the heart is a risk when using stiff wires,
when using extremely flexible ones there is a risk of *knotting*,
and this has been reported by Kimball.[398] Fortunately it has so
far proved possible to withdraw the electrode to the site of
entry into the vein and then remove it through a small incision.
Although extremely unlikely, the possibility cannot be ignored
that such a knot might form around the chordae tendinae of the
tricuspid valve and cause great damage when the wire is withdrawn.[779]

Perhaps the most tedious and the most common complication
of endocardial pacing is early displacement of the electrode tip
from contact with the ventricular wall. This occurred in 34 of
76 of our patients,[51] but in only 32 of 305 using Elema electrodes.[407] Pacing stops, as the threshold to pace with an electrode
within the ventricle, but not in direct contact with its wall, is
likely to be higher than the output of the pacemaker. X-ray
screening usually reveals obvious displacement, requiring repositioning. Fortunately, this complication is very rare after the
electrode has been in place for one or two days, as the insulated
wire when stable is probably trapped under a trabeculum of the
ventricular wall,[205, 407, 409, 413, 890] and soon becomes covered with
a filmy fibrinous sheath,[51, 134, 410] which may extend along the
course of the wire both in the heart and superior vena cava.[682]

Thrombosis along the wire within the great veins and the
heart has not proved to be a clinical feature even without anti-

coagulants, and we know of no confirmed report of pulmonary embolism with the venous technique. Clot along the course of the wire may be found at autopsy,[51, 575, 674] but death has not been attributed to it.

4. When Complete Heart Block Develops during Cardiac Surgery

In this case there is no problem of access to the heart, and a wire electrode should be stitched into the ventricular muscle and lead out through the wound to the surface in such a way that it can be pulled out without reopening the wound when pacing is no longer required.[17, 452, 454, 797] The wire is insulated except where it contacts the ventricular muscle. [75, 228] Most iatrogenic heart blocks occurring during operation recover within a few weeks,[757] but if complete block persists for three to four weeks, a more permanent pacing system should be established.[454, 486]

SUPPRESSION OF ECTOPIC VENTRICULAR ACTIVITY

Although electrical pacing of the ventricle has no effect during established ventricular fibrillation or tachycardia, it was clearly demonstrated by Zoll that, in patients with complete heart block, such episodes of ventricular arrhythmias would not occur, provided that the ventricular rate was maintained above a critical level; the elevation of ventricular rate could be carried out by electrical stimulation [837] or by the use of sympathomimetic amines.[461] The critical ventricular rate varies from patient to patient and from time to time in the same patient, but Zoll states that it is usually between 40 and 60 beats per minute.[831] Matthews [502] reported a patient who developed ventricular tachycardia whenever the ventricular rate fell below 50 beats per minute, and Haupt [311] described the abolition of ventricular arrhythmia following the implantation of a pacemaker by an increase in the pacing rate from 64 to 84 beats per minute. Similar observations that syncopal attacks due to ventricular tachyarrhythmia could be prevented by pacing above the critical rate have been made by Kantrowitz.[196] Escher [126] has found the critical rate to be as high as 120 beats per minute, and we have also had a similar experience.[719] We were able to extend the technique to patients not in heart block and have reported the long-term suppression of ventricular tachycardia by overdriving the ventricle with a pacemaker in one patient for a year;[713, 719] recurrent paroxysms of ventricular tachycardia following mitral valvuloplasty were also successfully suppressed by pacing in one patient without complete heart block by Eraklis.[211] The use of pacing with a transvenous catheter at a rate sufficient to suppress ventricular arrhythmias in two patients with intact conducting systems was reported by Johnson.[402] His group was able to prevent recurrences of ventricular fibrillation following cardiac arrest, and members of the group comment that their limited experience indicates this method was better than the use of procaine amide for the prevention of recurrent ventricular arrhythmias; Heiman and Helwig have reported similar experience in two patients.[876] We have employed the technique following cardiac infarction with some success,[715] but Chardack[125] was unable to suppress ectopic activity with pacing rates up to 100 beats per minute and prefers procaine amide. An interesting illustration of the importance of maintaining the ventricular rate above the critical level was reported by Robinson.[621] This patient was paced for four months with an implanted unit with a rate of 65 beats per minute, but developed ventricular extrasystoles followed by near-syncopal attacks due to episodes of ventricular fibrillation. These episodes were eliminated by pacing simultaneously with a second artificial pacemaker via a bipolar endocardial electrode with the production of an irregular pulse at a rate of 90 to 100 beats per minute. The ventricular rate was maintained above the critical level in this manner for three days, and the original implanted pacemaker was then changed for one with a discharge rate of 77 beats per minute, following which no further episodes of ventricular fibrillation occurred. This patient is particularly significant since the risk of pacemaker-induced ventricular fibrillation due to parasystole resulting from two artificial pacemakers was less than that from allowing the ventricular rate to remain beneath the critical level.

SUMMARY

The urgent treatment for a Stokes-Adams attack is the same as that of any other cardiac arrest. Ventricular fibrillation, which

can only be specifically diagnosed electrocardiographically, requires electrical defibrillation; and electrical pacing is not effective in rapid ventricular arrhythmias. If the heart does not recover
spontaneously sufficiently to produce an effective output, closed-
chest compression with suitable oxygenation can maintain an
adequate circulation, if necessary, for many minutes while await-
ing the apparatus for electrical pacing.

The listed indications for short-term pacing include its emergency use, and the apparatus for pacing should be set up prophy-
lactically to cover situations in which arrest is liable to occur.
The indications for and results of pacing to control various ventricular arrhythmias are considered. The three methods described
are: 1. with skin electrodes, an effective emergency method,
but requiring over 100 v and producing painful skeletal muscle
contraction and, if prolonged, skin burns; 2. with a percutaneous myocardial needle which avoids these complications and can
be maintained for a few days with little risk; 3. with an endocardial electrode passed via a vein to the right ventricle. This
technique, which is chosen when suitable x-ray equipment is
readily available, is described in detail. If the easily manipulated
stiff endocardial wires are used there is a risk of perforation of
the right ventricle, but this complication does not produce tam-
ponade or other serious sequelae.

Chapter 6

LONG-TERM PACING: INDICATIONS AND METHODS

INDICATIONS

LONG-TERM PACING is required in complete heart block when drug treatment fails to produce an adequate cardiac output or to prevent recurrent Stokes-Adams attacks. We do not consider a single attack sufficient to necessitate pacing, though others disagree with this view.[160, 570] When there is doubt whether the increased heart rate will result in an adequate output, a period of short-term pacing is tried. Cerebral symptoms, if they are to respond to pacing, will be relieved immediately, but the manifestations of congestive cardiac failure and of renal failure respond only slowly, requiring a trial period of pacing of several weeks before it is possible to judge whether worthwhile improvement is being obtained. A long period of observation may be required to decide whether drugs are preventing Stokes-Adams attacks, which may be infrequent even without treatment. If drug treatment produces a good rise in heart rate without variations in rhythm, and attacks have previously only occurred when not taking an adequate amount of a suitable drug, it is probably justifiable to rely on continued drug therapy and so avoid the risks and morbidity inherent in any system of long-term pacing.

METHODS

A system of pacing for more than a few days must not encumber the patient and must allow him to be ambulant and active. Electrodes, as with the short-term methods, can either make contact from within the heart or on its surface, permanent surface attachment requiring operative exposure of the heart. With these two types of electrodes, three arrangements of pacemaker can be combined—external, entirely implanted or apparatus both external and implanted as with the induction and radio frequency models.

Pacemaker	*Electrode*
1. External	a. myocardial or epicardial
2. Implanted	b. endocardial
3. Induction and radio frequency	c. skin

Methods 1a, 1b, 2a, 2b, 3a and 3b are illustrated in Figures 2 through 7.

External Pacemakers

There are obvious advantages in having a pacemaker outside the body: batteries can be changed readily; rate and power output adjusted to requirements of the moment. But a sudden pacing failure will have just as serious an immediate effect on the patient as when the unit is implanted. Our exerience is that wire breakages are more common with external wires, which are often subjected to greater strain than those embedded in the body. The advantages of rate control will be discussed under hemodynamics aspects (Ch. 10); a fixed rate has allowed greater variation in cardiac output than might be expected. The major disadvantage of any external apparatus is that patients cannot forget their dependence on electrical equipment, which in our opinion is a major consideration in weighing the advantages of implanted pacemakers.

1a. *External Pacemaker with Electrode on the Heart*

The *external pacemaker* with a wire running to *the electrode on the surface of the heart,* the first method practiced, is not now much used except for relatively short periods of pacing, for example, after the development of complete block during cardiac operations. Sepsis tends to track along the wire, leading to an inflammatory reaction around the electrode, which separates it from the responsive myocardium, thus increasing the threshold required to pace.[168, 440] This septic inflammatory reaction may be long delayed,[174, 207, 227, 248, 316, 452, 556, 646] and we have successfully paced patients by this method for up to three years, as has Senning [682] (see Table V). Landegren and Bjorck [413] also report on the use of this technique (20 patients up to 2 years). We consider that the only indication for the prolonged use of this technique is in the event of sepsis developing around an implanted pacemaker (Method 2a) requiring its exteriorization. If the threshold is not too high, pacing with the electrodes already in place can be continued for a useful period.

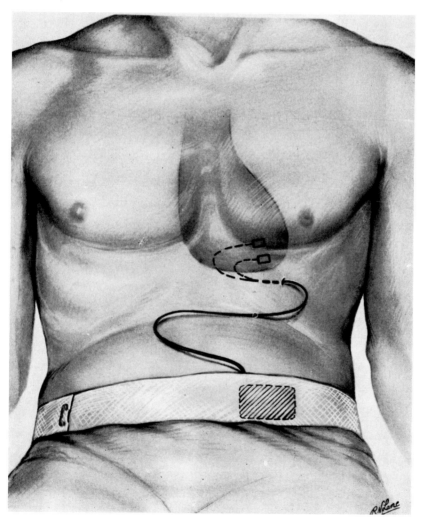

FIGURE 2. Method 1a: Pacing for long-term use. External pacemaker—myocardial electrode.

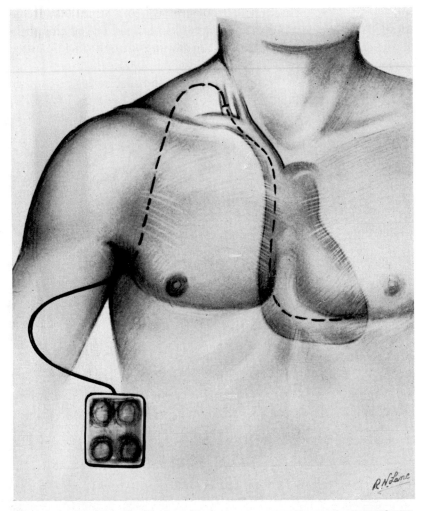

FIGURE 3. Method 1b: Pacing for long-term use. External pacemaker—
endocardial electrode.

1b. *External Pacemaker with Endocardial Electrode*

The *external pacemaker with endocardial electrode* method
was originated by the Montefiore Hospital group in New York,
and they showed that the use of the external jugular vein as the
entry site for the electrode catheter obviated phlebitis, which is
so prone to occur with an arm vein; they also reported that

threshold levels did not increase significantly after months of pacing.[674] Zucker [840] and Gordon [283] have each reported failure to pace in a single case from a rise of threshold which they attribute to a black coat of nonconducting material forming on the electrode within the heart (see p. 171). We too have seen a late rise in threshold with endocardial electrodes; it is however

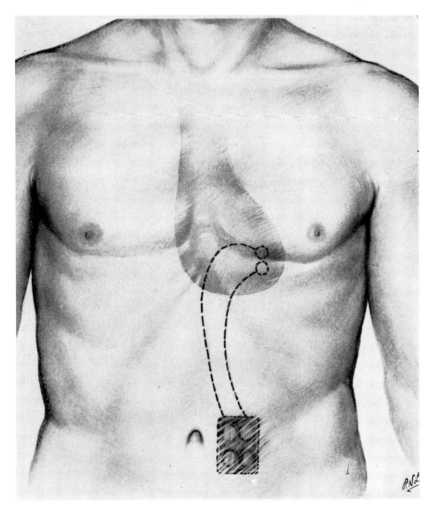

FIGURE 4. Method 2a: Pacing for long-term use. Implanted pacemaker— myocardial electrode.

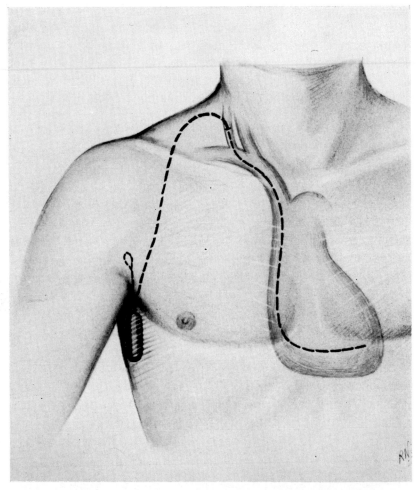

FIGURE 5. Method 2b: Pacing for long-term use. Implanted pacemaker—endocardial electrode. Reproduced from *Thorax*, **20**:128, 1965, by permission of B.M.A. Publishers.

exceptional and less common than with epicardial electrodes. The early complications of endocardial pacing have been discussed above under short-term pacing on page 59. If this method of pacing is used for more than three or four weeks with the wire brought through the skin close to its entry into the jugular vein, the incidence of bacteremia is high. Schwedel records bacteremia in one-third of his 85 patients,[672] but Furman [853] in a subsequent report from the same hospital says that infection was only troublesome in 14 of 116 patients paced for over four weeks; the infection was fatal in four. We have had three bacteremias in 27 patients paced by the venous route for more than four weeks.[687] It is sometimes possible to eliminate the infection by

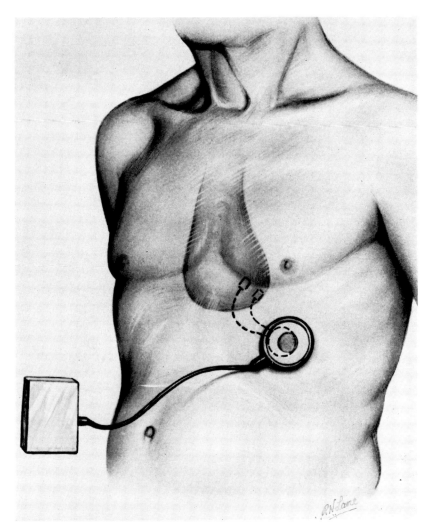

FIGURE 6. Method 3a: Pacing for long-term use. Induction or radio frequency pacemaker—myocardial electrode.

antibiotics without removing the electrode.[409, 673] A Swedish modification of the technique, running the wire for a long subcutaneous course from the site of neck vein entry before traversing the
skin in the groin, has reduced this risk.[37, 409, 413] Three (nonfatal)
septicemias in 100 patients have been recorded when this long
track modification was used.[410]

    For long-term pacing with an endocardial electrode the only

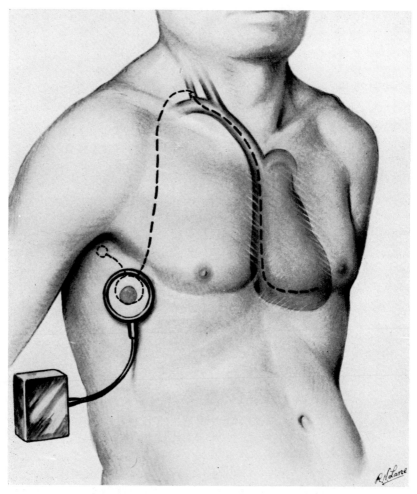

FIGURE 7. Method 3b: Pacing for long-term use. Induction or radio frequency pacemaker—endocardial electrode.

First Author	Reference Number	Year of Publication	Town	Country	Number of Patients	Number of Children Included	Postimplant	Later All Causes	Later Attributable to Pacing	Total	Months Since 1st Implant	Mean Months Pacing Survivors	Number Paced Over 12 Months	Survivors Continuing to be Paced by Same Method	Number of Reoperations	Number Make of Pacemaker (model number)
Method 1a — Epicardial Electrodes External Pacemakers																
Senning [682]		1964	{Stockholm / Zurich}	{Sweden / Switzerland}	12	(2)	1	2		3	30	3	7 over 2 yr			
Method 1b — Endocardial Electrodes External Pacemakers																
Lagergren [410]		1965	Stockholm	Sweden	100		11 with in 6 m	6	(1)	17	42		49			
Schwedel [682] [583] (Furman)		1964 1966	Montefiore Hosp. New York	U.S.A.	63					7			6 over 3 yr	23		
Siddons [687]		1965	St. George's Hosp., London	England	27					3	16					
Method 2b — Endocardial Electrodes Implanted Pacemakers																
Senning [682]		1964	{Stockholm / Zurich}	{Sweden / Switzerland}	50		4	3		7	19	15	15			Elema
Bluestone [51] (Siddons)		1965	London	England	49	(0)	1	2		3		10				Devices
Borst [57]		1965	Munich	W. Germany	43		3	2		5		7				Elema (137 +139)
Chardack [130,134]		1965	Buffalo	U.S.A.	20*		1	0		1	17	9 in 10 pat		17		Medtronic
Overbeck [860]		1965	Freiburg	W. Germany	15		0	0		0	11	6	0	15		Elema
Piwnica [863]		1965	Paris	France	11		1	0		1	5					{9 Medtronic / 1 Devices / 1 Elema}
				Total	188		10	7		17						
Method 3a — Induction																
Abrams [5]		1965	Birmingham	England	45	(1)	8	20	(3)	28	49			33		Lucas (England)
Widmann [807] (Glenn)		1964	New Haven	U.S.A.	17	(0)	0	8	(3)	8	37	15		16	3	Airborne (U.S.A.)
Cammilli [98]		1964	Florence	Italy	12	(0)	5	2	(0)	7	7	3				(Italy)
				Totals	74	(1)	13	30	(3)	43						

* Nineteen of these patients are included in Chardack's series on Table VI.

acceptable site for insertion of the wire is a jugular vein. In about 20 per cent of our cases we have been unable to find a suitable vein in the site of the external jugular, and therefore have used the internal jugular. This has also been the experience of Lagergren,[408] Chardack [134] and of De Sanctis.[182] The small diameter of the transvenous electrodes which we use is advantageous as it will pass into a much smaller vein than the other designs. The vein is exposed by dissection under local anesthetic, and the electrode inserted directly, care being taken that the patient remains flat throughout the whole procedure so that there is no possibility of an air embolism. In about one-third of our cases we had some difficulty in manipulating the electrode past the clavicular region. It may be useful in these circumstances to insert a soft plastic cannula into the vein alongside the wire and to inject 1 or 2 ml of a radiopaque medium. This will outline the course of the vein immediately in front of the electrode, and its clearance can be followed on the x-ray screen. It may also be helpful for the patient to move his arm horizontally or above the head and for finger pressure to be applied to the supraclavicular region.

When the electrode has been positioned successfully, so that its tip lies in the apex of the right ventricle, the external jugular vein is tied off and the wire attached to the deep tissues with one or two sutures. It is then ascertained that the electrode tip is stable and that the threshold for pacing is suitably low (see p. 157). The wire is then brought down past the clavicle to emerge after an extended subcutaneous course, and the Elema wire may be carried subcutaneously as far as the inguinal region.[409] We prefer to bring the wire deep to the clavicle, though others, particularly when using the more flexible wires, bring them anteriorly.

It might be thought that an electrode wire lying for a long period within the superior vena cava and the chambers of the right side of the heart would cause thrombo-embolic complications, or damage the heart. Clinical thrombo-embolism has been reported with other forms of pacing, but is remarkable by its absence with long term endocardial pacing, though anticoagulant treatment is not used. Nevertheless the finding of some clot on the wire at post mortem is not unusual. We know of no report of such clotting contributing to death. Lagergren,[890] from his experience of 21 post mortems, describes the thin coat of fibrin which forms around the wire within a week of insertion, and only saw any unsatisfactory tissue response in two cases; in these two cases stainless steel electrodes had been used and the reaction was confined to tissue around the electrode tips.

Lagergren, together with a number of European colleagues, has collected from five centers a series of 305 patients paced endocardially.[407] In 96 patients the pacemaker has been external throughout; in 74 patients the pacemaker was implanted after a period with it external; in the remaining 135 patients it was implanted from the start (Method 2b). The researchers did not separate the results with external units from those with implants, but the total mortality within six months was 12 per cent and overall 16 per cent; 98 patients were paced for more than one year (35 over 2 years). Only three reports are available of pacing ten or more patients specifically with an external pacemaker and endocardial electrode; the results are set out in Table V and include 100 patients of the 305 referred to above. Some of the figures in the table may include some short-term pacing experience, but the 66 patients paced by the Montefiore Hospital group [673] include three for over three years and two others for over four years.[351] We have maintained 27 patients by this technique for a mean period of 16 months with three deaths.[306, 307] The absence of other reports suggests that this technique is rarely used elsewhere except as a short-term method.

1c. *External Pacemaker with Skin Electrode*

In order to obviate having any buried apparatus including electrodes in or on the heart, Lord [478] has proposed a plastic operation on the anterior chest wall laying skin on the pericardium with no other tissue intervening. He showed that it was then possible to pace from outside with an electrode on this skin with currents which did not contract skeletal muscle and of which the patient was unaware. He records experimental work and a clinical trial in one patient.

Implanted Pacemakers

The total implantation of the pacemaker depended on the development of a small enough sterilizable pacemaker which would be inert in the tissues. Adequate miniaturization of the electronic components offered no great problem apart from the power source, which takes up nine-tenths of the unit. Mercury cells are now almost universally used for power, though the first pacemaker implanted used nickel-cadmium cells which could be recharged by induction from outside the body,[208, 682, 693] and research continues in this field.[319, 677] Recent experimental work [699] suggests that rechargeable nickel-cadmium cells with a life of 30 to 40 years may be available in the future. Furman [256] and Bonnabeau [55] have both designed pacemakers powered in this way and intended to be placed directly on the heart thus dispensing with wire electrodes. Bonnabeau found the life of the rechargeable nickel-cadmium cells inadequate and is investigating rechargeable mercury cells; others [385] remain skeptical of the long life predicted for these nickel-cadmium cells. Miniature mercury cells, which are not recharged, are used by all the standard models available commercially; they have an anticipated life of about four years, after which the pacemaker must be changed, involving its exposure by operation. The US Atomic Energy Commission has announced that their researchers are working on the development of a battery, powered by plutonium 238, which would have a much longer life.[771] The possibility of deriving power from a natural source in the body is discussed on page 216.

SUBSTANCES TO COVER. The most suitable *substances to cover* the implanted units are silicone rubber and epoxy resin, both of which can be prepared to a "medical grade" which is remarkably inert in the body. Polytetrafluoroethylene (PTFE or Teflon®) has been discarded by most manufacturers as it does not heat-seal satisfactorily. Some manufacturers use polyethylene as insulation cover for electrode wires.

SEPSIS. Any technique which involves the implantation of a foreign body such as a pacemaker must involve the risk of sepsis developing around the implant. None of the available pacemakers can withstand autoclaving, nor are they likely to stand up to

gamma irradiation. Ethylene oxide gas is the most popular sterilization technique, though formalin gas and various antiseptic
solutions have been used. Whichever sterilizing agent is used, it
should be thoroughly washed off. After sterilizing with ethylene
oxide it is advisable to leave the pacemaker for at least three
days before implantation, as some of the toxic sterilizing agent
is absorbed by the cover of the unit, and is only slowly released.
Zoll [828] has pointed out the necessity of the implant being washed
free of extraneous material which may cause an aseptic reaction;
he describes a complex technique of rendering the covering of
the pacemaker free of particulate matter.

The fullest sterile precautions are required for implantation,
though ideal conditions are not always achieved if the operation
is performed as an emergency, and particularly if cardiac arrest
occurs during the procedure. For this reason we strongly advise
establishing pacing on a temporary basis before anesthesia is
induced for the operation of implantation. Many reports mention
one or more implants becoming septic, and sepsis has usually,
but not always [46, 207, 408, 570, 682, 828] resulted in failure to keep the
pacemaker implanted. Sepsis may develop around the implant
as a late complication, and this has been described by van
Dijk [775] and ourselves [166] as resulting from an aseptic effusion
around the foreign material developing a sinus to the surface,
often many months after implantation. Once a sinus has reached
the surface, invasion by skin organisms results in sepsis. This
sequence of events was seen in four of 64 of van Dijk's patients [775]
and 23 of 55 of our early patients.[166] It has been recorded by
others,[6, 61, 408, 496] and may be due to the materials of the implants, their sterilization, or may be the result of a late blood-
borne infection. It is possible that aspiration of the fluid around
the implant and the use of steroids may prevent sinus formation
in some cases.

2a. *Implanted Pacemaker with Electrode on the Heart*

This method, using electrodes placed on the heart at operation and an implanted pacemaker, has been used more extensively
than any other. More than 1,500 cases have been recorded in the
literature, and the results collected from papers reporting ten or

more patients are set out on Table VI. These results are discussed in Chapter 8.

The procedure consists essentially of the exposure of the left ventricle and the fixation to it of one or more bare electrodes so that they just penetrate into the myocardium. It is usually recommended [136, 826] that insulated wires from two such myocardial electrodes are connected to the pacemaker which is implanted either in the abdominal or chest wall. We and others [116, 764] prefer, however, one myocardial electrode completing the circuit through the tissue fluid, and near the pacemaker a short tissue electrode, often called an indifferent electrode. At the operation we also place a second electrode on the heart with its wire buried at a suitable subcutaneous site so that it can be picked up as a spare in the event of failure.

ELECTRODE MATERIAL. It is advantageous to have as the electrode and its connection to the pacemaker a wire without any joint which might be a source of mechanical weakness or, if dissimilar metals were joined, other deterioration, including possible electrolytic change (see p. 160). Stainless steel has satisfactory mechanical properties to stand up to the constant movement of a wire leading to the heart, but, even if suitably balanced currents are used, fragmentation, presumably from electrolysis, may occur at a positive (indifferent) electrode of stainless steel [302, 641] (see p. 161). This electrolytic deterioration is avoided in some designs [105, 207, 277, 828] by using a platinum electrode attached to a stainless steel wire, at the expense of having a join of dissimilar metals. We know of electrodes of two different makes failing at such a join. Chardack [125, 128] uses a wire and electrode in one piece, but of platinum with 10 per cent iridium, which is electrolytically inert, though still inferior to stainless steel in its mechanical properties. The current Vitatron electrode depicted in the Appendix (p. 323) is also made of platinum-iridium throughout, but has good mechanical properties because the two helical spirals are set in solid silicone rubber and are not free to distort on stretching. We and others,[543] on the other hand, since electrolysis has only been observed at the positive electrode, have preferred to continue to use stainless steel for the negative electrode on the heart, but complete the circuit through the tissue fluid with a short electrode of platinum-iridium which is placed away from the heart and is not subjected to constant movement.[166] It has been reported [125, 128] that with an arrangement with both electrodes on the heart the threshold current required to pace is 10 per cent lower than with the negative electrode on the heart and the positive remote from it. We have not been able to confirm this threshold difference and do not regard a 10 per cent difference as a significant advantage in favor of the bipolar system. A cobalt-nickel alloy, "Elgiloy," (Elgin Watch Co.) has been recommended by Glenn [204, 278] for use as an electrode wire. In the form of a helical spring it is particularly well suited to stand up to the cardiac movement; it has, however, a high electrical resistance, is very brittle and is not suited as an anode, as it undergoes rapid destruction by electrolysis. Braunwald [68] has fatigue-tested this wire and found it mechanically superior to other types of electrode wire on the market, claiming also that it is more corrosion-resistant than stainless steel.

Some of the early designs of electrode used braided conducting wires, but metal fatigue resulted in failures, and it has become almost standard practice to use a helical spring form, the insulating cover usually being of silicone rubber.

SURGICAL EXPOSURE OF THE HEART. The standard approach is by a limited anterior thoracotomy dividing the 4th and 5th cartilages so that they can be separated to provide access to the anterior surface of the left ventricle. There are several detailed descriptions of the operative techniques.[136, 688, 828] The heart can be approached by other routes than the formal anterior intercostal thoracotomy. Some prefer to split the lower part of the sternum.[617, 860] If a previous incision anteriorly is septic, a posterior thoracotomy will allow access through a clean field. The approach to the pericardium ascribed to Sauerbruch, in which an incision by the xiphisternum allows access to the diaphragmatic surface of the heart without opening either pleura or peritoneum, has also been used and particularly recommended as a means of avoiding thoracotomy and its inherent complications.[321, 576, 750, 781]

ELECTRODE SITE. The heart will respond to a stimulus applied to any part of either ventricle, but electrodes are usually placed

TABLE VI

Method 2a

Epicardial or Myocardial Electrodes Implanted Pacemakers

First Author Reference Number	Year of Publication	Town	Country	Number of Patients	Number of Children Included	Deaths — Postimplant	Deaths — Later All Causes	Deaths — Later Attributable to Pacing	Deaths — Total	Months Since 1st Implant	Mean Months Pacing Survivors	Number Paced Over 12 Months	Survivors Continuing to be Paced by Same Method	Number of Patients Having Reoperations	Number of Reoperations	Number Make of Pacemaker (model number)
Chardack [134]	1965	Buffalo	U.S.A.	100*	(2)	9	18	(2)	27	60	25	72	70		61†	Medtronic
Zoll [827]	1964	Boston	U.S.A.	77	(1)	1	16	(1)	17	40		35	76	29	78	Electrodyne
Morris [530]	1965	Ann Arbor	U.S.A.	77		2	13	(5)	15	36	10	16	62		44	General Electric
Dack [160]	1965	Mt. Sinai, New York	U.S.A.	54	(1)	2	5	(1)	7	26			52	15 / 7	17 / 12	45 Medtronic / 9 Cordis synchronous
Dack [848]				(94)‡	(1)	(6)	(13)		(19)	(40)	(16.8)					
Kantrowitz [381]	1964	Maimonides Hosp., New York	U.S.A.	43	(0)	8	3	(0)	11	36	13		35	9	14	General Electric
Ellis [296] / Burchell [85]	1964 / 1964	Mayo Clinic	U.S.A.	43	(1)	4	2	(1)	6	30	11 in 31		38	8	8	28 Electrodyne / 3 Medtronic
Taber [751] / Taber [752]	1964 / 1965	Detroit	U.S.A.	38 / (91)	(3)	2	4	(1)	6	24 (33)			36	1	1 / (27)	Medtronic
Karlson [873]	1966	New York	U.S.A.	37	(0)	8	9	(1)	17	13			17	8	19	Medtronic
Zucker [841] (Parsonnet)	1965	Newark, N. J.	U.S.A.	31	(0)	1	4	(0)	5	34	15	17	30	12	26	Medtronic
Spear [721] / Nathan [545] / Center [116]	1965 / 1964 / 1964	Miami	U.S.A.	29	(0)	3	3	(1)	6	30			26	16	26	13 Medtronic / 16 Cordis synchronous
Lawrence [424]	1965	Seattle	U.S.A.	19		0	3	(1)	3	37			19	12	14	Electrodyne (TR14)
McGuire [857]	1966	Charlottesville	U.S.A.	18	(0)	0	1	(0)	1	48	12		17	3	3	16 Medtronic / 2 Cordis synchronous
Winters [816]	1965	Philadelphia	U.S.A.	13	(0)	2	2	(1)	4	18	10	6	9	2	2	Medtronic (5860)

Author	Year	City	Country													Devices
Parker [570]	1963	St. Louis	U.S.A.	12	(0)	2	1	(0)	3	25	13 in 7 pat		10	2	2	Medtronic / Electrodyne
Bruns [81]	1963	San Francisco	U.S.A.	10	(4)	1	0		1				9	4	4	Medtronic
Trimble [767]	1964	Toronto	Canada	37		3	6	(6)	9	33		37 over 6 mo	34	14	16	5 Electrodyne / 32 Medtronic (5860)
Allen [17]	1964	Vancouver	Canada	18	(0)	2	2	(2)	4	24	10.5	8	16	3	3	15 Medtronic (adjustable) / 2 Electrodyne
Buttigliero [91]	1964	London, (Ont.)	Canada	14	(0)	0	1	(0)	1	32			13	2	2	General Electric / Electrodyne
Johnson [368]	1963	Montreal	Canada	10	(0)	0	0		0	24	14.3		10	2	2	Medtronic / Electrodyne
Binet [46] (Mathey)	1965	Hôp. Laennec, Paris	France	160	(1)	7	3	(0)	10	39			154	46	60	15 Elema (137) / 35 Electrodyne (TR14) / 143 Medtronic (5860) / 6 Cotelec (French) / 4 Cordis synchronous
Ricordeau [617] (Dubost)	1964	Hôp. Broussais, Paris	France	80	(0)	3	5	(3)	8	30			77	13	19	1 Electrodyne / 11 Elema (137) / 68 Medtronic (5860)
van Dijk [775]	1964	Leiden	Holland	68		1	15	(4)	16	30			67		22	31 Elema / 107 Vitatron (Dutch) / 11 Medtronic
Siddons [689]	1965	London	England	62	(1)	8	16		24	42		9	Numerous			Numerous Devices
Lenègre [432] / Gerbaux [266]	1964 / 1964	Hôp. Boucicat, Paris	France	51	(0)	2	11	(1)	13			5	46	5	6	9 Elema / 8 Electrodyne / 19 Medtronic
Hallen [302]	1965	Uppsala	Sweden	47		2	3	(0)	5	37		16	45	32	60	Elema (137)
Effert [203]	1964	Dusseldorf	W. Germany	46	(1)	5	1	(1)	6	24			39	7	7	44 Medtronic / 1 Cordis synchronous

TABLE VI *Continued*

First Author	Reference Number	Year of Publication	Town	Country	Number of Patients	Number of Children Included	Deaths — Postimplant	Deaths — Later All Causes	Deaths — Later Attributable to Pacing	Deaths — Total	Months Since 1st Implant	Mean Months Pacing Survivors	Number Paced Over 12 Months	Survivors Continuing to be Paced by Same Method	Number of Patients Having Reoperations	Number of Reoperations	Make of Pacemaker Number (model number)
Courbier	[150]	1965	Marseilles	France	44		4	3	(3)	7	21		7	39	11	14	33 Elema, 9 Medtronic, 2 Cotelec (French)
Brück	[80]	1964	Stuttgart	W. Germany	34		5			5	32					13	9 Cordis synchronous
Gilgenkrantz / Faivre	[274] / [220]	1964 / 1964	Nancy	France	24		3	2		5	19			21	5	5	16 Elema, 6 Medtronic (5860), 1 Medtronic (5870)
Cole	[144]	1964	Auckland	New Zealand	24	(2)	5	1	(0)	6	22	12		19	7	10	4 Medtronic (5850), 17 Medtronic (5860), 2 Medtronic (5870), 3 Elema (137), 1 Devices
Welti	[800,801]	1964	Hôp. Tenon, Paris	France	23	(0)	1	3	(2)	4	18			Numerous	Numerous		Elema, 19 Elema in 5 pat
Castberg	[110]	1965	Copenhagen	Denmark	23		4	3	(1)	7	31	17	12	19	12	24	22 Medtronic in 18 pat, 1 Devices
Senning	[682]	1964	Stockholm / Zurich	Sweden / Switzerland	18		1	1		2	30		10	14	Several		Elema

	Year	City	Country													Make
Overbeck [860]	1965	Freiburg	W. Germany	17	(0)	3	1		4	35	21	13	12	10	14	Elema
de Gasperis [174]	1962	Milan	Italy	15	(0)	0	1		1	17	6		15	3	3	Electrodyne (TR14)
Senn [680]	1965	Bern	Switzerland	14	(0)	1	0		1	10+			13	4		{13 Elema, 1 General Elec.
Primo [603]	1964	Brussels	Belgium	13	(0)	2	0		2	12			11	2	2	Medtronic
Derom [178]	1963	Ghent	Belgium	12		1	1		2	21			Numerous			Elema
Kieny [397]	1964	Strasbourg	France	12		1	0		1	18	8	2	11	4	7	{5 Elema, 9 Electrodyne
Perasalo [590]	1963	Helsinki	Finland	11	(0)	0	0		0	14	6		11	4	4	Elema
Hahn [301]	1965	Lausanne	Switzerland	11	(0)	1	0		1	11+	6		10	9	15	{Elema (137), Vitatron (Dutch)
Johansson [367]	1963	Malmö	Sweden	10		2	0		2	18		1				{1 Elema, 9 Medtronic
Totals				1499	(17)	112	163	(38)	275							
Percentage					(0)	7.5	10.9		18.3							
Bouvrain § [62]	1965	Hôp. Lariboisière, Paris	France	139	(0)	15 related to pacing	8		23	31			105 over 6 mo		42	{18 Elema (137), 35 Electrodyne, 118 Medtronic, 6 Cotelec (French), 1 Cordis synchronous}

* One hundred includes 19 endocardial also given on Table V.

† Sixty-one pacemaker replacements and 15 rethoracotomies.

‡ Dack's 94 not included in totals as information is incomplete and 5 patients had endocardial electrodes.

§ This series of 139 of Bouvrain is excluded from the totals as it overlaps with Binet's 160 patients.

Since this table was compiled the total experience up to April, 1965 of all surgeons in France (including that tabulated above) has been collected and analysed,[884, 886] 784 patients had 965 implants with 77 post-implant deaths.

on the anterior surface of the left ventricle, which is easy of access and in which fixation sutures can be put without penetrating the endocardium. Should sepsis develop around the electrodes they can be removed from the surface of the thicker left ventricle with little danger of hemorrhage. Parsonnet [576] has suggested that there is some theoretical advantage in stimulating the right ventricle, as it is less likely to become the site of an infarct which would render the muscle unresponsive. However, a considerable amount of hemodynamic study in dogs has been devoted to the selection of the optimal site for stimulation, and the consensus of opinion clearly favors the left ventricle. Meijler [507] studied the site at which the normal ventricular contraction commences in dogs and concluded that it is where the bundle of His approaches the epicardium most closely, namely a point just to the right of the descending coronary artery. That this site is the first part of the ventricular muscle to be depolarized has also been shown electrocardiographically.[200, 507] Meijler measured the pressures in the femoral artery and the left ventricle, and the oxyhemoglobin level of the blood in the aorta and in the coronary sinus, in complete heart block when pacing with electrodes at various sites, and concluded that a stimulus at this same site just to the right of the descending coronary artery produced the most efficient heart beat. Another technique for measuring contractility with various electrode sites was used in dogs by Vagnini.[772] A polyethylene balloon was introduced into the left ventricle of dogs on total cardiopulmonary bypass, and filled with known volumes of saline. The heart was then paced at different rates from nine locations on the right and left ventricles. The best ventricular epicardial pacemaker site in terms of myocardial contractility was found to be the anterior aspect of the apex of the left ventricle. William-Olsson and Anderson [811] were, however, unable to confirm any advantage from stimulating at this site rather than various other sites, using as their criteria cardiac output measured by a dye dilution technique. Klotz [403] investigated the optimum site for pacing when block occurred during a right ventriculotomy. From studies of the ECG, pressures in the right ventricle and aorta and dye-curve output estimations he selected two optimal sites, the apex of the left ventricle anteriorly and the base of the left ventricle posteriorly. Work from the same laboratory [372, 468] on dogs who had not undergone right ventriculotomy suggested that there was 100 per cent difference between the optimal sites low on the left ventricle as opposed to the least effective site, which was on the right ventricle. From a study of the timing of the spread of the depolarizing wave, they deduced which part of the ventricular muscle was activated directly through muscle and which part via the Purkinje system when stimulated at various sites. Woolfolk [818] stimulated the hearts of dogs with surgically induced block at various sites on the right and left ventricles. He found that when the conduction system was intact or when right bundle branch block was present, stimulation at different ventricular sites produced small variations of up to 13 per cent in the LV pressure and up to 25 per cent in the RV pressure. Following Purkinje net destruction with Lugol's iodine, pressure variations of up to 41 per cent in the left ventricle and 31 per cent in the right ventricle were found, with stimulation in the region of the pulmonary conus producing the worst results. They noted, however, that the differences were greatest for one stimulated beat, and tended to disappear with continuous pacing. It appears to be hemodynamically preferable to stimulate as much as possible of the muscle mass through the Purkinje system,[808] and so obtain the sequence of spread of muscular contraction from area to area as occurs physiologically.[275] This sequence was recorded by Lewis in 1915.[444] Finney [225] recently carried out a thorough experimental investigation of the hemodynamics in dogs when pacing at different sites, measuring the tension developed and the maximal rate of development of tension as well as other parameters, and he concluded that with the electrode on the left ventricle, the heart beat was clearly more efficient than with it on the right ventricle. His results also favored pacing from the apex of the ventricle rather than the other sites tested. So far these canine hemodynamic studies favoring the left ventricular site have not been confirmed in man. Benchimol and Dimond,[29] measuring cardiac index, stroke index, blood pressure, ejection time and ventricular power in 26 patients stimulated in both left and right ventricles at inflow tract, midventricular and outflow tract sites, were unable to show any significant statistical differences. However, an anterior site on the left ventricle is recommended,[207, 367] and at this site there is usually an adequate area of muscle free from the larger coronary vessels where the electrode can be sutured, obtaining good contact with a minimum of bleeding. Tissue damage and too many sutures at the electrode site will lead to reactive fibrosis and, in due course, a rise of the threshold required to pace, a complication which must certainly be minimized.

If the course of the coronary vessels requires the most suitable site for an electrode to be close to the phrenic nerve, the nerve can be separated from the electrode with absorptive surgical sponge [574, 724] or dissected free from the pericardium and re-routed.[63, 423, 687] Stimulation of the nerve produces intolerable pulsation of the diaphragm. If necessary this can be stopped by crushing the nerve in the neck.[306, 572]

PACEMAKER SITE. The pacemaker itself has been implanted at various sites. An early method was to implant it in the rectus sheath behind the muscle, and we have used this site for most cases. However, others [136] place the pacemaker subcutaneously anywhere convenient in the abdominal wall. Lillehei [450] has advocated putting it under the external oblique, well down in the left iliac fossa, so that it cannot move further from the heart. This method thus avoids the risk of wire fracture due to pacemaker migration. Courbier [151] places it under the internal oblique at the level of the umbilicus. Furman [254, 255] has drawn attention to the strain put on the wires from changing position, particularly from the arched back of yawning to stooping to tie shoes. It seems that these difficulties can be avoided by implanting the pacemaker in the chest wall [423, 827, 828] rather than the abdomen. Parsonnet [893] has reduced the incidence of wire fracture from 13 with abdominal implantation to 3 per cent with a chest wall site. In a woman the unit can be hidden by the breast, and in an adequately covered man there is usually comfortable room low in the axilla between the pectoral and latissimus dorsi.[828] The pacemaker should be sited away from the incision so that the foreign body does not interfere with skin healing.

THRESHOLD RISE. Threshold is discussed fully in Chapter 9, but it must be noted here that there is always some rise of threshold of current required to pace in the first few weeks after placing the electrodes. This can be measured if the procedure is carried out in two stages: bringing the electrodes out through the skin when they are first implanted; and delaying a few weeks before implanting the pacemaker. Before experience had accumulated, this seemed a practical procedure, but now that the likely level of the maximum threshold can be forecast sufficiently accurately, pacemakers are designed to stimulate with an adequate margin of power, and implantation can be carried out at the time of plac-ing the electrodes, thus avoiding a two-stage operation which might increase the risk of sepsis.[138] It is unusual for the threshold to rise further after about four weeks unless sepsis develops, in which case a considerable rise can be expected to a level likely to be above the output of the standard pacemakers. However, Parsonnet [574] had pacing failure from rise of threshold certainly in three and possible in two more of his 85 patients, Kaiser [889] has reported it in 9 of 36, and Morris [530] has reported it in 14 of 77 patients.

POSTOPERATIVE COMPLICATIONS. This method of pacing must involve operative exposure of the heart, and, however skillfully it may be performed, the associated postoperative complications cannot be entirely avoided. There are specific complications such as pleural effusion, pericarditis and the postpericardiotomy syn-drome,[60, 180, 193, 828] but more important are the commonplace sequelae of such an operation in the elderly,[219, 306] including pul-monary infections, atelectasis, deep vein thrombosis and pulmo-nary embolism.[144, 617] Sudden postoperative death has been re-ported frequently. Ricordeau [617] estimates that 11.5 per cent of patients with implants die an early death, and we suggest that the local cardiac reaction to the operation may be an important fac-tor in rendering the heart susceptible to serious arrhythmias, which must account for a considerable portion of these deaths. With the heart in an irritable state postoperatively, the stimuli of the pacemaker are more likely to provoke ventricular fibrilla-tion than at other times.[716, 755] Thus it is important to design pacemakers with the power output as low as is compatible with the anticipated threshold, and experimental work from Ann Arbor suggests that the output from some commercially available im-plantable pacemakers is insufficient to cause fibrillation in normal dogs' hearts.[136, 561, 570] Postoperative mortality is considered again on page 137.

Although the establishment of pacing with electrodes on the surface of the heart requires a considerable operation, replacement of the pacemaker, in the event of failure from battery exhaustion or other defect within the unit itself, is a minor procedure which can be done under local anesthesia. The results of pacing with electrodes on the surface of the heart and an implanted pacemaker, and the diagnosis of failure with this system, will be discussed in Chapters 7 and 8 (see also Table VI, page 80).

2b. *Implanted Pacemaker with Endocardial Electrode*

The combination of an implanted pacemaker with a transvenous endocardial electrode became our standard method in 1963,[692] and was developed independently in Sweden in the same year.[409] Zucker also recorded its use in one patient in the same year.[840]

The outstanding advantage of this method over 2a and 3a is that it avoids operative exposure of the heart; our early mortality has been considerably less with this method.[306] The method accepts the difficulty of obtaining stable contact of an endocardial electrode within the right ventricle, and proved impracticable in 8 cases out of 200 attempted, owing to inability to maintain a satisfactory contact with the endocardium (see the reports shown on Table V, together with Rodewald's experience).[622] Perforation of the heart can be avoided by using a soft endocardial wire, as has been indicated under 1b; thrombosis and embolism have not proved significant complications even without anticoagulant cover. By implanting the entire system the risk of septicemia is avoided.

PROCEDURE. The technique for passing the endocardial electrode by the external or, if necessary, internal jugular vein is as described on pages 56 and 74. When the electrode is stable near the apex of the ventricle at a site with a suitably low threshold, the wire is fixed with sutures in the neck. In the Swedish technique the wire is then run by a subcutaneous course to the abdomen, where it is connected to the pacemaker implanted subcutaneously. If it is thought desirable to use an external pacemaker for a period, the wire is brought through the skin in the groin, and at a later stage it can be picked up as it traverses the subcutaneous tissue of the abdomen and the pacemaker attached and implanted.[409, 410] We have adopted a rather different technique, implanting the pacemaker in the axilla or beneath the breast instead of the abdomen. There is usually ample room in the axilla for the small pacemakers which we use, though the skin over the implant has necrosed in two thin patients. We regard it as important that the incision for axillary implantation is made over the pectoralis major so that this muscle will eventually separate the pacemaker from the skin incision. The whole of this implantation procedure can be carried out under local anesthesia, but we have usually given a general anesthetic once the endocardial electrode is stable in the ventricle. If for a week or so an external pacemaker is preferred, the endocardial wire is coiled in the axilla before coming through the skin; if implantation of the pacemaker has been delayed, we have not encountered sepsis or other difficulty. For the reasons discussed in Chapter 9, "Threshold," we prefer a unipolar endocardial electrode, and we complete the circuit with a tissue electrode making contact with axillary fat. A site must be chosen by trial and error where skeletal muscle twitching does not occur, and if the axillary part of the operation is done under general anesthesia, muscle relaxants must not be used as they will temporarily prevent twitching.

COMPLICATIONS. Some of the difficulties and complications associated with endocardial pacing have been considered in Chapter 5, "Short-Term Pacing." These are, notably, the difficulty of getting the electrode tip stable and the risk of perforation of the heart if a rigid wire is used; these are difficulties in establishing pacing and are not specifically associated with its long-term use. The risk of bacteremia inherent with the electrode wire traversing the skin should be eliminated with this technique when the pacemaker is implanted. We have had one troublesome complication using the C50 endocardial electrodes, which were not designed for long-term use; eight *fractures* occurred in 40 patients over a mean period of pacing of eight months. The common site for fracture was in the neck outside the vein, and it usually occurred after several months of use.[51] Parsonnet, using bipolar electrodes for short-term pacing, had three fractures in 40 patients.[582] With

the early Medtronic design of endocardial wire, which contained
a stainless steel stylet, fracture tended to occur first in the stylet
and subsequently at the same site in the conducting filament.[130,]
[134] This complication has not been reported with these flexible
Medtronic wires if the stylet is removed after introduction, as is
now recommended by the manufacturers, nor has it been reported
with the Elema wires, though the insulation failed in 13 of 305
patients.[407]

ᐯThis endocardial technique with an implanted pacemaker has
been gaining popularity mainly because it avoids a thoracotomy.
ᐯIt is now used as the method of choice by Chardack,[130, 134] a number of Scandinavian surgeons,[410, 665, 682] some German surgeons [57,]
[622] as well as ourselves.[51] Results in series of over ten patients are
set out on Table V, which perforce omits Lagergren's [407] large
series of 305 patients, as he did not differentiate between results
with an external pacemaker (1b) from those with an implanted
system (2b). Furman's [853] series of 39 is also omitted, as his report does not specify follow-up information excepting that seven
patients have died since their implants.

3a. Induction and Radio Frequency Pacemaker with Myocardial Electrode

The induction and radio frequency techniques with myocardial electrodes have some appealing features.ᐯThe power source
is outside the body and can be renewed without operation.ᐯRate
and power can be controlled easily, the latter being of particular
value should the threshold rise. Bakulev in Russia [22] recommends
the induction method for intermittent block. The implanted apparatus is not unduly complex, and in Abram's design is particularly simple.[9] The disadvantages are those mentioned above common to all methods with external apparatus, together with the
ᐯnecessity for a thoracotomy to implant the receiver and electrodes.
ᐯAs so little of the energy transmitted is picked up by the receiver,
the power required is considerable; as a result, the external apparatus requires frequent battery changes or must be of considerable size.ᐯThe external transmitter has to be located accurately
on the surface in relation to the implanted receiver, and it has

been reported that some patients cannot manage the external apparatus,[531, 701] resulting in occasional dangerous loss of pacing control and in at least one case in death.[94]

Stimulation of excitable tissue within the body by means of electromagnetic induction has been used as an experimental technique since 1933.[119, 479] The scientific basis and early clinical applications of this technique have been reviewed by Mauro.[503] Experimental work in dogs on the induction method for heart stimulation has been reported from various centers.[339, 340, 664, 736] The main advantage of the induction system is the extreme simplicity of the implanted apparatus, while the radio frequency system involves implantation of several electronic components. The radio frequency systems, however, allow complete control of the impulse wave form and duration. Several centers have developed induction techniques (Abrams of Birmingham, England,[5, 9, 562] Huo Luan-Ch'iang of Shanghai, China,[349] and Suma of Tokyo, Japan;[870] other centers prefer radio frequency transmission (Cammilli of Florence, Italy,[97, 98] and Glenn of the Yale School of Medicine [204, 278, 279, 439, 807]). These techniques, excepting Cammilli's, employ wires leading to the electrodes on the heart. Breakage of these wires has proved an important potential source of failure, which led Cammilli [96, 97, 601] and Schuder [663, 664, 736] to design very small receiver units which are placed directly on the heart surface to obviate the use of any internal wires. The greater depth of the receiver in the body requires more power from the external transmitter, the positioning of which becomes critical. In Glenn's and Abrams' technique the receiver coil is subcutaneous, and the foreign material so close under the skin may be a factor leading to ulceration and sepsis. Glenn usually places the receiver in the axilla, and Abrams on the anterior chest wall.

These induction methods have not been widely used, and too few results (74 cases; see Table V) have as yet been reported in the literature for evaluation, which, as with all methods, must depend on the proven reliability of the implanted apparatus over a long period. However, Glenn [855] has now paced 42 patients with this method and is well pleased with the performance of his apparatus (Airborne).

3b. Induction Pacemaker with Endocardial Electrode

Abrams, who originated one of the induction techniques, recently modified it for use with an endocardial electrode, thereby avoiding a thoracotomy.[7] Glenn [855] has recently paced eight patients in this way. Barr [24] has developed a similar induction technique using radio frequencies and has employed it on dogs.

EXTERNAL CONTROLS OF IMPLANTED PACEMAKERS

Some pacemakers can, when implanted, be switched on and off, speeded and slowed, or have their power output altered. The three techniques in use for this are: (a) a magnetic switch; [36, 63, 105, 530, 749, 794] (b) electrical induction; [163, 277, 386] (c) The use of a needle screw inserted through the skin into a socket in the implanted pacemaker (Medtronic).

Whichever method is used, rate control must render the pacemaker more complex, and it has been argued that this must increase the risk of breakdown of the implanted unit.[91] Some of the advantages of rate control and the ability to switch the unit on and off are partly illusory. For instance, it is not safe in a patient who has had Stokes-Adams attacks to switch off when block gives way to sinus rhythm, for this change is no guarantee of cessation of the attacks.

The optimum heart rate is discussed in Chapter 10. Hemodynamic studies show that patients with good ventricular function can increase their output to meet the requirements of exercise with a fixed rate, provided this is not too low. In a minority of patients with poor myocardial function, however, an increase of rate above 70 to 75 may provide for some increase in maximal output. Patients with rate-controllable pacemakers do not prove good judges of when to adjust their heart rate.[207] Moreover, if the rate control is to be adjusted every time the patient exerts himself, his dependency on the pacemaker is likely to prove psychologically undesirable. On the other hand, increasing the rate in the postoperative period may be of real value, particularly to avoid interpolated beats, and thus reduce the risk of ventricular fibrillation. Kantrowitz [381] and colleagues [194, 530] recommended raising the rate for this purpose and advocated the General Electric pacemaker, which has an induction control. Since the impulse energy delivered by this pacemaker is a function of rate, the threshold for stimulation can be checked at any time by increasing the rate with the external control until pacing ceases. At a heart rate of 60 beats per minute, the pacemaker delivers approximately 60 µj each impulse, and at a rate of 120 beats per minute this has been approximately halved; as the relationship between these two rates is approximately linear it is possible to measure the cardiac threshold from a knowledge of the rate at which pacing ceases. There are two disadvantages to this method of threshold measurement, apart from the fact that it is, of course, only applicable to pacemakers of this type. Firstly, the threshold for cardiac stimulation will normally be well below 30 µj (see Chapter 9), and it is not practicable to turn the pacemaker rate control up to the necessary high levels for pacing to cease. Secondly, the sudden cessation of pacing during rapid tachycardia is particularly prone to result in prolonged asystole (see p. 113). Although pacing can be resumed easily when the measurements are being carried out at a pacing center, the maneuver would be potentially dangerous elsewhere. This type of pacemaker can also be controlled by means of high frequency, low energy pulses introduced from an externally applied induction-coupled control unit. This control unit, known as a threshold analyzer (see p. 164), rapidly provides information concerning the myocardial threshold and the presence of faults in the pacemaker.[371, 602]

ATRIAL-TRIGGERED PACEMAKERS

The first papers referring to experimental pacing by means of pacemakers which are triggered by the P wave of atrial contraction have been mentioned in the historical section on page 6. Folkman and Watkins'[234] work was elaborated by Stephenson[526, 730, 732, 733] and Battye.[25] By 1963, both Nathan[547, 548] and Bonnabeau[54] had developed atrial-triggered pacemakers which were small enough for implantation. The first clinical report was on the use of Nathan's instrument, the "Cordis Atricor" pacemaker, appearing later in the same year,[117] and this has been followed by other reports [115, 116, 545, 546] which refer to the technique as "synchronous pacing." Carlens [103] and Lagergren [891] have reported on the clinical use of a Swedish-made implantable P wave stimulator (Elema EM 141).

A pacemaker which follows the atrial rate and supplies impulses to the ventricle after a suitable delay (PR interval) has obvious physiological advantages, which are more fully discussed in the section on hemodynamic aspects on page 190. The most important of these advantages are that variation in cardiac output according to demand is allowed for by change of rate as well as stroke volume, and that the ventricular contraction is suitably timed after atrial filling. Although atrial-triggering will theoretically avoid artificial stimuli falling during the vulnerable period of a T wave, it has been reported that ventricular beats triggered the P wave circuit, and the resulting pacemaker stimulus fell during the vulnerable period with the risk of ventricular fibrillation.[543, 891] For use in clinical practice, atrial-triggered pacemakers must have a basic inherent rate at which they will take over if no atrial impulse is detected, either as a result of an electrical fault or of atrial asystole. At the other end of the scale they must guard against too high a ventricular rate, such as may be created by atrial fibrillation or flutter. One of the difficulties in developing this technique has been that the electrical potential of the P wave is often small relative to the ventricular and other potentials detectable in the area. With the Cordis Atricor this has proved a practical difficulty.[540]

Chardack [124, 125, 133] has argued that the physiological advantages of atrial-triggered pacing, including ventricular filling from atrial contraction, are negligible in elderly patients with narrowed coronary arteries. He stated that such patients should not be permitted to overexert themselves. He claims that an increase in cardiac output is very costly in terms of energy if achieved by an increase of rate, as opposed to increased stroke volume.

The P wave can be picked up in a variety of ways. Nathan's technique has been to suture, at thoracotomy, an extra electrode to the surface of the left atrium.[117] Bonnabeau [54] intended to use one of the pacing electrodes sutured on to the left ventricle, and Lillehei [447] noted that this technique would enable patients to have fixed-rate pacemakers replaced by atrial-triggered units when the batteries were exhausted; however, this design of atrial-triggered pacemaker has not been used clinically.[449] Carlens,[103] who paced with venous endocardial electrodes, has placed at mediastinoscopy a detector-electrode outside the pericardium, between the atrium and the esophagus. Rodewald,[623] who also paced endocardially, used a second venous electrode with its tip within the right atrium.

Experience with these atrial-triggered pacemakers is as yet limited, though the Cordis model has been available since 1963. The originators report in 1965 [115] having implanted their "new" model in 36 patients with one postoperative death and one fractured electrode; in two other patients ventricular capture was lost. Pacer pocket infections occurred only in those undergoing reimplantations. Brockman [882] inserted 19 Cordis synchronous pacemakers and records his experience with these and 15 fixed rate units. He states that the complications were fairly evenly distributed between fixed rate and synchronous units. There were seven wire fractures and five unit failures in the 34 patients. Lagergren [891] has used the Elmqvist atrial-triggered pacemaker in association with endocardial electrodes in 20 patients, six of these having been paced with it for more than six months. In three it proved necessary to readjust the site of the mediastinal pick-up electrode and two electronic failures necessitated a change of pacemaker. His paper gives evidence of hemodynamic improvement in patients changed from fixed rate to atrial-triggered pacing.

Atrial-controlled pacemakers have particular appeal for those patients in whom the stroke volume does not adjust to allow adequate output to meet the varying demands for reasonable activity, for patients in sinus rhythm and for younger patients with disease confined to the conducting tissue. It is reasonable to suppose that sudden postoperative death, which is more common in patients in sinus rhythm than in block,[716] and is presumably sometimes due to pacemaker-induced arrhythmias, while not totally eliminated, will occur less often with atrial-triggered than with fixed-rate pacemakers. Continuing use will show whether the more complex apparatus is associated with more frequent breakdown,

"ON DEMAND" PACEMAKERS

More than a quarter of all patients requiring pacing for the threat of Stokes-Adams attacks are in sinus rhythm [85, 716, 826] and only require ventricular stimulation when an attack of complete block supervenes. The pacing requirements of this group are well served by a pacemaker which only fires when the ventricle fails to beat on its own. The first external pacemakers used at our hospital were of this type,[426] and use of pacemakers to achieve this end have also been reported by Johansson,[366] by Effert,[202] by Nicks,[556] by Sykosch,[749] by Fortin [239] and by Lemberg.[429] We are aware of four versions of fully implantable demand pacemakers (also known as "standby" or "ventricular-inhibited" pacemakers) of which 2 are being developed by the Cordis Corporation, one by the American Optical Company [885] and one by the Department of Medical Physics at Gröningen University in Holland. In addition a fifth unit is under development by Devices Ltd. in England and similar work is progressing in Italy.[883] Most of these pacemakers detect spontaneous ventricular activity and do not produce a stimulus unless the R-R interval exceeds a pre-set limit but one, the Cordis Ventricor 3, utilises a different principle. This unit which has been used by Neville [892] has been modified from the Cordis Atricor; the stimulus is normally triggered by a spontaneous R wave so that it falls in the absolute refractory period but if the R-R interval exceeds the limit the pacemaker functions as a fixed-rate unit. This system has the advantages that an ECG instantly reveals the unit to be functioning and that the pacemaker can be triggered at any desired rate by small external stimuli.

The other demand pacemakers do not produce impulses continuously but only stimulate when the ventricular rate falls below the pre-set limit.

Satisfactory function can be assessed for the American Optical unit, the Gröningen University unit and the Devices unit by application of an external magnet which temporarily converts the pacemaker to a fixed-rate continuously stimulating pacemaker. The heart rate must be slowed below the pacemaker rate for confirmation that the Cordis Ventricor 2 is functioning satisfactorily and this can usually be achieved by massage of the carotid artery.

We have found that an intravenous injection of 1-2 mg edrophonium chloride (Tensilon ®) is an excellent test for a demand pacemaker as it produces transient slowing of the heart and allows two or three paced beats to occur. The most comprehensive report so far available on fully implanted demand pacemakers is that of Parsonnet [894] who describes satisfactory results with the Cordis Ventricor 2 for periods of up to one year. Our own experience is still too scanty for firm conclusions to be drawn but we have implanted units which are functioning successfully after several months.

SUMMARY

The indications for long-term pacing have been briefly stated. The methods depend basically on whether the pacemaker itself is to be implanted, whether electrodes are to be placed by operation on or in the myocardium, as opposed to the use of the endocardial electrode passed via a vein, and whether induction techniques with power outside the body but with some implanted receiving apparatus are used. Combinations of these techniques have resulted in six methods which are in general clinical use, and these are described in detail. With increasing clinical experience, the various methods have been modified from time to time; the results reported in the literature and in our own clinical practice are tabulated and discussed, though the results of pacing with an implanted pacemaker and a myocardial electrode, the most widely practiced method, are discussed more fully in Chapter 8. The risks specific to each method have been considered, for example, those of operative exposure of the heart required when using myocardial electrodes and those of thromboembolism and bacteremia when using the venous endocardial electrodes.

Many technical problems have been considered. The most suitable materials for electrodes and their wires are as yet unsettled. While platinum does not undergo electrolysis, it does not have ideal mechanical properties, and various alloys have been tried; some designs use only the negative electrode on the heart, in which case a material of suitable mechanical properties can be used, as electrolysis is not a problem at the cathode. The optimum site at which to place electrodes at operation, as judged from experimental work on cardiac efficiency and practical surgical access, is an area free from coronary vessels near the apex of the left ventricle. Although most pacemakers have been implanted in the abdominal wall, the chest wall is now usually favored, particularly as there is less strain on the wires.

Induction methods are not very widely used, but have some appealing features, especially the ease of control of rate and power and the simplicity of renewing batteries, which, with the implantation methods, requires a minor operation every few years. Some implanted pacemakers can be switched on and off and their speed and power controlled from outside the body. This has been achieved in many different methods by a magnetic switch, an electrical induction control or the use of a needle screw inserted through the skin.

The most sophisticated of pacemakers are atrial-controlled (synchronous), the heart benefiting from physiological atrial filling. By timing the ventricular impulse in relation to the P wave, the possibility of the stimulus following in the vulnerable phase of the cardiac cycle is avoided, and it is hoped that this will reduce the risk of ventricular fibrillation.

"On demand" pacemakers only emit a stimulus to the ventricle when there has been a preset delay since the previous QRS complex. They are of particular value for patients in sinus rhythm who are liable to paroxysms of complete heart block or Stokes-Adams attacks.

Chapter 7

LONG-TERM PACING: COMPLICATIONS AND FAILURES

EXTRANEOUS ELECTRICAL APPARATUS INTERFERING WITH PACEMAKERS

THERE ARE TWO WAYS in which currents capable of producing ventricular fibrillation can reach patients being paced artificially: first, when an external pacemaker is connected to the main power line and is inadequately earthed; and second, when the patient comes close to apparatus setting up radio frequency waves which may be picked up by the pacemaker apparatus.

1. A patient with an electrode making contact with the myocardium always risks developing ventricular fibrillation due to stray electric currents passing through the heart; the risk is greater when the electrode contact area is small,[792, 804] probably because of the resulting high current density. The risk is particularly high if a line-powered pacemaker is connected directly to the heart, and some other line-powered apparatus, such as an electrocardiograph, is also connected to the patient. Small leakage currents may then possibly pass through the heart even when neither piece of equipment is turned on and, the hazards of inadequate earthing of line-powered equipment in this respect are now recognized.[84, 726] Ventricular fibrillation has been recorded in this manner in three patients,[525, 558] and in three other recorded patients, fatal ventricular fibrillation may have originated similarly.[674] We recommend that all external pacemakers be powered by batteries to avoid this potential risk.

2. The possibility of apparatus picking up radio frequency waves is very real with some designs of external pacemakers.[446] It is also theoretically possible with fully implanted pacemakers, although the electrical coupling is different when the unit is implanted, and the risk is remote.[134] Models designed to receive

power from outside might be expected to be the most susceptible, but it is claimed by the users of the two most popular models that they have tested out their apparatus in various situations, including proximity to radio broadcasting stations and in aircraft, and that pacing is not affected.[94, 559, 806] Cammilli [94] has stated that his model would be affected only inside a very powerful radio station. Carleton [105] states that the magnetic external control of his dual-rate pacemaker is unaffected by automobile electric components, commercial electrical generating stations and diathermy. Lichter [446] pointed out that the surgical diathermy is the apparatus emitting radio frequency waves, which is most likely to come into close proximity to patients. He observed fibrillation in two patients when the diathermy (American Cystoscope Co.) was switched on, and carried out tests showing that the *external* pacemaker being used at the time, I.M.E. model G.V. 2371 (G.U. Mfg. Co.), was particularly liable to interference from radio frequency waves, and produced fibrillatory currents as a result. It was also adversely affected by Hyfrecator diathermy (Birtcher Corp.), short-wave diathermy (Liebel Flarsheim Co.), U.V.L. machines (Fitzgerald Mfg. Co.), broadcasting stations and neon advertising lights. Of the other pacemakers tested in this way, an Elema implantable pacemaker was the only one affected, and this was less sensitive than the external pacemakers tested; the Elema unit was adversely affected at 6 ft from the U.V.L. machine and at 4 in from the neon light. The experimental arrangement has been heavily criticized by the manufacturers [759] because the unit was not implanted, a factor which is of great importance in the electrical coupling; it is the arrangement of the electrodes and their wires which is the critical factor in susceptibility to this form of interference.[320, 877] A Medtronic unit, a Devices unit and a Corbin-Farnsworth pacemaker were not affected by surgical diathermy in their experimental setup. Lichter attributes the lack of sensitivity of these units to their design, in particular that the pulse "generator" is separate from the pulse "shaper." Electrosurgical transurethral prostatectomy has been carried out on patients with implanted units (both Medtronic and General Electric) without interference with pacing.[405]

Three pacemakers, one of which was purchasable on the market (type not specified, but Chardack [134] states that this was a Medtronic model), have been tested out by Carleton [106, 107] with an oscilloscope and camera in a large number of situations in which it seemed possible that interference might occur. The only situations in which the pacemakers were adversely affected were as follows: within 6 cm of an automobile distributor; within 8 cm of the spark plugs of a lawn mower; within 30 cm of a commercial diathermy (13.5 to 27 megacycles); and when held in a bath of saline 6 cm and 31 cm away from the paddle-electrodes of a cardiac defibrillator. The commercially available pacemaker was stopped permanently by an AC defibrillating current, but was unaffected by a DC shock; the other pacemakers were affected by both currents. Chardack [134] suggests that an automobile ignition system and lawn mower spark plug would not have affected the pacemakers had they been completely implanted. He found that Medtronic units were adversely affected by electrocautery coagulation within 2 in and by exposure to diathermy, but not by electrocautery currents, external defibrillation shocks or x-radiation at diagnostic or therapeutic levels of exposure.

There is insufficient evidence from other sources regarding the effect of defibrillatory currents on implanted pacemakers for firm conclusions to be drawn, though Norman [559] states that successful defibrillation has been carried out with the Lucas induction pacemaker *in situ,* without damage to it; he has also shown experimentally that the General Electric pacemaker will usually stand up to AC and DC defibrillatory shocks.[560] Kantrowitz [382] records successful defibrillation by countershock with an implanted General Electric pacemaker, and Cole [144] records that a Medtronic 5860 pacemaker worked satisfactorily as an external pacemaker after it had been in a patient treated with a 750 v DC countershock, though the patient succumbed. Norman [560] describes a patient under the care of Dr. Austen at the Massachusetts General Hospital in whom a pacemaker discharged at a rate of 900 beats per minute following defibrillation. Fortunately, the patient survived. Keller [392] states that Cordis has incorporated in their circuitry a bypass so that if the atrial pickup carries more than 3 v or the ventricular lead more than 8 v, the current bypasses the unit itself, and is led off to the indifferent electrode. He has also ascertained that pacemakers implanted in patients within a jet aircraft are unaffected by the pilot's controls. [546]

The magnetic field used for charging nickel-cadmium cells of implantable pacemakers has been shown to be powerful enough to stop units of the Medtronic type.[699]

PACEMAKER-INDUCED ARRHYTHMIAS

When considering arrhythmias induced by artificial pacing, it is important to distinguish between two main groups. The first group is composed of instances in which the discharge rate of the pacemaker increases and the ventricle continues to follow the pacemaker, initially with a 1:1 response, but usually developing varying degrees of block subsequently so that ventricular capture becomes intermittent. This situation is now called the "runaway pacemaker." The second group of pacemaker-induced arrhythmias includes instances in which a stimulus from a pacemaker, which may be functioning normally or abnormally, falls in the vulnerable period of the cardiac cycle [400, 810] and provokes ventricular tachycardia or fibrillation.

The "Runaway Pacemaker"

Early models of several types of pacemaker were designed so that an increase in the rate of discharge indicated impending battery exhaustion,[136, 701, 828] but it later became apparent that in its original form this was an undesirable feature, since failure of certain electronic components can result in secondary battery exhaustion, with the production of a rapid ventricular tachycardia; the pacemaker discharge rate may become extremely fast and we are aware of units which discharged at over 1,000 beats per minute with intermittent ventricular capture. At rapid pacemaker discharge rates, the impulse energy may become insufficient to stimulate the myocardium, so that ventricular response becomes intermittent and may cease altogether, at which time an idioventricular rhythm may or may not reappear. If the ventricle follows the pacemaker, the rate may become fast enough for the development of ventricular fibrillation. The circuitry of many implanted pacemakers is now designed to produce a decrease in stimulation rate when the batteries become depleted, but failure of critical components may, nevertheless, result in a dangerous tachycardia, and Chardack [134] points out that the additional circuitry itself may be the cause of pacemaker failure.

A "runaway pacemaker" usually presents as an emergency complication with ventricular fibrillation as a frequent development.[16, 123, 621, 713, 817, 828] In less severe instances, chest pain is one of the dominant clinical features. This was present in five of our first eight patients with this complication, as well as featuring prominently in the presentation of other cases.[817] The development of pain at rapid ventricular rates in these patients is not surprising, since both we [713] and others [546] have shown that relatively minor increases in pacing rate up to 90 to 100 beats per minute may result in the production of anginal pain. In the case of one of our patients with a "runaway pacemaker," the chest pain was so severe that he was diagnosed and treated with large doses of morphia for four hours as having had a cardiac infarction, his electrocardiogram being interpreted as showing ventricular tachycardia secondary to infarction. Other clinical features produced by a "runaway pacemaker" are weakness, palpitations, dyspnea, orthopnea and clouding of consciousness which may amount to semicoma; the blood pressure is unduly low, and Stokes-Adams attacks may develop.

Table VII lists a number of reports of "runaway pacemakers" appearing in the literature. These reports represent only a small proportion of the total incidence of this complication, and we are aware of many cases which have not been reported and which have occurred with almost all the commercially available implantable units. Because of the inadequate information available, it is not justifiable to draw statistical conclusions from the table, but the danger of the "runaway pacemaker" is emphasized by the fact that, of these 34 patients, 12 died. The treatment of the complication is now clear, and the malfunctioning pacemaker should be urgently disconnected from the heart. This is usually carried out by cutting the electrode wires in the subcutaneous tissue, pacing being continued by attachment of another pacemaker to the myocardial end of the cut wires or possibly by

TABLE VII

THE RUNAWAY PACEMAKER

First Author	Year	Rate	VF	Outcome
Aldridge [16]	1965	336–750	VF	Died
		80–150		Survived
Bouvrain [61]	1963	110		Died
Costeas [148]	1965	300		Died
Derom [178]	1963	140		Died
Effert [203]	1964	180		Survived
Faivre [220]	1964	130		Survived
Furman [252]	1965		VF	Died
Gaal [260]	1964	400		Survived
Glass [277]	1963	140		Survived
Harris [309]	1963	135		Survived
Hoffman [331]	1965	440		Died
Kieny [397]	1964			Survived
Langendorf [415]	1965	300–600		Survived
Nash [542]	1964	400		Survived
Nathan (Center) [116]	1964	⎰ 600		Died
		⎱ 400		Died
" [117]	1963			Survived
" [546]	1964	90–120		Survived
Norman [560]	1965	up to 900		Survived
Parsonnet [577]	1963	120		Survived
Robinson [621]	1965	120	VF	Died
Siddons [687]	1963	150		Survived
Sowton [713]	1963	130		Survived
		175		Survived
		136		Survived
		140	VF	Died
		108		Survived
		110		Survived
		100		Survived
		140		Survived
Welti [802]	1965	250		Died
Wisoff [817]	1965	288	VF	Survived
" [123]	1964	150	VF	Died

application of external skin electrodes or needle electrodes in the chest wall. Disconnection of the "runaway pacemaker" and substitution of a normal pacing rate usually results in a dramatic clinical response, and one of our patients awoke prematurely from an anesthetic when this was done. If the ventricular rate is only moderately elevated, there may be time for a transvenous electrode catheter to be passed to the right ventricle for subsequent control of the heart rate when the faulty indwelling pacemaker is removed, and Langendorf and Pick [415] have suggested that paired stimulation of the ventricle via this catheter would provide a means to control the ventricular tachycardia (see p. 212). We cannot recommend this procedure, which is likely to allow periods of breakthrough of rapid ventricular tachycardia [614] and which has caused ventricular fibrillation in several of our animal experiments. It may rarely be possible to inhibit the discharge of certain types of implantable pacemaker by the application of external induction or radio frequency signals,[163, 371] but these techniques are applicable only to specific pacemaker models and require the use of apparatus which is not generally available outside pacemaker centers. Antiarrythmic drugs are useless in this complication.[864]

Pacemaker-induced Ventricular Fibrillation

The threshold for production of ventricular fibrillation by electrical stimulation during the vulnerable period is normally between 10 and 30 times the threshold for ventricular contraction when the stimulus is applied during the nonrefractory part of diastole,[77, 197, 250, 605] but it has been shown that the threshold for fibrillation can be lowered under many circumstances. Myocardial ischemia is associated with considerable lowering of the fibrillation threshold,[76, 810] and a similar effect is produced by vagal stimulation.[77] The threshold for fibrillation can be lowered to a level barely exceeding the level for contraction by small amounts of epinephrine,[77] and similar effects can be produced by sympathomimetic drugs, anesthetics, digitalis and other agents.[54, 273, 393, 488, 810] Other factors also influence the relation between the fibrillation threshold and the contraction threshold; Zoll and Linenthal[831] reported that the normal safety factor, 10 to 20, was lowered to about 7 when the impulse duration was increased from 5 milliseconds to 20 milliseconds in dogs, thus confirming previous reports that the threshold for ventricular fibrillation increased as the impulse duration decreased.[329, 330, 605] The fibrillation threshold is higher when the stimuli are applied near the base of the heart than when the electrode site is near the apex,[566, 776] and the fibrillation threshold is increased as the electrode area is reduced.[153]

Brooks[77] reported that no period was ever found during the cardiac cycle when the minimum effective stimulus provoking contraction would cause ventricular fibrillation in a normal animal's heart, and Chardack[136] has confirmed that ventricular fibrillation in dogs did not follow stimulation at up to 100 v and

250 ma during stable pacing; during the vulnerable period, impulses of 30 to 68 ma were needed before short bursts of ventricular fibrillation were produced.

It is apparent that in paced patients the stimulus can fall in the vulnerable period in two situations only: when spontaneous ectopic beats arise; or when a second focus is present with the production of parasystole. Johansson [367] analyzed the relationship between pacemaker stimuli and spontaneous ectopic beats occurring in patients with complete heart block and a basically stable paced rhythm. He found that the distribution of pacemaker stimuli was not uniform; most stimuli appeared during the ectopic systole and very few appeared during the last part of the T wave or during diastole. He suggested that the most probable explanation was that the artificially induced (paced) beat depolarized both the myocardial muscle and the conducting system. This observation suggests that the risk of a pacemaker stimulus falling in the vulnerable period of an ectopic beat in a patient with otherwise stable paced rhythm is very low indeed. The situation is quite different when parasystole is present due to the return of A-V conduction so that competition occurs between the artificial pacemaker and the sinus rhythm. Under the conditions commonly found in clinical practice, about 4 to 6 per cent of pacemaker impulses fall into the vulnerable period of patients in sinus rhythm,[367, 713] and there will be approximately 3,000 pacemaker impulses potentially able to cause ventricular fibrillation in 24 hours. The safety factor between the threshold for fibrillation and the threshold for contraction is normally large, and many authorities hold that the risk of pacemaker-induced fibrillation is negligible.[136, 367, 561, 831, 843] Some support for this view was provided by Parker,[570] who produced parasystole in a dog without heart block by pacing the heart by a right ventricular catheter, and was unable to provoke ventricular fibrillation, despite alterations in the pacing rate and the stimulus current. Whalen,[804] on the contrary, also paced the hearts of normal dogs anesthetized with choralose, and found that ventricular fibrillation was caused when a 30 ma impulse of two milliseconds duration fell during the vulnerable period. This fibrillation current was lowered progressively as the respirator was stopped for longer periods of time, until fibrillation could be produced by a current of 17 ma. Similar findings were reported by Rothfeld,[639] who produced competitive pacing in 20 dogs for at least 30 minutes without provocation of ventricular fibrillation. Following intravenous injection of quinidine (5-10 mg/kg), however, 14 of the 20 animals developed ventricular arrhythmias, although no such arrhythmias occurred in a control group in whom the catheter was present but pacing was not carried out. This demonstration that competitive pacing can provoke ventricular fibrillation when the fibrillation threshold is artificially lowered is substantiated by an investigation carried out by Nathan,[549] who applied stimuli of the types provided by contemporary indwelling pacemakers (2 msec biphasic, 0.1-17 ma) to dogs' hearts during the vulnerable period. The results showed that hypoxia reduced the fibrillation threshold considerably and that circumflex artery occlusion had the same effect, so that repetitive ectopic beats and ventricular tachycardia could be produced easily by stimuli of low intensity. The stimulus magnitude needed to sustain a tachycardia was less than that for initiation, and the vulnerable period could be shifted in the direction of the ST interval by repetitive stimuli following occlusion. The vulnerable period in human subjects has been directly investigated by Castellanos.[112] Fourteen patients with complete heart block were paced with transvenous catheter electrodes, and test impulses were inserted during different portions of the ventricular cycle. When the test impulses fell close to the peak of the T waves, multiple extrasystoles occurred in two patients, repetitive firing in three and ventricular fibrillation in one. The intensity of the testing stimulus was never less than four times the threshold for contraction, with voltages varying between 2.4 and 6.7 (see also reference no. 847).

Several other reports are available of repetitive firing induced in human subjects by pacemaker stimuli falling within the vulnerable period,[54, 187, 197, 207, 429, 448, 625, 682, 713, 731, 768] and the particular importance of digitalis in this syndrome has been reported by Lewis.[442] A well-documented case in which several periods of proven ventricular fibrillation were induced by pacemaker stimuli falling in the vulnerable period was reported by Tavel, and

Fisch [755] and other authors have reported similar experiences.[448,] [543] As would be expected from the results of animal experiments, the risk is high in patients with myocardial ischemia, and Julian [374] noted pacemaker-induced fibrillation when pacing a patient who had developed a complete heart block following myocardial infarction. The suspicion that pacemaker-induced ventricular fibrillation might be occurring in our own series led to the analysis of the death rate in our first 58 patients treated for more than six months with implanted pacemakers; [718] we found that the death rate among patients with parasystole was five times higher than that among patients with paced rhythm only, although there was no other significant difference between the groups, suggesting that pacemaker-induced fibrillation might be occurring. The possible occurrence of this complication is also suggested by reports in the literature describing paced patients who died unexpectedly and in whom no pacemaker malfunction nor cause of death could be found at autopsy. In such reports, parasystole from sinus rhythm was often present, and one such example is given by Lawrence,[424] who noted that one paced patient in sinus rhythm developed temporary ventricular fibrillation one hour after pacemaker implantation. At the follow-up visit after three months, the patient was well, and the electrocardiogram continued to show competitive pacing; the patient died suddenly one and a half hours later, but no cause for death could be found at autopsy. Trimble [768] also reports death from ventricular fibrillation three hours after insertion of a pacemaker; this was in a 49-year-old patient with sinus rhythm, but he was considered to have had progressive coronary arterial disease. Parker [570] reports that severe coronary arterial disease was also found at autopsy in a paced patient with sinus rhythm dying from cardiac arrhythmia. Ventricular fibrillation may well develop in some patients with ischemia with no relation whatever to artificial pacemaking, but it also seems possible that the actual development of the arrhythmia may be precipitated finally by a stimulus falling at a vulnerable period in a patient with a low fibrillation threshold. Kohler and MacKinney [405] reported the development of ventricular fibrillation in paced patients in sinus rhythm with successful defibrillation and replacement of the unit.

Indeed, suspicion that this iatrogenic arrhythmia occurs occasionally is becoming widespread.[323, 573, 864] A particular type of parasystole is that produced by two functioning artificial pacemakers, and development of the pacemaker-induced ventricular fibrillation in this situation has been documented by Robinson [620] and us.[718]

Table VIII lists the rather incomplete information available on 42 patients reported in the literature in whom there is at least a high degree of suspicion that rapid ventricular arrhythmia was triggered by the pacemaker stimulus falling within the vulnerable period. In almost every case in which the information is available, pacemaker parasystole, usually due to sinus rhythm, was present, and it will be noted that 35 of the 42 patients died. It is significant that many of the instances occurred in the immediate postoperative period, a finding very noticeable in the six patients of our own in whom we were able to document rapid ventricular arrhythmias occurring during pacing.[718] This finding is only to be expected, since when the arrhythmia occurred after the patient had left the hospital it would be unrecognized; but the high incidence in the first 48 hours postoperatively is particularly noticeable. The fibrillation threshold may be lowered by the inflammatory reaction around the site of electrode attachment to the heart, while the inevitable pericardial reaction may also have a similar effect; there may be an unusually high concentration of blood catecholamines following an operation, and various drugs may have been given. The threshold for contraction is very low at the time of attachment for electrodes to the heart (see p. 157), and so the stimulus strength is likely to exceed the threshold for contraction by a larger proportion at this time than subsequently, when the contraction threshold has increased to its final plateau.[127, 324]

The differing opinions held by various workers on the likelihood of pacemaker-induced ventricular fibrillation presenting a significant risk to the patient in sinus rhythm may be partially due to the differences in stimulus strength provided by different pacemakers. A pacemaker electrode system in which the stimulus strength is only slightly above the threshold for myocardial contraction should very rarely be associated with pacemaker-induced

TABLE VIII
PACEMAKER—INDUCED FIBRILLATION

First Author and Reference No.	Year	Parasystole or Multiple Ectopic Beats	Possible Predisposing Factors	Time Since Operation	Outcome
Allen [18]	1964			6 wk	Died
Bonnabeau [54]	1963	+	VF before pacing	1 dy	Died
		+	VF before pacing	1 dy	Died
Bouvrain [62]	1965	+	Aortic stenosis: Starr valve	3 dy	Survived
					Died
					Died
Castellanos [112]	1966	+	Fallot repair	During investigation	Survived
Cole [144]	1964			7 dy	Died
Crastonopol [155]	1964	+++		2 wk	Survived
Dittmar [187]	1962			11 dy	Died
Elmqvist [207]	1963		Severe cardiomegaly	8 dy	Died
Gerbaux [266]	1964	+			Died
Jensen [356]	1966		Recent infarct	After 6 wk endocardial pacing	Died
Julian [374]	1964				Died
Lawrence [422]	1964	+	Recent infarct	In "postoperative" period	Died
Lemberg [429]	1965	+++	Isoprenaline, digitalis		Died
Nathan [543]	1965		Isoprenaline, digitalis, myopathy	In "postoperative" period	Died
Overbeck [860]	1965	++	Recent cerebrovascular accident	3rd dy	Died
				3rd dy	Died
Parker [570]	1963	+	Aortic stenosis	6 wk	Died
Portal [598]	1962		Pulmonary emboli	7 dy	Died
				2 dy	Died
Ricordeau [617]	1964		Old infarct		Died
Robinson, D. S. [620]	1965		Old infarct		Survived
					Survived

TABLE VIII—Continued

First Author and Reference No.	Year	Parasystole or Multiple Ectopic Beats	Possible Predisposing Factors	Time Since Operation	Outcome
Robinson, J. S. [621]	1965	+	Diabetes, prepacing VF, 2 pacemakers	4 mo	Survived
			Diabetes, change pacemaker	2 dy	Died
			Quinidine, digoxin, change pacemaker	12 mo	Died
Senning [682]	1964			1 wk	Died
				6 mo	Died
Sowton [718]	1965	++++		2 dy	Died
			Recent infarct	2 dy	Died
				4 dy	Died
		+++++		7 dy	Survived
			High impulse energy	1 dy	Died
Spear [721]	1965			8 mo	Died
				1 wk	Died
				1 wk	Died
Tavel [755]	1964		2 mo after insertion Starr valve	1 dy	Died
Trimble [767]	1965	++	Gross coronary artery disease		Died

ventricular fibrillation, while a high energy output pacemaker should carry a greater risk. The patients initially treated in our series had pacemakers delivering approximately 200 μj at each stimulus, and the threshold with the myocardial electrodes then in use was about 20 μj. The stimulus intensity was thus about ten times the contraction threshold, and so approached the fibrillation threshold. Since the output energy of these pacemakers was reduced to two or three times the contraction threshold, we have been unable to find any incident suggesting pacemaker-induced ventricular fibrillation in our patients. At the same time, the area of myocardial electrode contact was reduced, and the impulse was considerably shortened. Our current view is that there is very little danger from pacemaker-induced ventricular fibrillation in patients with sinus rhythm treated with most commercially available pacemakers and matching electrodes. The important factor is not the absolute impulse current or energy provided by the pacemaker, but the degree to which this exceeds the threshold for contraction; a pacemaker with high energy output may present little risk with one type of myocardial electrode, but be delivering stimuli of near fibrillation-threshold levels with electrodes of different design. Such risk as exists is probably maximal in the early postoperative period, and is higher in patients with known myocardial ischemia. We consider sympathomimetic drugs to be contraindicated in paced patients because of their known effect in lowering the threshold for ventricular fibrillation.

Some of the features affecting the risk of pacemaker-induced ventricular fibrillation are shown in Table IX.

ASYSTOLE FOLLOWING PACING

If the ventricles of an experimental animal with complete A-V block are paced at a rapid rate and pacing then ceases suddenly, the idioventricular pacemaker becomes depressed and is unable to initiate a spontaneous rhythm until a latent period has elapsed. This effect was first reported by Erlanger [212] and has been used as a method for the experimental production of ventricular asystole.[720] Brockman [74] pointed out, on the basis of dog experiments, that ventricular asystole was not an invariable

TABLE IX

FACTORS INFLUENCING PACEMAKER-INDUCED VENTRICULAR
FIBRILLATION

Factors associated with low risk	*Factors tending to increase risk*
Normal myocardium.	Abnormal myocardium.
Stimulus intensity just above threshold for contraction.	Low threshold for ventricular fibrillation:— particularly due to ischemia hypoxia sympathomimetic and other drugs anesthetic agents post-surgical inflammatory reaction
Absence of non-paced ventricular activity.	
Short impulse duration, (less than 3 millisec.)	
Small contact area between electrode and myocardium.	Parasystole.
	Multiple ectopic (non-paced) beats.
	Stimulus intensity many times threshold for contraction i.e. x 10
	Long impulse duration (over 5 millisec.)
	Two simultaneous stimulation sites.
	Electrode site near apex.

sequel to cessation of pacing, but that it might offer an explanation of the mechanism of some Stokes-Adams attacks in man. The length of the ventricular asystole is often dependent upon the preceding pacing rate being longer when pacing ceases from a rapid rate.[136, 137, 464] Rogel [626] points out that in dogs adequate myocardial oxygenation and a satisfactory circulatory condition are probably more important than the pacing rate. The phenomenon was noted in patients by Furman and Schwedel.[258] In our patients [713] we have found that the period of the asystolic gap may vary in the same patient from day to day and often from minute to minute, so that one failure in pacing may result in immediate idioventricular contractions, while a second failure a few moments later may precipitate asystole for 20 seconds. Chardack [125, 128] has made use of this asystolic period by temporarily switching off the pacing control of patients when fixing electrodes onto the heart, the momentarily still heart allowing easy electrode fixation. In investigating the effects of drugs on this phenomenon, Edelist [201] showed that, on three patients, the period of ventricular asystole following cessation of pacing at rapid rates was considerably lengthened when the patients were digitalized; treatment with isopropylnorepinephrine counteracted this effect of digitalis.

When idioventricular rhythm rapidly follows the cessation of ventricular pacing, the heart rate may initially be the same as the previous pacing rate, with a later reduction to its slow idioventricular rate. This effect was first noted in animals by Hyman in 1932,[352] and occasionally occurred in our own patients.[718] It is presumably due to the adequate myocardial oxygenation during pacing giving way to a new steady state with a poorer coronary flow during complete heart block.

When using external or other rate-control pacemakers, should it become necessary to stop pacing temporarily, it is wise to slow the rate gradually until the inherent pacemaker takes over; by this means the asystolic episode can be avoided.[71, 713]

REVIEW OF THE COMPLICATIONS OF VARIOUS METHODS

Before considering the results of long-term pacing and the choice of method, it is helpful to reiterate some of the complications inherent in the various techniques.

Exposure of the heart, as in Methods 1a, 2a and 3a, requires an operation, the risks of which, in the age group requiring pacing, are significant. Exposure from the epigastrium through the diaphragm may reduce both the operative mortality and morbidity, but no comparable figures are yet available to show this. Sudden death, sometimes shown to be due to ventricular fibrillation, seems more common in the postoperative period than at the similar stage when venous endocardial electrodes are used; and it is possible that placing electrodes in the pericardium may be a factor in lowering the threshold to fibrillation.

Any method which entails the use of wires traversing the skin (1a, 1b) involves the risk of sepsis tracking along them. With epicardial electrodes, after months of pacing, this usually raises the threshold too high to pace, and an epicardial abscess is in itself serious. The risk of bacteremia when an electrode wire runs directly from the surface to a vein seems to have been much reduced by the use of a long subcutaneous track between the skin opening and the vein entry.

There is some risk of sepsis with any technique using implanted units, and even an aseptic reaction resulting in an effusion around the implant, if it is complicated by the formation of a sinus, is likely to result in the need to remove the implant.

It is now established that an electrode wire within the heart and great veins (1b, 2b, 3b) is not associated with a significant risk of clinical thrombosis or embolism, even without anticoagulants. Some thrombus formation on the wire has, however, been observed at autopsy, and there is therefore a potential risk, which is greater if the positive electrode is in the blood stream.

The great advantage of the endocardial method, its avoidance of a thoracotomy, far outweighs the minor disadvantages, the time-consuming technique of placing the electrode tip correctly and the occasional need to reposition it within the first day or two. Stiff electrode wires are liable to perforate the right ventricle, but, though this complication has been reported many times, provided the patient is not under anticoagulant treatment, it has not proved a serious matter. More flexible wires are usually directed by a stylet or enclosing tube [682] which can be withdrawn, but a larger vein entry site is often needed.

PACING FAILURES

Causes of Failure

Failure to continue pacing may be due to a rise of stimulus threshold required or failure of the apparatus to continue delivering a suitable stimulus.

1. A rise of threshold above the output of the stimulus is most commonly due to the physical separation of the electrode from the nearest responsive myocardial fibers. The implantation procedure may have been faulty (not obtaining permanent mechanical fixation), or sepsis may have been introduced, and this, in the presence of the electrode as a foreign body, is likely to persist. There is always some aseptic fibrotic reaction to the electrode and the sutures fixing it, which may be sufficient to result in the current being too diffused before it reaches the myocardium. It had been hoped that endocardial pacing with the electrode in the blood stream would avoid trouble from threshold rise, but

we have recently had experience with failure to pace from this cause.[51]

2. Failure of the pacemaker system to deliver a suitable impulse may be due to battery exhaustion, an electronic fault in the pacemaker itself or a breakdown of the electrode wire or connection.

Since the life of all batteries is limited, whether they be rechargeable or not, implantation of the power source accepts the necessity of a subsequent operation when the battery becomes exhausted. The battery life of the early pacemakers proved to be less than the three or four years predicted by the manufacturers, but in practice battery exhaustion has not proved to be the commonest cause of pacing failure, and it is to be hoped that the occasional premature battery exhaustion will be even less common now that the manufacturers (Mallory Inc.) are supplying batteries to a special "pacemaker specification." The failures have been distributed between all types and all available makes of pacemaker. In a survey conducted by Lawrence,[424] 60 surgeons were asked why they had changed from one make of pacemaker to another. This change had been made by 10 on the grounds of component failure and by 20 because of fractured electrode wires, and the reliability of the electrode wires has frequently been criticized.[12, 381, 424]

The Reliability of Electronic Equipment

The reliability of electronic equipment has been defined [11] as the probability that a system will perform its intended function for a specified time under specified conditions of use, and Glass [276] has defined failure of a pacemaking system as having occurred when a second surgical intervention is necessary within the expected lifetime of the batteries or if the patient dies as a result of interruption of the electrical stimulation to the heart. Each component of a pacemaking system has its own reliability, which is expressed as a percentage of failures occurring in every 1000 hours of use. The total reliability of the system is the sum of the individual reliabilities.[108] Probably the simplest circuit for an implantable pacemaker is the complementary transistor type [277, 386, 606] described by Suran.[742] Reliability figures for components in the pacemaker of this type have been given by

Glass [276] as 0.01 per cent per 1,000 hours for each of two transistors, two condensers and five batteries, as 0.001 per cent per 1,000 hours for each of four resistors and as 0.0001 per cent per 1,000 hours for each of thirty solder joints. The overall reliability of the pacemaker as regards the electronic components alone is the sum of these figures, 0.097 per cent per 1,000 hours, which indicated that, of 100 pacemakers brought into use, only one should fail from electronic component failure within one year. Kantrowitz has claimed [383] that a pacemaker he uses has only six different components, but a published circuit of the General Electric pacemaker [386] shows that, including batteries, a minimum of 11 components are used, and when the necessary soldered joints are taken into account, the overall electronic reliability is probably of the same order as that described by Glass. The more complicated blocking oscillator circuits [105, 163, 288] entail additional components, and in particular may include a transformer in the output stage. From an analysis of components which have actually failed, Greatbatch [290] has determined that the reliability for a transformer was 0.16 per cent per 1,000 hours, and for the batteries 0.025 per cent per 1,000 hours; he reported that the overall electronic failure rate, excluding the electrode wires, was actually found to be 1.2 per cent per 1,000 hours. Comparable figures for other types of pacemaker are not available.

Electrodes

Electrodes, wires and their connections have given more trouble than was anticipated, but reliability has varied from design to design. Many report this as the most common cause of failure with *epicardial* pacing. The helical spring type of wire appears to be able to stand up to the cardiac movement, though where the spring leaves a fairly rigid electrode mount there is a point of weakness. The widely used Chardack electrode,[122] supplied with the Medtronic pacemaker, has a very good reputation, but a few fractures have been reported,[46, 125, 617, 752, 767, 873] usually at this point of strain. The Vitatron spiral electrode wire (see p. 323) has proved satisfactory, and we have had no fracture with wires designed by Davies [116, 691] and manufactured by

Devices, nor has any fracture been reported to the manufacturers after the sale of 1,000 pacemakers. Reports suggest that the multistrand wire, until recently supplied with the Electrodyne pacemaker, which is not of the helical spring type, is more susceptible to fracture,[46, 741] as is the braided wire initially supplied by General Electric;[380, 530] fatigue fracture occurred after 15 months in the multistrand wires which we used initially. With Elema electrodes the weakest point has proved to be the means of attachment of the disc electrode onto the heart. On the basis of figures quoted by Chardack, Glass[276] has estimated the reliability of one type of myocardial lead as 0.06 per cent per 1,000 hours, or, when considered over the period of anticipated battery lifetime, four years, the reliability figure for the leads may be expressed as 2 per cent per four years.

The strains and movements of an *endocardial* wire and electrode are different from those on the surface of the heart. Although experience of the long-term use of endocardial electrodes is not so extensive as with surface electrodes, it appears that fracture within the heart or venous system is extremely rare. We had a number of fractures outside the vein,[51] and we attribute these to the use of rather rigid wires which are angled as they turn from the axilla to enter the jugular vein. Moreover, full arm movement is partially transmitted along the wire up to its site of entry, where it is relatively fixed. More flexible wires are now available, and Lagergren[407] has reported the use of Elema endocardial electrodes in 305 patients collected from five centers without wire fracture.

Overall Reliability of Pacemaker System

The *theoretical* reliability figure for implantation of a pacemaker of the Chardack type is about 18 per cent per four years, indicating that 18 out of every 100 pacemaker implantations may be expected to fail within the battery lifetime. The *actual* figure for the General Electric pacemaker is a failure rate of 3 per cent per 1,000 hours, or 18 per cent per year, quoted by Hayes;[313] this figure includes a low value for electronic failure but a high incidence of electrode wire failure; the introduction of a new helical coil multistrand lubricated electrode wire (see Appendix p. 301) should improve the overall reliability figures considerably, since accelerated life testing in the laboratory has shown a new lead to be intact after 300 times as many flexions as cause fractures of the old leads.[384]

The translation of these various estimates of reliability represents only one aspect of the clinical practice of pacing patients, whose health and life also depend on numerous other factors, not the least of which is basic disease process which necessitates pacing. The clinical results are considered in the next chapter.

Methods of Improving Reliability

The electronic components used in the manufacture of pacemakers are highly selected, but the cost of a super-reliability component may be 50 times that of the standard commercial component,[276] and since the electronic reliability is only one factor in the overall reliability, it is apparent that at some point it will become uneconomic to improve reliability by selection of components, since the cost will increase greatly, but the overall reliability will be hardly affected. It is of more practical value that extensive production and preimplantation testing be carried out and all pacemaker manufacturers now apply extensive tests to their components and completed units. The procedure followed by the Electrodyne Corporation has been outlined by Steigle;[869] all components undergo a heat test for seven to ten days before use and must meet the original specifications at the end of this time. The whole circuit is then assembled and the rate checked, following which the heat test is again applied for ten days and the rate checked again; if the discharge rate has altered by more than $\pm$ one impulse per minute from the original value, the component which has drifted is identified, replaced, and the heat test is repeated for a further seven to ten days, after which the rate is again checked. Heat-testing at 40 C is also recommended by Glass,[276] and most pacemaker manufacturers have their own similar test procedures. Every completed pacemaker should be bench-tested under load for a considerable period (14-28 days), since the possibility of failure is much higher during the early period of the life of electronic components. The importance of this testing being carried out at body temperature[306] and under conditions of 100 per cent humidity [291] is apparent, and a further precaution utilized by the Medtronic Corporation [291] is for x-rays to be taken of all units at the end of one month's load-testing to determine the state of the batteries. In the future, manufacturers are likely to design pacemakers with redundant circuits so that, should one circuit fail, a reserve will take over.[276, 880]

Clinical Manifestations

Failure, if sudden, may result in a Stokes-Adams attack (see p. 112). Some sudden deaths may have this basis, but, more often, after a period of unconsciousness or dizziness, the idioventricular rhythm takes over.

The patient is usually aware that he is not being paced and seeks advice at once. In other cases, when failure is impending, there is a change in rate which should lead to full investigation. Since the tachycardia from a speeding pacemaker can prove dangerous (see p. 102), most pacemakers are now designed to slow rather than speed when the battery is nearly depleted, although the appearance of other electronic faults may nevertheless result in dangerous tachycardia. It is very valuable for pacemaker patients to be taught to take their own pulse at least once a day and to report to their doctor if the rate varies by more than three beats a minute. For this precaution to be useful, it is essential that the pulse be correctly counted over a full minute and that a variation in rate reported by a patient should be checked as soon as possible.

In our experience, the commonest presentation of a failure is intermittent pacing. The patient reports transient dizzy spells, but when examined is found to be pacing normally. The tendency to attribute such symptoms to occasional extrasystoles resulting in a few dropped beats is tempting but dangerous, and a story of dizzy spells, even if transient, requires full investigation.

Organization of a Pacemaker Clinic

Patients with artificial pacemakers may suffer from purely medical disabilities or from problems associated with malfunction of the artificial pacemaker or from a combination of both these, so that the aftercare of paced patients presents a difficult administrative and clinical problem. The most satisfactory solution is for a special pacemaker clinic to be organized where both medical and electronic facilities are available and where the follow-up procedures can be carried out in a routine manner; we describe here our own practice in this respect.

One or two days before the patients leave the hospital after implantation of the pacemaker, control values are established for subsequent comparison; the apex rate is accurately measured; a prolonged recording of one ECG lead is made to detect ectopic beats; penetrated PA and lateral chest x-rays are taken to establish the position of a transvenous electrode if pacing is being carried out by this method; x-ray of the implanted unit for future assessment of battery exhaustion is taken; and photographs are taken of the impulse displayed from limb leads on the screen of a calibrated oscilloscope for the measurement of impulse duration, wave form and height of stimulus deflection in millivolts. On discharge the patient is given a card stating that he is being treated with an artificial pacemaker, that pulse rate should be fixed at "x" beats per minute; the card notes the telephone number of the hospital for use in emergencies.

The patient is told to return to the pacemaker clinic at any time if he is worried about the integrity of his pacing system or if any one of the following criteria apply: (a) syncopal or near-syncopal attack; (b) pulse varies more than five beats per minute from the control rate; (c) palpitation or missed beats; (d) pain around the pacemaker site; (e) evidence of infection of the pacemaker system.

In the absence of any such complication, patients are asked to return to the clinic, initially one month after discharge from hospital and subsequently at three-month intervals. At each visit a history is taken and clinical examination carried out, and drug therapy is reassessed with particular reference to the need for diuretics or digitalis. Any external wires or apparatus are carefully examined and external batteries checked or replaced. A chest x-ray is taken for clinical assessment and to confirm the site of a transvenous electrode, and at alternate visits the state of the batteries is assessed by x-ray also. The pacemaker rate is checked for a full minute, and a prolonged strip of ECG taken to confirm stable pacing. Measurements of the impulse duration, stimulus amplitude and wave form are taken at each visit.

Comparison of the results obtained at each outpatient attendance with the control values before leaving hospital frequently provides advance information concerning pacemaker failure. Progressive alteration in impulse duration, reduction in stimulus amplitude, alteration in rate or unduly rapid battery depletion, particularly if the various cells alter unevenly, are all indications for early pacemaker replacement. As a result of the continuing improvement in reliability of implanted pacemakers, together with the information provided from a pacemaker clinic, it is now rare for paced patients to present as emergencies.

Investigation of Pacing Failure

There are now several publications describing the techniques adopted at various centers for the tracing of pacemaker faults.[46, 53, 175, 176, 283, 381, 404, 424, 577, 717] The approach from each of these centers is broadly similar and essentially depends on an assessment of the changes found on electrocardiograms, x-rays and, if necessary, threshold measurements.

Electrocardiographic Changes

For the maximum information to be obtained from ECGs recorded during possible pacemaker failure it is essential that a comparison be made with ECGs recorded when the pacemaker is known to be functioning perfectly, and for this reason all patients should have routine ECGs recorded as soon as possible after pacemaker implantation and at frequent intervals during follow-up. Records made with apparatus with a high frequency response, such as a photographic recorder, or obtained from an oscilloscopic trace are more valuable than those obtained with direct writing machines. For some applications, records should be taken at reduced sensitivity in order that the entire pacemaker stimulus may be clearly shown, and a sensitivity of 1mv/mm is recommended. For more specialized investigation of the ECG, photographic records taken from the screen of the measuring oscilloscope with a time scale of 1 msec/cm are satisfactory. It should be noted that the height of the stimulus record on the ECG will depend on, among other factors, the separation between the two pacing electrodes and the lead used for the recording. When bipolar electrodes are in use the stimulus spike will be small and may not be noticeable at all on certain leads in which the stimulus vector is at right angles to the axis between the exploring leads. As the position of the heart and electrodes usually varies somewhat with respiration, the height of the stimulus spike on the electrocardiogram may show a cyclical respiratory variation, and this normal finding should not be interpreted as due to pacemaker malfunction. When pacing is being carried out with a unipolar electrode on the heart and an indifferent electrode elsewhere in the body, the height of the stimulus spike should be considerably greater than that seen with bipolar myocardial electrodes, and although the respiratory change may still occur it is unlikely to cause confusion. It is recommended that short records be taken of all standard and chest leads, and long strips are then recorded of those which show the stimulus spike clearly. For unipolar myocardial electrodes with the indifferent electrode in the abdominal wall, Standard Lead II or III is usually satisfactory, but if the indifferent electrode is in the axilla, Standard Lead I is usually the better choice.

Rate

Perhaps the simplest and most important measurement which can be obtained from the ECG is the pacemaker discharge rate. A transistor radio placed close to the implanted unit and tuned out from broadcasting stations will click audibly with each impulse, and has proved, outside the hospital, a particularly useful method of ascertaining that the pacemaker is still functioning and showing its rate. A "pacemaker monitor" for this purpose is commercially available from Vitatron. Even when an ECG is available this may be a valuable test as it will demonstrate a functioning pacemaker even when there is no contact with the tissues to produce a stimulus spike on the ECG. The rate at which a pacemaker discharges after implantation in the patient is rarely identical with that found during testing in the laboratory, although it should be very close. The variation is probably due to differences in pacemaker temperature and in load impedance between the test conditions and those pertaining after implantation, and for this reason it is more satisfactory to regard the heart rate at the time the patient is discharged from hospital, rather than the test rate of discharge in the laboratory, as the standard against which subsequent comparisons are made. Any significant variation in rate on this control value should lead to a more extensive investigation of pacemaker function,[53] and most authors agree that a fixed-rate pacemaker which has altered its rate by more than ± five beats per minute should be replaced.[134] Most of the fixed rate pacemakers currently available are designed to slow when the batteries are nearing the end of their life and in some instances clearly defined alterations in rate occur with failure of individual cells,[139] but as the usual fall in rate when one cell fails is of the order of 10 per cent adoption of the rule that a pacemaker slowing by five beats a minute should be changed will cover this situation.

A pacemaker speeding to a rate of over 110 has proved to be very dangerous, and the "runaway pacemaker" has been considered on page 102. We recommend that if a pacemaker fires at over 110 the wires should be exposed and cut as a matter of urgency. If a replacement pacemaker for implantation is not available immediately, an external unit can be used temporarily.

The General Electric pacemaker speeds up in the event of an increase of resistance as occurs with fracture of strands of the electrode wires.[642] As this also reduces the total energy per pulse, this particular defect is not likely to cause fibrillation. The ECG tracing resembles that due to AC mains interference, but the cycle timing will not be that of the line supply (60 cps in the USA or 50 in the UK).

Missing

From a simple electrocardiogram it is also possible to detect the occurrence of "missed beats" in which a pacemaker stimulus is not followed by a QRS complex. The only situation in which this is acceptable is when the pacemaker stimulus falls during the refractory period; the presence of even one pacemaker stimulus falling outside the refractory period but failing to provoke a ventricular contraction calls for a full investigation to determine the cause.

Stimulus Spike

The next point to be considered should be the height of the stimulus spike on the ECG; if only the record of a direct writer is available, little significance can be placed upon variations between different records, although it may be possible to demonstrate a progressive diminution in the height of the stimulus on serial tracings as noted by Parsonnet.[577] If ECG records taken from a measuring oscilloscope are available, the height of the deflection can be measured and changes used to assess the output of the pacemaker.[166, 167, 404] The height of the stimulus deflection depends upon the amplitude of the pacemaker impulse and the projection of the impulse vector in the particular ECG lead recorded. The deflection is usually small when bipolar electrodes are in use, since the dipole is small, but values of several hundred millivolts can be recorded when a unipolar electrode is in use and the indifferent is placed at some distance from the heart. Control measurements are made in this manner in all our patients before discharge from the hospital, so that subsequent comparisons can be made. It should be noted that the height of the stimulus spike gives no information as to the voltage actually applied at the myocardial electrode, and several authors have reported cases in which fracture of the insulating material as well as the electrode wire has resulted in a full-sized stimulus deflection on the ECG with failure of ventricular capture.[577] If the insulation of the electrode wire is faulty but the wire is essentially intact, the effect may be to produce an alternative current pathway avoiding the heart; this is particularly prone to happen when a unipolar pacing system is in use. In this case the height of the stimulus spike on the ECG may be normal, but the ventricular response may be completely absent or only intermittent, and this situation is likely to be mistaken for that due to a high cardiac threshold. Theoretically, the frontal plane vector loop of the stimulus deflection should provide the differential diagnosis between these possibilities, but in our experience this has been a disappointing investigation. The construction of equipotential lines on the body surface [303] is very time consuming but has been used successfully in the investigation of electrode fracture by Dekker.[175, 176]

Polarity

The ECG record can also be used to check the polarity with which a unipolar pacemaker has been connected, provided that two leads have been recorded with a photographic or oscilloscopic machine. If the pacemaker has been inserted in the usual manner with the negative electrode connected to the heart and the positive indifferent electrode in the abdominal wall, then the initial deflection due to the pacemaker stimulus will be negative in Standard Lead I and positive in Standard Lead III. If the pacemaker has been incorrectly attached so that the positive terminal is connected to the heart, then the initial deflection due to the pacemaker stimulus will be positive in Lead I and negative in Lead III, and reexploration of the pacemaker site will be necessary for the connections to be corrected.

Wave Form

A more sophisticated examination of pacemaker function can be carried out by analysis of the wave form of the pacemaker impulse as displayed upon a measuring oscilloscope screen from external limb electrodes. The peak voltage and impulse duration can be directly compared with previous records, and Davies [164] has pointed out that the rate of decay of the impulse wave form from peak voltage is an indication of the impedance in the pacemaker circuit. The importance of observations of this type with regard to indirect measurements of myocardial threshold is considered on page 165. Oscilloscopic analysis of pacemaker wave form has also been used by Sloman.[404] Skin electrodes were used, and ECG Leads I, II, III displayed upon a calibrated oscilloscope; sequential measurements of impulse duration and the amplitude of the stimulus deflection were made in ten subjects. Sloman was able to show significant changes in impulse duration as well as in stimulation rate in three cases. Similar techniques have been used by Nickel.[555]

X-ray

X-rays taken in the investigation of possible pacemaker failure should be "overpenetrated" and, as with the ECG, should be compared with previously taken records soon after the onset of artificial pacing. The most satisfactory way to detect malposition of an endocardial electrode is for two x-rays to be superimposed so that the diaphragmatic shadows and the apex of the heart are coincidental. It will be apparent at once if the endocardial electrode has altered its position. This technique is less likely to cause confusion than the alternative method of superimposing the bone landmarks on repeated x-rays or superimposing the outlines of the course of the catheter, since movement of the heart with respiration may lead to the erroneous conclusion that significant movement of the electrode has occurred. We find it is essential that a stable position be found for the electrode so that the tip is not influenced by respiration, coughing, exercise or body position, and we feel that the technique of utilizing the bipolar system with the electrodes lying free in the right ventricle is acceptable only for very short periods with an external unit (see p. 57).

Fractured Wire

The diagnosis of a broken electrode wire should be suspected when a patient gives a history of intermittent pacing related to alterations in body position. General palpation along the course of the electrode wire may bring the two broken ends of the wire into contact and so restore steady pacing temporarily. It is often possible to confirm the diagnosis from the x-ray,[53, 577, 628] but failure to demonstrate a broken wire by this method does not invalidate the diagnosis.

State of Batteries

It is possible to estimate the state of the mercury batteries [133] in artificial pacemakers from an x-ray of the unit, and this technique is used by several pacemaker manufacturers in their final testing procedure (see Fig. 8). Although it is considerably more difficult to carry out this test satisfactorily when the pacemaker is implanted in a patient, it is possible to position the patient by

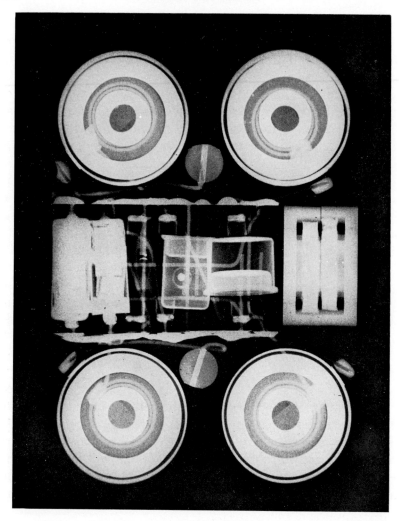

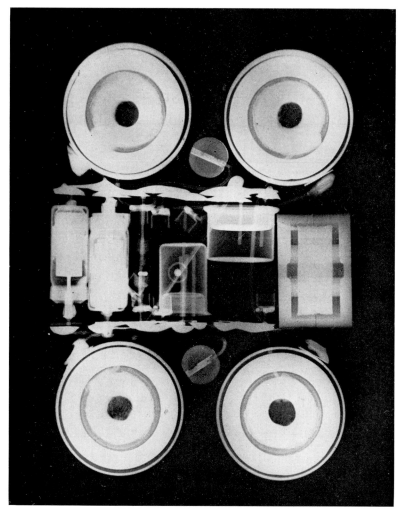

FIGURE 8. X-rays of pacemakers with new and partly exhausted batteries, showing the partial obliteration of the dark ring between the two opaque cores. *Left:* new battery. *Right:* battery sufficiently exhausted to justify replacement.

preliminary screening so that suitable x-rays can be obtained.[16,][167] Lillehei has described in detail the technique required (for regular overhead films, Bucky 100 ma, 2 to 2.5 sec and 80 to 90 kv; for spot films, 200 ma, 0.5-1 sec and 120 kv) and has emphasized the necessity of fluoroscopy to obtain films in exactly the long axis of the battery. He recommends taking a film postoperatively for comparison with subsequent six-month films, and cites three patients in whom this technique proved of practical value.[451] This method of assessing the state of pacemaker batteries has proved in our experience of less value than the measurements made from high frequency ECGs previously described.

Electrolysis

Many of the pacemakers currently available utilize stainless steel electrodes, and from time to time failures of artificial pacing are caused by fragmentation and electrolysis of one electrode, almost invariably the anode (see p. 161). A diagnosis of this fault may be made from the x-ray when the positive electrode cannot be seen.

Threshold Measurement

If a pacing failure is established it is necessary to operate and expose the pacemaker. At this operation the pacing threshold should be tested with a pacemaker with variable output control. The problem of threshold and its measurement is discussed in the section on electronic aspects, page 145.

DRUGS AND THRESHOLD

A rise in threshold usually shows up as intermittent pacing, and while arranging for threshold measurement, it is worthwhile trying the effect of corticosteroids, potassium and isoproterenol (isoprenaline). The Ann Arbor group have described this threshold rise as "exit block," and, using General Electric pacemakers, have developed a technique by which they were able to study the effect of drugs on threshold. They concluded that corticosteroid therapy reduced the threshold.[535]

Levowitz [440] recommended the correction of postoperative acidosis and sympathomimetic amines when the heart did not follow the stimulus. Haywood [314] found that giving isoproterenol (isoprenaline) and ephedrine resulted in pacing in three patients who were not following pacemaker stimuli; whereas potassium by mouth or intravenously resulted in only intermittent pacing action. Walker,[782] Burchell [85] and Guyer [298] have each found that potassium restored pacing in various circumstances. For fuller discussion of the effects of drugs on threshold, see page 168.

REPAIRS AT SURGICAL OPERATION

As failing pacemakers must be replaced and connected to wires already implanted, it is necessary to have a means of making these connections under sterile operative conditions. Some prefer to join wires with a crimping tool and cover with fresh insulation.[607, 826] Dow-Corning produce a medical adhesive (Medical Adhesive, A. Dow-Corning Corp., Midland, Michigan) for use with silicone rubber insulation, which can be autoclaved in its tube; when expressed, it hardens as a result of exposure to moisture. We have preferred to rely on a mechanical join to the replacement pacemaker, a nylon screw pressing the exposed end of the wire to a metal plate within the unit. In the General Electric, Electrodyne, Vitatron and Cordis models, the leads are attached by a simple plug-in arrangement, allowing immediate connection even under sterile conditions.

SUMMARY

The Hazards of Pacing

With an electrode in direct contact with the heart there is a risk of transmitting lethal fibrillatory currents to it. Such currents have leaked through faulty apparatus from the main power line, and it is recommended that all pacemakers should be battery-powered. A second possible hazard arises, since an implanted apparatus with its wire electrodes can act as an aerial picking up radio frequency emissions from the neighborhood, surgical diathermy being the most likely apparatus to come into close contact with the patient.

Should a pacemaker develop a fault increasing its rate above 110 ("runaway pacemaker"), there is a serious risk of ventricular fibrillation, and the urgency of this situation has been stressed.

Ventricular fibrillation has also been precipitated by a pacemaker working normally; the various circumstances in which this risk is great include the presence of parasystole as with artificial pacing in sinus rhythm, the use of the more powerful pacemakers and various factors associated with the postoperative state.

Pacing Failures

Pacing failures have been broadly divided into two groups; firstly, those resulting from a rise in threshold required to pace, often attributable to tissue reaction to the electrodes or sepsis; and secondly, those resulting from a failure of the pacemaker to continue delivering a suitable impulse, which may be due to the unit itself, including its batteries, or to failure of the wires and electrodes. An attempt has been made to determine the reliability of the electronic equipment which makes up a pacemaker and from this to calculate the degree of reliability that can be expected of the overall pacemaker system.

It is recommended that patients with artificial pacemakers should attend a pacemaker clinic organized to check the normally working implanted pacemaker and to investigate faults in pacing. A very elaborate routine is required at regular intervals. It includes checking with an ECG, with x-rays and with a measuring oscilloscope. These techniques have been described in some detail, indicating particularly the significance of changes in rate, of "missing," of the size of the stimulus spike and its wave form as seen on the oscilloscope.

Chapter 8

CLINICAL RESULTS OF PACING

SYMPTOMATIC RELIEF

EFFECTIVE PACING AT A suitable rate is a guarantee of the prevention of Stokes-Adams attacks. It also provides immediate relief of the cerebral symptoms resulting from inadequate blood flow. When symptoms are due to cardiac failure or to renal failure, relief is slow and may be incomplete.

PREVENTION OF ARREST DURING OPERATIONS

One of the outstanding values of pacing the heart is its use to cover anesthesia in patients liable to cardiac arrest at operations of any description. Quite apart from the operations for pacemaker implantation, many patients in complete heart block require surgical procedures for cancers, for prostatic enlargement,[405] for aortic stenosis,[4] for carcinoma of the bronchus [425] or for other conditions.[399] It is recognized that for patients in complete heart block the risk of arrest [774] or serious arrhythmia during such procedures is considerable, and it can be avoided by artificial pacing. A patient in sinus rhythm, in whom a previous unexplained incident of cardiac arrest has been recorded, should not undergo any further similar procedure without having suitable electrodes applied so that pacing can be started immediately if arrest occurs. Childbirth has been recorded with an implanted pacemaker,[83, 828] but also in complete block without a pacemaker.[589]

RESULTS WITH LONG-TERM PACING

The patient in whom a battery-powered pacemaker was first implanted still survives. The implantation was performed by Senning in 1958,[681] and the patient is working in 1966.[760]

Interpretation of Reports

There is now a considerable accumulation of reports on artificial pacing by Method 2a, that is, with epicardial electrodes and an implanted pacemaker. Experience with Methods 1a, 1b, 1c, 2b, 3a and 3b is more limited and has been considered in the previous chapter. In analyzing these results of pacing by Method 2a, only reports of ten or more patients have been considered, since, by eliminating reports of fewer cases, the bias resulting from the tendency to record a few cases if successful, but not to record small numbers if unsuccessful, is partly avoided. The results as published in 1499 cases from 42 different centers are set out in Table VI. As each paper tends to set out results in a different manner, the figures are not always strictly comparable, and some of the figures on the table have been obtained by deduction rather than from a precise statement. The relevant facts which are often missing in these reports include the mean period for which patients have been paced; from some of these reports it is possible to deduce from the date of publication an approximate period of observation, and, if so, this has been given. Since follow-up cannot always be up to date at the time of publication, the figures given will tend to indicate too long rather than too short a period of pacing. In spite of this it is immediately obvious that most of the reports have been made when the mean observation period of paced patients has been very short, often under six months. The figures for reoperation and the late mortality must be considered in association with these provisos.

Failures with Different Pacemaker Models

It must also be emphasized that the relatively few reports which cover several years of practice are of experience with early designs of pacemaker, and it is reasonable to assume that the failure rate with these earlier models will prove higher than with the latest models. There are no figures available which allow a strict comparison of the various apparatus available. In the few cases in which one center reports experience with more than one make of pacemaker, it is usually made clear in the report that, after experience with one make for perhaps a year or so, a change was made to a different make; thus, though the clinical material may have changed little, the comparison is between an early model of one manufacturer and a more up-to-date model of the second manufacturer. Moreover, the period of observation of results with the newer model is inevitably shorter. These weaknesses in comparison are evident, for instance, in the large series reported by Binet from Paris. He implanted 15 Elema pacemakers with 60 per cent failure, 35 Electrodyne pacemakers with 63 per cent failure and 143 Medtronic with 15 per cent failure. The Elema models were of an early model (EM137) implanted before November, 1962. The Electrodyne models (TR 14) were implanted up to October, 1963 and the Medtronic after November, 1963. This paper is particularly valuable in indicating the incidence and type of failures, but the comparison is not that of the up-to-date models of the three manufacturers, and the differing length-of-observation period must result in a higher failure rate in the model implanted in the first series. Bouvrain [62] has also analyzed pacing failures in 139 patients, many of whom overlap with the patients reported by Binet.

The Medtronic pacemaker has proved the most popular, and, in 1965, Chardack [134] reports that 8,000 units have been produced, and he gives figures for their reliability based on information obtained by the manufacturers. The failure rate of units was 10 per cent after 15 months of implantation. Medtronic Inc. have advised that all their units manufactured up to January 1964 be changed after this period of use, the company allowing appropriate credit (prorated on a 3-yr basis) on the purchase of the replacement unit. More favorable figures for up-to-date models have been reported to us. Of the current model of the Medtronic pacemaker, 90 per cent are satisfactory after two years,[291] and 95 per cent of the current Elema model (EM139) are satisfactory after one year.[760] The Dutch Vitatron MIP 100 has been available since April, 1965, and, in the ensuing 12 months, 367 units were sent out for implantation for a mean period of just under 5 months. Only two are known to have developed electronic faults, and it is believed that, owing to a close follow-up, these figures include almost all the failures.[879]

Apart from strictly electronic breakdown of the unit, there

are a number of other causes of clinical failure, particularly those arising in connection with the implantation procedure. The apparatus may be contaminated with foreign material (e.g., ethylene oxide or talcum powder), or the surgeon may attach the myocardial electrodes incorrectly to the heart, or the pacemaker may be rejected by the patient's tissues, either because of sepsis or as a reaction to a foreign body. As a result, clinical reports indicate a failure rate higher than that of the pacemaker itself. Chardack, in his own practice with units manufactured from January, 1962, to January, 1964, had 16 failures in 76 implants (21%) after 3 to 21 months of use.[160] Dack [160] had to reoperate 18 times for generator or electrode failure in 45 patients in whom he had implanted Medtronic pacemakers between November, 1962, and November, 1964, his mean period of follow-up being eight months. Trimble,[767] treating 32 patients from April, 1962, to September, 1964, with Medtronic pacemakers found that the average time of failure was at 15 months. Five failures were due to tissue fluid accumulating in the power pack, resulting in wire corrosion.

Few significant figures regarding the expected life of other pacemaker models are available. Bjork,[49] reporting on 36 surviving patients who probably overlap with those reported by Hallen (see Table VI), gave the average Elema (Model EM 137) unit life as 9.4 months (4-15 mo).

Two reports [301, 775] have discussed the relative merits of the Elema (Swedish) and the Vitatron (Dutch) models, finding that the Elema wires were more reliable but that the Vitatron pacemaker batteries lasted longer. One [775] of these reports considered the Medtronic (USA) electrode wires superior to both, and the Medtronic pacemaker appeared to be the most reliable of the three, but again the comparison was made between the newest Medtronic model against the Elema and Vitatron of previous years.

Spear [721] implanted 29 pacemakers using approximately an equal number of fixed rate units and of synchronous units. He reported an equivalent failure rate of over half in both groups, but he did not indicate whether the two groups were observed for the same length of time, nor how long the observation period was. Dack, in the paper quoted above,[160] compared the reoperation rate with 9 Cordis synchronous implants with his 45 Medtronic implants. Out of the 9 synchronous models, which were of the earliest synchronous pacemakers to be made, 7 required reoperation, as compared with 15 patients having reoperation out of 45 Medtronic implants.

A later report (October, 1965) from the same hospital [783] reports 74 patients having implants of various pacemakers between October, 1962, and May, 1965. Failures occurred in 30 (40%) of the patients (using 55 pacemakers); of these, 28 were electrode breaks (12 in the myocardium) and, in 12, increased energy was required to stimulate the heart (4 being associated with polarization from a DC leak). Our own experience involved the use of 143 units in 79 patients from April, 1960, to September, 1964, when we were developing the pacemakers now manufactured by Devices Ltd. in England. This series included some patients paced by means of endocardial electrodes.

Conclusions regarding the reliability of these various systems based on the clinical reports reviewed above and shown in Table VI must be guarded, for the number observed for more than a few months is small. An electronic apparatus may fail at any time; the earliest reported was within five minutes of implanting [109] and the longest implants of which we are aware are over four years.[222, 875] Reliability of newer pacemaker models continues to improve, and better clinical results are no doubt now being achieved with many different models. As clinical experience extends, there are likely to be, in the next few years, many further reports substantiating this hope.

Early Mortality

The overall postoperative mortality using an implanted pacemaker with electrodes on the surface of the heart is seen in Table VI to be 112 in 1499 patients, 7.5 per cent. This has been due largely to the basic cardiac condition, the complications of a thoracotomy and sudden death sometimes known to be caused by ventricular fibrillation. It also includes a few deaths from technical failures, including those in whom the threshold has risen above the output of the pacemaker. In those who die suddenly within a fortnight of starting pacing, there is often no good explanation at autopsy, and the electrical apparatus and its contacts appear intact. In a number of these cases, arrhythmias have been reported prior to death and in some the mode of death has been proved to be ventricular fibrillation.

A detailed study of the reports from which this overall picture was obtained suggest that there are a significant number of deaths which are directly dependent on the thoracotomy; we believe that these include not only those due to chest complications, postoperative sepsis, etc., but also a proportion of the sudden deaths. Unfortunately, the number of reports of patients paced on a long-term basis by techniques which do not involve a thoracotomy are few. The numbers are insufficient for a valid statistical comparison, particularly when there is inadequate evidence of clinical similarity between the two groups of patients. Our own postoperative mortality with methods involving thoracotomy was 8 in 59 patients,[306] as opposed to 1 in 49 patients paced with implants associated with endocardial electrodes.[51]

Later Mortality

The figures in the table for late mortality are only of significance when the period of follow-up is known; and, as will be seen, this information is lacking in many reports. A proportion of these deaths were from carcinoma and other unrelated conditions.

Reoperation

A fault in the electrode on the heart or in its wire within the chest requires a second thoracotomy, and this is a much more serious matter than one that can be repaired by exposing only the pacemaker, a procedure usually done under local anesthesia. The papers from which Table VI was prepared do not always indicate how often a further thoracotomy proved necessary. At least one of the rethoracotomies proved fatal.[424]

Children

The reports comprising Table VI, which were selected because they covered ten or more patients, include only 17 children. Lillehei[455] and Michaëlsson[511] have reported their experiences pacing respectively eight and three children, and many others have reported on single cases.[271, 283, 335, 376, 534, 859] Martin has reported an implant in an infant of four months.[874] In children, particular problems are involved, because very prolonged pacing may be required and because of the relatively large size of the pacemaker for small patients.

The Authors' Current Choice of Technique

Early in 1965 we analyzed our experience with long-term pacing in 102 patients.[687, 690, 691] When complications had arisen in an individual patient with one technique, we had tended to switch to another method, so that a number of our patients had been paced by two or more means; thus, after using many techniques we accumulated appreciable experience of three different methods. The three groups treated by these three methods are not strictly comparable, particularly as our early experience was mostly with epicardial electrodes, and more recently we have preferred endocardial electrodes. Nevertheless, this somewhat varied experience in 102 patients was the basis on which we developed our practice.

The *endocardial* technique with an *external* pacemaker (1b) was complicated by septicemia in 3 of the 27 patients who were paced from 1 to 32 months (mean 16 mo) by this method. Septicemia did not occur in the later patients in whom the electrode wire ran a long subcutaneous course before entering the vein. Though we feel that most patients are psychologically better with a totally implanted apparatus, this method proved remarkably safe and 24 of the 27 patients survive.

Our results with the *epicardial* electrode and an *implanted* pacemaker (2a) were less satisfactory than both our other groups and as compared with published series from other hospitals chiefly because of the high rate of rejection following aseptic sinus formation, leading to sepsis entering from without. The longest period of pacing in the 62 patients was three and one-half years; 24 of the patients have died and only 6 continue to be paced by this method.

Forty-nine patients were paced with an *endocardial* electrode and an *implanted* pacemaker (2b), the longest pacing period of

21 months and the mean 10 months. Three have died and 31 continue to be paced by this technique.

From a study of the potentialities and this practical experience with the various methods of long-term pacing we have reached various tentative opinions on which we base our current practice. Such opinions are continually being changed as electronic apparatus and techniques improve, and as understanding of the problems develops.

All pacing methods are subject to failures and should be avoided if drug treatment will have as good a result. The endocardial electrode technique is preferable to one involving an operation to place electrodes on the heart. Obtaining a lasting contact for the electrode within the heart is a complex procedure requiring skill and experience, and the ideal electrode wire for this purpose is yet to be devised. The reoperation or failure rate with all methods involving implantation remains undesirably high. The method which requires the least operative procedure is an external pacemaker with an endocardial electrode. The risk of blood stream infection with this method appears to have been reduced by running the electrode wire through a long subcutaneous course. If it were not that external apparatus is undesirable, particularly psychologically, this method would suit most patients, and it has proved to have the lowest morbidity and mortality of the methods we have used. The desirability of implanting the entire apparatus has to be weighed against its reliability.

Of the implantation techniques, we currently use the endocardial venous electrode method with a fixed-rate unit in the majority, thereby avoiding the early mortality and morbidity associated with operative exposure of the heart.

Owing to the inevitable complexity of atrial-triggered pacemakers we were reluctant to implant the earlier models, but we are hopeful that the failure rate of the new atrial-triggered models will prove low enough for us to feel confident in using them more often, particularly in younger patients.

COMPARISON OF PACED AND UNPACED PATIENTS

There are no comparable figures for prognosis with and without artificial pacing. The figures for survival from the published papers shown in the tables can only be compared with those pre-dating the advent of artificial pacing, or alternatively with those for patients with complete block or Stokes-Adams attacks selectively managed by means not including pacing; this selection inevitably produces two groups with differing prognoses. There are only a few reports of a considerable number of patients with complete heart block, with or without Stokes-Adams attacks, in which there has been an adequate period of observation to judge the expectation of life. These reports cover a period when the modern sympathomimetic drugs and resuscitative techniques were not available, but they provide some background for comparison of the results of pacing.

Penton in 1956 [589] reviewed 251 cases of complete heart block from the Peter Brent Brigham Hospital,[589] and Rowe and White in 1958 [640] followed up 191 cases from the Massachusetts General Hospital. Curd [159] from Houston, Texas, has more recently reported a series of 130 A-V block cases which included a high proportion of children. He does not indicate how many of the total he was able to follow up, but estimates that 47 per cent survived two years.

These and other authors have not only provided evidence for the overall expectation of life after the onset of complete block or of Stokes-Adams attacks, but have attempted to show which clinical features are associated with a good or bad prognosis. Unfortunately, the results are often inconsistent, and there is very little evidence to indicate which patients with block are likely to do well without pacing or in which it is essential. Most reports have attempted to correlate prognosis with etiology from which, as would be expected, it is clear that the outlook is worse for those with acute myocardial infarction than for the rest,[366, 419, 589, 640] though Gilchrist [273] and Zoob [839] pointed out that those who survive a few days usually revert to sinus rhythm and have a reasonable prognosis.

Both Penton's [589] and Rowe's [640] series suggest that the outlook for those with valvular disease is better than for the remainder, most of which were thought to be due to coronary disease with or without hypertension. As indicated above (p. 10) only very few prove at autopsy to have gross coronary disease, and etiology can rarely be established in life.

For patients with complete block the presence or absence of Stokes-Adams attacks does not seem to influence survival materially. Penton and Rowe found the mean survival time for those with attacks was somewhat longer than those without, but as Friedberg [245] has pointed out, often there were complicating factors causing early death in those without attacks.[419] He thought Stokes-Adams attacks affected the outlook adversely. Penton's overall mean survival time was 42 months; and in Curd's series 59 per cent of those with attacks survived 12 months. In Friedberg's series of 100 cases with attacks, 50 survived a year. Johansson's 42 cases [366] also had a 50 per cent survival rate for one year. Most of the deaths in these series were sudden and presumably occurred in Stokes-Adams attacks. Penton [589] points out that sudden death is three times as likely in those with a history of attacks.

The following points are also brought out in these papers. A history of attacks for a period of over six months carries a better prognosis than for a shorter period.[245] Unstable block (as opposed to established complete block) is usually considered to be an unfavorable feature. However, in Friedberg's series the established block cases did not survive quite so long as the others, and neither Cosby,[147] Penido [862] nor Lau [419] were able to show an association between the presence or absence of changing block and prognosis. The outlook is not greatly different for those whose mechanism of Stokes-Adams attack is asystole as opposed to a rapid ventricular rhythm.[366] There is a tendency for attacks to decrease in frequency, but in 7 of Johansson's 19 survivors, attacks continued throughout the ten years or more of follow-up.

Cosby's analysis [147] of 100 unselected patients with complete heart block is particularly pertinent, as 50 were seen prior to and 50 after the advent of permanent pacing. The clinical features which they found to be critical factors in prognosis were myocardial infarctions, diabetes and uremia. Age and congestive failure were not significant in this respect. In patients without prior or new myocardial infarction, a striking improvement in mortality was noted in those paced (60 to 80% before and 10% with pacing).

This view contrasts strongly with that of Curd,[159] who, in analyzing his 130 cases, concluded that "optimum pacemaker therapy would have altered the prognosis in less than 10% of the total patients."

Chardack[134] has compared his results in 50 patients started on pacing more than two years previously with Curd's 55[159] and Friedberg's[215] 100 unpaced patients. At two years, 71 per cent of Chardack's patients survived, while under 60 per cent of the patients in the other two series survived one year.

Other authors, in reporting their paced patients, mention the outlook without pacing. Cammilli saw four patients who were not paced; all of them died. Bruns[81] records that 8 of 22 unpaced patients died. Lawrence[423] reports 49 patients with arteriosclerotic complete heart block managed without pacing since 1944; nine lived nine to fourteen years; 20 per cent died suddenly; one in ten who underwent surgery for other conditions died. Lau[419] has also compared 100 paced patients with 50 treated before pacing had been introduced and found that pacing improved the outlook, though prognosis depended on the severity of cardiorenal and metabolic complications.

Vookles[780] compared 20 paced patients, all of whom had complete heart block with Stokes-Adams syndrome or intractable congestive failure, with 25 in complete heart block who did not have these added features and were therefore not paced. Two of the 20 paced patients died in the hospital, compared with 14 of the 25 unpaced patients. On reviewing this experience, Vookles advocates widening the indications for pacing in emergency resuscitative situations and in some situations of asymptomatic complete heart block. Penido,[862] in comparing 10 patients with implanted pacemakers with 23 unpaced, recorded that those paced survived more than twice as long as the unpaced.

SUMMARY

Although more than 1500 paced patients have been written up in the literature and different pacemakers of various manufacturers have been used, it is not possible to draw firm conclusions regarding their relative reliability. Those reports recording details of more than ten patients have been tabulated in Tables V and VI (pp. 73, 80), but many of the reports do not provide significant relevant information, such as the length of follow-up, which must be short in many cases; those reports with a follow-up of more than a few months inevitably refer to the use of pacemaker models now out of date. With due regard to these shortcomings, a postimplantation mortality of 7.5 per cent in 1499 patients with implanted pacemakers using myocardial electrodes is noted, and tentative conclusions are drawn regarding the present choice of technique.

There is no doubt that successful pacing transforms the life of an incapacitated patient in complete heart block. It is probable that pacing prolongs life, but there are difficulties in comparing paced and unpaced patients, since strictly comparable series are not available. Some of the relevant figures obtained from the literature are discussed. It is remarkable how little indication of prognosis can be obtained from ECG and similar investigations.

Chapter 9

THRESHOLD FOR STIMULATION

THE THRESHOLD FOR electrical stimulation of the heart may vary according to the type of electrode, the site of stimulation, the period during the cardiac cycle at which the stimulus is applied, the polarity and wave form of the stimulating impulse, the impulse duration, the state of the myocardium, variations in body electrolyte concentration and certain drugs the patient may be taking. Values are also influenced by the heart rate, the apparatus and technique used for measurement and whether voltage, current, charge or energy levels are being considered. The threshold for initiation of contraction is usually a little higher than the level which just maintains steady pacing, but in the present discussion threshold values refer to those measured when stimulus strength is slowly reduced until one or more stimuli are not followed by ventricular contraction, since this is the usual method employed in clinical practice for the measurement of cardiac threshold. At very rapid pacing rates more powerful stimuli are needed than at rates within the physiological range, but over the range of heart rates normally met with in pacemaker practice there is no significant difference in threshold values.[168]

METHODS OF MEASUREMENT

Apart from special techniques which will be discussed later, threshold measurements in patients are carried out by detection of the point at which stable pacing ceases when the stimulus intensity is progressively reduced.\The threshold point usually can be identified clearly when ventricular capture becomes intermittent; in most instances, pacing ceases completely and suddenly as the intensity is reduced. Occasionally, every alternate stimulus will provoke ventricular contraction, or contractions will follow only occasional stimuli, and under these circumstances the thresh-

145

old level should be considered to be that at which the first failure of ventricular capture occurs.

For direct measurement of threshold values an adjustable pacemaker is connected to the myocardial electrodes, and this may entail surgical exploration of the site of an implanted unit so that temporary connection can be made between the electrodes and the adjustable pacemaker. Approximate threshold measurements can be obtained from the calibrated dials of many adjustable pacemakers, but for accurate readings it is essential that a calibrated triggered oscilloscope be used. The wave form of the pacemaker stimulus at the threshold point is displayed upon the oscilloscope screen and photographs taken for subsequent analysis. Measurements can then be made of the voltage applied to the heart and of the current flowing as well as the impulse duration; the energy transferred to the load and the charge transfer can then be calculated from these measurements. The impulse wave form of many pacemakers is such that the voltage and current are considerably larger at the beginning of the impulse than at the end, and in considering threshold values care should be taken to establish whether "leading edge," "mean" or "trailing edge" figures have been reported. In general, "mean" figures are implied in the present discussion.

The point at which pacing ceases can be determined from an electrocardiogram which may conveniently be displayed on the screen of either a separate or the measuring oscilloscope. A potential source of error in the measurement of threshold when bipolar myocardial electrodes are in use is that one lead of the pacemaker and the right leg lead for the ECG provide a common earth with the measuring oscilloscope, so that the system may be partially converted into a unipolar stimulating arrangement.[849] This error may be avoided if the threshold point is identified by means of an independent battery-driven pulse indicator or by palpation of the patient's radial pulse so that only one piece of line-powered equipment (measuring oscilloscope) is connected to the patient. As in all instances when line-powered equipment is used on patients with artificial pacemakers, great care must be taken to avoid the passage of any leakage current along the myocardial wires which might produce ventricular fibrillation (see p. 99).

In the presence of infection around the attachments of the electrodes to the heart or of an intermittent fault in the pacing circuit, there is no clear end-point, and it is impossible for threshold values to be obtained accurately.

STIMULUS POLARITY

The normal depolarization potential of the heart is mimicked by cathodal (negative) stimulation,[328, 613] and the fact that pacing could be carried out with lower stimulus strengths when a negative stimulus was applied to the heart than when the stimulus was positive has been noted since early reports on artificial pacing.[674] In our own patients[168] comparison of thresholds with different polarities showed that up to 16 times more energy was needed to initiate ventricular contraction when the initial stimulus polarity was positive (anodal) than when it was negative (cathodal). An investigation of the excitability of the dog's ventricle to anodal and cathodal stimulation carried out by Van Dam [773] showed that the relative efficiency of positive and negative stimuli varied according to the point within the cardiac cycle at which the impulse was applied. Although cathodal excitability was lower during most of the cycle, there was a period immediately following the absolute refractory period at which the excitability for anodal stimulation reached its maximum, and at this point the ventricle was more sensitive to anodal than cathodal stimuli. In clinical practice, the initial polarity of the pacing impulse is invariably negative, and it is apparent that during stable pacing the stimulus cannot be applied immediately following the absolute refractory period unless non-pacemade activity is occurring or the pacemaker rate is extremely rapid.

PHASE OF CARDIAC CYCLE

It is usually accepted that the electrical threshold for ventricular contraction is not constant throughout the whole of the cardiac cycle, but falls progressively as the stimulus is applied later during the relative refractory period until a low constant level is reached, which then persists throughout the remainder of diastole; Linenthal and Zoll,[463] however, found that in their patients the threshold continued to fall throughout the whole of diastole. The absolute refractory period in human subjects is of the order of 250 milliseconds after the onset of electrical activity and occupies approximately the first third of the cardiac cycle. The relative refractory period occupies approximately the next 5 per cent of the cycle and corresponds to the initial portion of the T wave on the ECG; at this time, a contraction can be produced by a stimulus of greater intensity than that needed to provoke contraction later in diastole.[223, 442] The refractory period of the ventricle in human subjects was reported by Burchell [85] to be abnormally short (200 msec) in the immediate postoperative period after pacemaker implantation but to increase to its final value of about 300 milliseconds after two or three days. The QRS complex on the ECG was noted to be bizarre during the time that the refractory period was changing. Feldman [223] reported that, during the relative refractory period, the latent interval between the stimulus and the myocardial response was double that found when the stimulus was applied after the end of the relative refractory period, but Lewis [442] was unable to detect prolonged latency at any point during the cardiac cycle.

Variations in the threshold at different phases of the cardiac cycle have little clinical importance in the management of paced patients, and the threshold for regular pacing with cathodal stimuli is lower than that found when isolated stimuli are applied at any point in the cardiac cycle.[223] For a full discussion of stimulation during the relative refractory period, reference should be made to standard works on electrophysiology.[77, 327]

SUPERNORMAL EXCITABILITY

The existence in man of a supernormal phase of recovery of myocardial excitability was deduced by Scherf and Schott,[659] who observed the pattern of dropped beats in two patients with partial heart block. Burchell [85] has pointed out that, under certain abnormal conditions, pacemaker stimuli, which are normally subthreshold, may initiate ventricular contraction. Similar observations were made by Linenthal and Zoll [463] and Dressler.[198] This supernormal period is by no means invariably present, and Feldman [223] was unable to detect the effect in any of his ten subjects with intracavity right ventricular electrodes, while Lewis [442] found the phenomenon to be the exception rather than the rule. When present, the supernormal period is related to the termination of the T wave in the ECG, and the phenomenon is most commonly observed during the investigation of failure of pacing; when pacing has ceased because of a rise in threshold or a fall in the output of an implanted pacemaker, it is common practice for control of the cardiac rhythm to be obtained by means of a temporary transvenous right ventricular catheter electrode. It will then sometimes be found that the stimulus from the implanted pacemaker causes a ventricular contraction when it falls following the T wave of a ventricular contraction stimulated by the electrode [85] (Fig. 9). Dressler [198] was able to demonstrate the supernormal phase in five patients in whom implanted units had failed because of fractured wires; the implanted unit stimulated the ventricle only following an artificially paced beat. The subthreshold stimulus from the implanted unit was usually effective only when it fell at the end of the T wave, and the period of supernormal excitability began earlier with faster ventricular rate. A somewhat similar situation can arise in which a low-intensity stimulus from an implanted pacemaker causes ventricular contraction following an idioventricular beat.

SUB-THRESHOLD STIMULI FROM IMPLANTED PACEMAKER

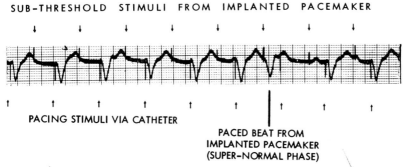

PACING STIMULI VIA CATHETER

PACED BEAT FROM
IMPLANTED PACEMAKER
(SUPER-NORMAL PHASE)

FIGURE 9. Supernormal phase. Pacing is being carried out via a transvenous electrode catheter in a patient with a faulty implanted pacemaker. Stimuli from the faulty unit cause contractions only when they fall during the supernormal period near the end of the T wave.

UNIPOLAR AND BIPOLAR STIMULATION

Myocardial stimulation can be carried out with two electrodes on the heart (bipolar system) or with one electrode on the heart and one situated elsewhere in the body (unipolar system); this second electrode is usually referred to as the "indifferent," "remote" or "tissue" electrode, and care should be taken that the "indifferent" electrode is connected to the positive pole of the pacemaker when this system is in use. Several early reports claimed that bipolar electrodes were considerably superior to unipolar electrodes for long-term pacing and resulted in thresholds which stabilized sooner and at lower levels.[135, 347] Other workers were unable to show any significant difference in the sensitivity of the heart to unipolar or bipolar stimulation.[391, 452, 828] It is probable that the superior performance of early bipolar electrodes was due to the high current density resulting from their shape and was not related to their bipolar properties;[136] our own experience[168] and that of Thalen[879] is that threshold values are almost identical when stimulation is carried out with bipolar electrodes or with only one cardiac electrode and an indifferent electrode.

There are several considerations apart from the threshold values which influence the choice between unipolar and bipolar stimulation. When emergency pacing is necessary, the use of a bipolar transvenous electrode passed to the right ventricle is recommended, since ventricular capture can always be attained by increasing the stimulus strength, provided both electrodes remain within the right ventricular cavity; the time lost in positioning the unipolar electrode so that contact is made with the endocardium and in attaching an indifferent electrode may be vital. When transvenous pacing is used on a long-term basis, both we and others[182, 283] feel that both bipolar and unipolar catheters must be positioned to make permanent contact with the endocardium for satisfactory results, and as early models of bipolar transvenous electrodes proved considerably less reliable than unipolar electrodes,[166, 283] we have mainly used the unipolar system for endocardial pacing. We have found that with commercially available pacemakers, ventricular capture is intermittent when the electrodes of a bipolar system lose direct contact with the endocardium. With the advent of new reliable electrode wires,[129] the inconvenience of providing a separate indifferent electrode may no longer be necessary. Another argument against the use of both electrodes within the heart is the risk of clot forming around the positive electrode. There is experimental evidence that clot is more likely to form on a positively charged surface,[616] perhaps as a result of an electrophoretic mechanism, and at autopsy clot has been found around endocardial wires,[259, 821] particularly at the positive electrode.[575, 581, 673] Fortunately, the anticipated risk of extensive clotting around a wire within the veins and the right ventricle with resultant pulmonary embolism has not materialized, and anticoagulants are not required; indeed, they carry their own inherent risks.[673]

When intramural or epicardial electrodes are attached to the heart, the advantages of unipolar stimulation include the fact that only one electrode need be attached to the myocardium (though a second electrode can be left as a spare) and that, since the indifferent electrode is the anode (positive), tissue damage due to standing DC current leaks or due to electrolysis are likely to be confined to a small area well away from the heart. A further advantage of unipolar stimulation is that the deflection on the electrocardiogram due to the pacemaker impulse is many times larger than when bipolar electrodes are in use, so that frequent checks on the state of the pacemaker by ECG analysis can be performed more easily.[167, 404]

A major advantage of a bipolar system is that, should breakage or failure of the stimulating electrode result in pacing failure, there is little difficulty in converting to unipolar stimulation.[828] An advantage of a bipolar system which appears to have escaped notice hitherto has been pointed out by Hill;[320] the degree to which an implanted pacemaker system will pick up electromagnetic radiations is greatly influenced by the total area enclosed within the electrical circuit, and it seems possible for bipolar electrodes to be arranged side by side throughout their course in such a manner that the entire system is symmetrical and that very little area is enclosed between the wires. By contrast, the usual unipolar system with one electrode in the heart and the indifferent electrode in the abdomen represents an excellent dipole and would be expected to pick up radiation with possible resulting interference to pacemaker function (see p. 99). Van Dam [773] has pointed out another theoretical complication with bipolar stimulation. Investigations on dogs showed that there may be two fronts of activation from the cathode and anode simultaneously, and this leads to favorable conditions for reentry so that it may be significant in determining the vulnerable period and the susceptibility to ventricular fibrillation. In clinical practice, this point seems of little, if any, importance and both unipolar and bipolar systems are in widespread use with equally satisfactory results. The situation is quite different if two electrodes on the heart are both connected to the negative terminal of the pacemaker so that unipolar stimulation occurs simultaneously at two ventricular sites; the conditions where the two activation fronts meet are likely to favor the development of ventricular fibrillation.

IMPULSE WAVE FORM

Stimuli may be monophasic, in which case current only flows in one direction throughout the whole of the impulse duration, or biphasic, in which case there is a reversal of current flow at some point. Most commercially available cardiac pacemakers provide biphasic impulses in which the wave form is balanced so that there are equal areas enclosed above and below the baseline although these two areas are not of identical shapes. There is some evidence that symmetrical biphasic wave forms result in less tissue damage than monophasic,[456] but this point is still not finally settled. In theory, "area-matching" should result in the transfer of equal amounts of electricity during the two phases of the impulse so that there would be no net charge transfer, but the changes produced during the first part of the impulse may influence current flow during the second part. As Weinman [795] has shown, the use of biphasic impulses does not result in a symmetrical current flow nor in the development of comparable voltages on the electrode during the positive and negative phases.

The influence of the stimulating wave form was investigated by Angelakos and Torres,[20] who found that pulse duration was more important than pulse shape in determining threshold requirements for dogs' hearts under the conditions of their experiments. Rectangular pulses produced excitation with lower currents than triangular pulses of the same duration, but the total electric charge for stimulation was less with triangular than rectangular pulses. The total energy required for stimulation was lower for triangular pulses, and they concluded that this was probably the most efficient wave form for cardiac stimulation. Unfortunately, their results cannot be applied directly to clinical practice since the apparatus and techniques they used differ considerably from commercially available pacemakers, and their silver/silver-chloride stimulating electrode is not in clinical use. Zoll [828, 831] has also investigated different wave forms and has concluded that a monophasic, rounded impulse is the most effective for use in human subjects.

Commercially available pacemakers provide impulses of several different types, but the most common are either the so-called "square wave" or the "condensor discharge" wave forms (Fig. 10). Impulse durations as long as 40 milliseconds [769] or even 100

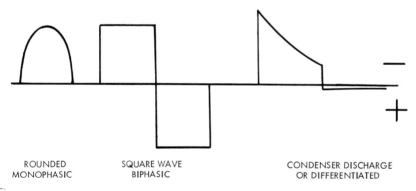

ROUNDED   SQUARE WAVE   CONDENSER DISCHARGE
MONOPHASIC   BIPHASIC   OR DIFFERENTIATED

FIGURE 10. Wave forms. Theoretical wave forms used clinically for artificial pacing; the pulse shape is altered when the pacemaker is attached to a patient. Most pacemakers produce impulses with an initial short negative portion followed by a prolonged positive recovery phase so that there are equal areas above and below the baseline ("area-matching").

milliseconds [732] have been recommended in the past for clinical use, but most commercially available pacemakers now provide impulses between 1 and 2 milliseconds in length, although the

range extends from 0.5 milliseconds to 6 milliseconds; the shortest impulse with which we have been able to pace a patient's
heart was 3 microseconds,[168] and it is likely that on this occasion
cardiac conducting tissue was being directly stimulated via a
right ventricular endocardial electrode.

ELECTRODE MATERIAL

During stimulation with metal electrodes situated in tissue
fluids an interface appears between the electrode and the electrolyte, and since the electrode properties are influenced by this
interface, these depend also upon the metal from which the
electrode is made. The relation of this effect to artificial pacemaker electrodes has been studied by Greatbatch[289] and by
Weinman,[795] who have demonstrated that the effective stimulus
delivered to the heart varies considerably according to the electrode material. When a noble metal, which cannot be destroyed
by electrolysis, is used and repetitive positive voltage pulses are
applied, the electrode impedance increases with each additional
pulse as a function of stimulus frequency.[795] In his study of different pacemaker electrode materials, Greatbatch clearly demonstrated the importance of the metal-tissue interface and showed
the superiority of a platinum-iridium alloy over stainless steel as
a stimulating electrode (see also p. 78).

MYOCARDIAL EQUIVALENT CIRCUIT

From the above considerations it is apparent that the equivalent electrical circuit of the heart will be influenced by the
type and material of electrodes used as well as by the impulse
duration and type of pacemaker employed for the measurements.
The myocardial interelectrode impedance has been shown[494] to
increase approximately logarithmically with pulse duration when
either a constant current or a constant voltage stimulator was
used. The impedance also varied inversely in logarithmic fashion
with electrolyte ion concentration, and Mansfield and Cole[494]
suggest that the impedance is higher in myocardium than in normal saline because the cells act as relatively low-conducting
material; they postulate that extracellular fluid may move to the
intravascular compartment when the intravascular pressure sud-

denly falls, and since this shift results in an increased percentage of low-conducting material in the extravascular compartment it results in a time-dependent increase in impedance. Their results indicate that with their cone electrodes of 0.0725 sq cm surface area in viable myocardium the impedance was 2200 ohms at the end of an 0.5 millisecond, 1 ma pulse; when the same electrodes were immersed in normal saline the impedance was about 1500 ohms. Because of differences in technique and equipment, only approximate comparisons can be made between reports from different centers, but estimates of the impedance across pacemaker electrodes connected to the human heart are usually between 200 and 400 ohms.[167, 207, 687, 701] In these reports the electrodes used all had considerably greater contact areas with the heart than that used by Mansfield and Cole, and much of the discrepancy between the values is probably accounted for by this factor.

Various equivalent circuits approximately representing the load presented to the pacemaker have been described,[167] but since these are influenced to such a large extent by electrode design there is little value in discussing the details of the circuits. In general the equivalent circuit consists of a resistance shunted by a capacitance and connected to a series resistance. At high frequencies such circuits may be considered fundamentally resistive.

STRENGTH-DURATION CURVES

Whether the threshold is measured as voltage, current or energy, the results are related to the duration of the stimulating impulse, and if the threshold intensity is plotted against the impulse duration, a strength-duration curve is obtained. If linear scales are used, strength-duration curves are usually hyperbolic in shape (see Fig. 11). There are many differences in strength-duration curves reported from different centers, and these are probably due to the very different techniques in use, and to the fact that the shape of strength-duration curves is dependent upon the position of the electrode on the heart.[661] In general, the results may be divided into two groups. The first type of curve is produced when the conditions of measurement are such that a constant quantity of electricity produces the necessary potential

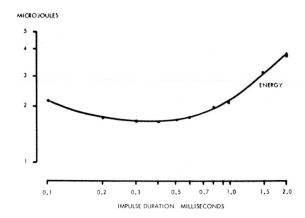

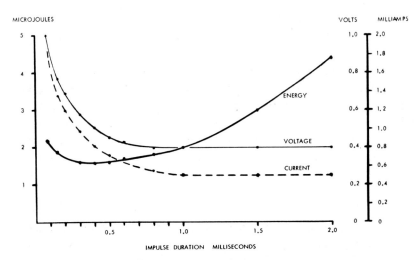

FIGURE 11. Strength-duration curves from a 65-year-old man with complete heart block paced via a C50 U.S.C.I. electrode catheter in the apex of the right ventricle and a coiled platinum indifferent electrode in the neck. Measurements were made immediately by the catheter had been positioned. The upper graph shows the energy curve with log-log scales for comparison.

difference for stimulation over a range of impulse durations.[14] The second type of curve is produced when a constant amount of electrical energy is needed for stimulation over a range of impulse durations.[77] The differences in shape between these two types of curve are only apparent when the results are plotted on log-log scales, and the situation is complicated by the fact that "mixed" curves can be obtained easily when measurements are made on pacemaker patients. Tolles [763] reviews this field and concludes that when the cell impedance is principally resistive at the pulse lengths used, a "constant energy" strength-duration curve will be recorded, but where the cell impedance is principally capacitative, a "constant coulomb" type of curve will be found.

Under actual clinical conditions in paced patients the most usual finding has been that "constant energy" criteria apply, so that over a fairly wide range of impulse durations the threshold can be expressed in microjoules.[14, 167, 168, 341, 380, 609] The values for threshold energy reported by various workers vary considerably according to the technique used for measurement and the type of electrode employed, but approximate values are 5 μj for high-efficiency intramural electrodes [134] and up to 20 μj for low-efficiency epicardial electrodes,[168] although values as high as 280 μj have been reported for intramural electrodes.[223] Thresholds obtained with small intracavity electrodes are about 5 μj. These values refer to the energy threshold when electrodes have been in place on the human heart for a few weeks; initial values were about one-tenth of the final values in our patients.[168] Final values for current thresholds with other electrode systems have been reported as three or four times the initial values.[122, 828]

For clinical purposes the energy threshold can be simply calculated from measurements taken from the screen of a calibrated oscilloscope on which the stimulus wave form at the threshold point is displayed. The energy delivered to the load during each pacing impulse is represented approximately by the product of the simultaneous values of voltage, current and impulse duration. For convenience, the mean values of voltage and current are taken, and phase angle between them is ignored. We have found that accurate calculations involving planometric integration of the current and voltage wave form traces and allowance for phase difference affect the calculated energy values by less than 2 per cent.[168]

When the impulse-duration is very short no contraction can be produced even though the stimulus strength is increased to very high values. As the impulse-duration is increased the threshold falls until it reaches a plateau on which it stays constant, regardless of the length of the stimulating impulse, so that this plateau value (rheobase) represents the minimum impulse intensity at which stimulation can occur. Investigations on our patients indicate that the rheobase values increase by two to three times during the first three weeks after attachment of the electrodes, but then remain stable for long periods. Final values with Devices epicardial coil electrodes were about 2.3 v and 3.5 ma, and final values for long-term right ventricular endocardial pacing with C50 or C51 electrodes were 1.5 v and 0.8 ma.[168] The term *chronaxie* is used to describe the impulse duration at which a stimulus of twice the rheobase value will just cause contraction. Our investigations indicate that the value for chronaxie when the electrode had been in position for several weeks was not appreciably different from the initial value, but wide variations in chronaxie values for the human heart have been found by workers using different techniques. The range varies from less than 0.25 milliseconds for right ventricular endocardial stimulation [168] to 3 milliseconds for intramural myocardial electrodes.[223] Angelakos and Torres [20] found that the threshold energy required for stimulation of dogs' hearts with their technique fell to a minimum with an impulse whose duration corresponded to the chronaxie. An impulse duration equal to the chronaxie (2 msec) was also chosen by van den Berg,[844] who found little difference between values with electrodes in the wall of the left ventricle and transvenous right ventricular electrodes.

POLARIZATION AND OVERVOLTAGE

The two electrodes necessary for cardiac pacing are situated within tissue fluid and, as this is an electrolyte solution, current is conducted by ions which may be discharged at both electrodes. Until the voltage between the electrodes reaches a critical value known as the "reversible cell voltage," no current will flow.[600] The amount by which the voltage across the electrodes exceeds this reversible cell voltage is known as the "overvoltage" or "overpotential" and is made up of three components.

1. *Ohmic component*: This is the result of electrolyte resistance and follows Ohm's law (current $= \dfrac{\text{voltage}}{\text{resistance}}$).

2. *Concentration component*: This voltage is related to a concentration gradient between the ions immediately around the electrode and those in the bulk of the solution. It occurs when current density is such that the rate of electrolysis of the electrolyte in the solution exceeds the speed at which ions are brought to the electrodes. For a given voltage a steady state of current flow is reached when the ion concentration near one electrode is zero.

3. *Activation or decompensation component*: This is a property of the electrolyte, the electrode material and the rate of removal of ions from the bulk of the solution. It is a logarithmic function of current at moderate current densities, although the current-voltage relation may be regarded as fairly linear at very low current densities of up to 1 ma/sq cm.

At the start of a stimulating impulse the three components of the overpotential are all zero, but all increase in a nonlinear manner during the duration of the impulse. The overvoltage appearing across pacemaker electrodes depends upon the impulse length, and when electrical impulses of short duration, such as those provided by artificial pacemakers, are applied to electrode systems of the type in clinical use, the current-voltage values never attain a steady state. Weinman [795] has demonstrated that the same total charge delivered by impulses of various lengths will be associated with different overvoltage, and this implies that the electrochemical processes at the electrode are functions of the impulse duration. When stainless steel electrodes are immersed in 0.9 per cent saline solution and constant current impulses passed between them, the overvoltage for a positive pulse is considerably higher than for a negative pulse of the same duration.[793] This suggests that damage is much more likely to occur to the positive than to the negative electrode in pacemaker patients.

The overvoltage produced at pacemaker electrodes is also a function of the current density, and it has been shown that a stimulating electrode of 0.5 mm diameter delivering a current of 1 ma produces a current density of approximately 500 ma/sq cm; [600] this high current density results in a high concentration voltage being produced around the electrode. Tolles [763] points out that the current density is not uniform over the surface of pacing electrodes, but will be highest in regions adjacent to the smallest radius of curvature. Under conditions of such high current density the overvoltage across the electrode may become unstable and attain different values for the same current density, while electrochemical reactions between the electrodes and the products of electrolysis may further influence the overvoltage. Electrochemical asymmetry will occur around stainless steel electrodes during positive and negative stimulation whether the pacemaker is of the constant current or constant voltage type.[795]

ELECTROLYSIS

When two metal electrodes are immersed in an electrolyte and a potential difference is maintained between them, there will be a steady flow of current which is associated with an accumulation of different ions around the two electrodes. If the electrodes are made of a non-noble metal, electrochemical reactions may occur which eventually lead to the destruction of the electrodes. The amount of metal removed will be directly related to the net charge transfer between the electrodes. A net charge transfer between pacing electrodes results when monophasic impulses are used for stimulation or when a standing DC current is present, a fault which can occur during pacemaker failure. The situation was investigated experimentally by Rowley,[641] who used stainless steel electrodes in the leg muscles of dogs and attempted to pass 10 ma constantly for five days (equivalent to the charge transfer which would be expected during 10 yr of pacing with monophasic impulses). He found that stainless steel electrodes failed within six hours during these accelerated tests, although platinum-iridium electrodes remained unaffected after the full five days. He was able to demonstrate by microscopy that failure of stainless steel electrodes was due to electrolysis and that electrode material had been deposited in the surrounding myocardium. Even when no standing DC current is present, a net charge transfer can occur when monophasic stimulating impulses are used, and excessive corrosion of a stainless steel anode would then be expected.

An investigation into electrode changes during continuous and intermittent pacing in dogs was reported by Townsend,[766] who used bipolar stimulation. Stainless steel positive electrodes were rapidly eroded during continuous pacing with unidirectional (monophasic) impulses, but this effect was not seen with biphasic impulses. Platinum-iridium needle electrodes remained in good condition with both monophasic and biphasic impulses, but the positive electrode showed slight changes in one dog paced with monophasic impulses for 571 days.

It is interesting to note that Zoll [828] reports that one of two stainless steel electrode pins in use often became useless. One of the two stainless steel electrodes utilized by Stoeckle and Schuder [736] in dogs who were paced by means of apparatus producing monophasic stimuli also failed, and they pointed out that this pin erosion was related to the total duration of pacing. It is usually assumed that with "area-matched" biphasic impulses there is an equal charge transfer in each direction with no resulting net transfer, so that any injury caused to the tissue should be minimal, but it has not yet been demonstrated that this assumption is valid. The foregoing discussion on electrochemical changes occurring around pacemaker electrodes indicates that even with biphasic impulses of the type produced by most commercially obtainable pacemakers, electrolytic destruction of the positive electrode could occur occasionally.

In our own series, there were three instances of electrolytic destruction of stainless steel positive electrodes in the first 60 cases (Fig. 12), although "area-matched" biphasic impulses were provided by the pacemakers, and we are aware of similar instances occurring with most other units commercially available (see p. 130). The "sterile reaction" around the indifferent electrode described by Glenn,[279] the "autogenic abscess" described by Ford [236] and the electrode destruction reported by Dittmar,[187] by Nicks [556] and Thalen [879] probably all have a similar explanation. Early pacemaker electrodes were often made from stainless steel, [168, 347, 348] but the almost universal use of platinum-iridium or of gold-plated electrodes, at least for the anode, has led to

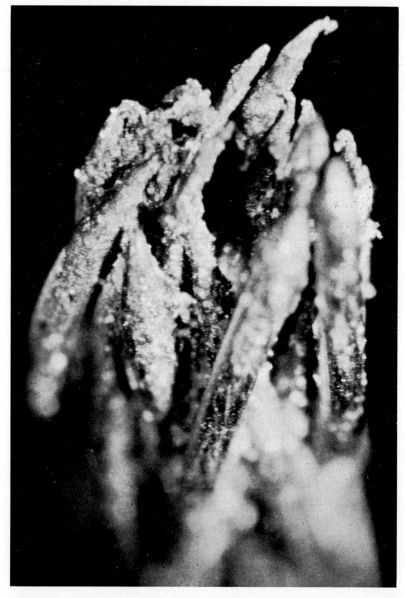

FIGURE 12. Electrolysis of anode. Destruction of stainless steel braided wire indifferent (positive) electrode by electrolysis three weeks after implantation. X30. Reproduced by permission of British Insulated Callender's Cables Ltd., from *Research Report No. C.Me/T 190*, Nov., 1962.

the virtual disappearance of this complication. It remains to be seen if electrolytic damage of tissue in the region of an anode made from noble metal will appear as a complication of pacemaker failure in the future. The better mechanical properties of stainless steel have led us to retain this material for the cathode which is attached to the myocardium, but we use a platinum anode as the indifferent electrode; theoretically, this practice leads to a standing DC current since the dissimilar metals in a common electrolyte will have a potential difference between them. A similar situation exists in the patients described by Hageman [300] who have an Elgiloy cathode in the myocardium with a platinum anode in the subcutaneous tissues, as well as in those treated with other units commercially available.[36, 548] Direct measurements with a high impedance valve voltmeter on several of our patients have shown that the potential difference is of the order of 0.001 v, the myocardial electrode being negative with respect to the indifferent electrode. The tissue impedance is fairly high, and any current flowing is so small as to have no ill effect, particularly as the anode is electrochemically inert. In practice, we have experienced no trouble from this source.

INDIRECT METHODS OF THRESHOLD MEASUREMENT

The problem of measuring the long-term threshold with different electrode systems in human subjects is normally met by one of two methods. Pacemaker implantation can be carried out as a two-stage procedure, the myocardial electrodes first being led through a subcutaneous tunnel before emerging to be attached to an external pacemaker, so that threshold measurements can be repeated frequently until a stable plateau is reached; [168, 380, 701] alternatively, measurements can be made whenever nonfunctioning pacemakers are surgically removed.[166, 168] The disadvantages of both these methods are considerable. With the former there is a fairly high risk of infection which may track along the electrode to the heart and even result in an abscess of the myocardial wall [713] (Fig. 13); even if there is no clinical evidence of infection at the site of electrode attachment to the heart, the threshold measurements may be affected by the presence of subclinical infection. With the second method, only occasional measurements

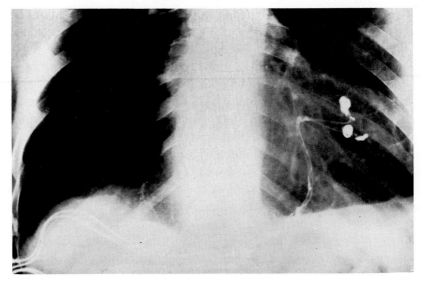

FIGURE 13. Myocardial abscess. Infection around platinum disc electrodes. Radiopaque medium has been injected along the wires and outlines two abscesses in the myocardium.

can be made and the time of measurement cannot be selected. Alternative approaches to the problem of multiple threshold measurement in patients with implanted units have been made by taking advantage of the design of particular pacemakers in which induction or radio frequency coupling can be utilized to obtain information about the load presented to the pacemaker *in situ.*

The Ann Arbor group [602] has applied one such technique to the development of a "threshold analyzer" for use with the General Electric pacemaker. This instrument utilizes a detector coil (7,000 turns of No. 33 magnet wire) on the skin surface above the pacemaker unit and measures the impulse duration from the current wave form induced in this coil; the threshold analyzer also introduces a high-frequency (2,000 cps), low energy (1.45 μj) signal into the implanted pacemaker by induction into the receiving coil which is contained in this design. This high frequency signal prevents the discharge of the output condenser of the implanted unit, and the amplitude of each pacemaker stimulus is inversely proportional to the number of suppression pulses produced so that the output energy per pulse can be suppressed down to 2½ per cent of normal. The stimulation rate of the implanted pacemaker can be maintained constant during this procedure or can be varied from 60 to 120 pulses per minute so that threshold measurements can be made at several rates on many occasions with very little disturbance to the patient, the entire electrical analysis being performed externally in less than one minute. Measurements made with this technique indicate that the interelectrode resistance (General Electric myocardial wires) of human patients increases during the first three months after implantation but thereafter does not change. The initial increase is attributed to changes in the electrode surface and fibrosis in the myocardium surrounding the electrodes. In applying the method to clinical investigation of pacing failure, the authors were able to diagnose battery failure in eight patients, in five cases while the myocardium was still responding to the pacemaker stimulus. They also diagnosed breaks in the electrode in five cases, and in one further unit a short circuit between the electrodes was diagnosed. In discussing failure of pacing due to an increase of the myocardial threshold to a level above the pacemaker stimulus, workers from the Ann Arbor group [602] refer to this situation as "exit block" and report that there was a high correlation with a rapidly rising interelectrode resistance but no correlation with high absolute values of interelectrode resistance. They were able to diagnose exit block in 11 patients, and their findings concerning the influence of drugs on myocardial threshold are discussed later (see p. 168).

Tissue resistance can also be measured repeatedly in patients who have implanted radio frequency pacemaker receivers by the use of a specially designed reflectometer described by Holcomb, Anagnostopoulos and Glenn.[334] In this instrument, the primary coil normally used for radio frequency transmission to the implanted pacemaker (Airborne) is replaced by one with an established high Q, and the primary circuit is tuned to the optimum frequency for the secondary RF implant receiver. An RF voltage is then applied to the probe and its wave form displayed on the screen of a calibrated oscilloscope. The wave form obtained depends upon the secondary load to which the probe is coupled and thus depends upon the unknown physiological load between the implanted pacemaker electrodes; the reflectometer probe is calibrated by comparison with a model system in which the secondary loads are known. Experience on dogs with well-functioning RF pacemaker systems showed that the interelectrode resistance was about 300 ohms, and in one dog where the resistance was measured to be 1600 ohms, subsequent examination of the implant revealed failure of a welded connection between the electrode lead and a platinum cardiac button caused by electrolysis at the anode. Investigations on patients with well-functioning RF implants several months postoperatively showed that the interelectrode resistance increased postoperatively but that normal values could range from 100 to 1,000 ohms. The reflectometer probe has also been used to investigate wire breakage and electronic component failure in patients with this type of RF pacemaker.

The common feature between the threshold analyzer used with the General Electric pacemaker and the reflectometer probe used with the Airborne Instruments RF pacemaker is that implanted coils originally intended for reception of externally applied signals have been utilized for the detection of the pacemaker load impedance, and it seems likely that in the future implantable pacemakers will be specifically designed so that sequential measurements of myocardial threshold can be made by induction or radio frequency coupling to an externally applied measuring instrument. It will probably be necessary for a signal to be applied to the coil of the implanted unit in the same manner as the signal is applied by the General Electric threshold generator and by the Airborne Instruments probe, and this in turn may result in a stimulus appearing across the myocardial electrodes; under the worst possible conditions the current version of the RF probe results in stimuli of 50 μa occurring in impulses of 500 microseconds duration every 17 milliseconds, and this is equivalent to impulses of 0.00025 μj being applied every 17 milliseconds. Because of the electrical coupling between primary and secondary circuits, the effective stimulus delivered to the heart by activation of the reflectometer probe will be slightly different from this value, but these stimuli induced by the measuring system itself are very far below the cardiac threshold. Use of the General Electric threshold analyzer also results in a stimulus being applied to the heart when the apparatus is in use, but this is also a low energy stimulus of 1.45 μj, which is well below the threshold for cardiac contraction via the electrodes normally used with this pacemaker system, provided that the electrodes have been in place for some time. Use of the threshold analyzer on dogs during the first postoperative week resulted in production of a tachycardia of about 200 beats per minute due to the dogs' hearts responding to the high frequency suppression pulses as well as to the regular pacing impulse and showed that in the immediate postoperative period the cardiac threshold was lower than 1.45 μj; in all dogs studied, the threshold level had risen above 1.45 μj by 14 days after pacemaker implantation.[371] This effect was not produced on human subjects in over 700 determinations, even when the threshold analyzer was used only two days postimplantation, but Judge [371] recommends that the instrument should not be used for the first two weeks after surgery.

A certain amount of information can be obtained by utilizing the electromagnetic signals emitted by implanted cardiac pacemakers of different design from those discussed previously. Sprawls [723] has used a coil of 25,000 turns of copper wire to monitor the electromagnetic signals emitted by Medtronic and Electrodyne pacemakers, although this report covered only experimental information obtained when the pacemakers were not implanted. He concluded that the signal produced directly over the pacemaker originated in the oscillator or timing circuit, and had little value other than to indicate that the circuit was functioning. He also concluded that the signal produced from the electrode leads was of value in indicating a rise in the interelectrode resistance. Similar electro-magnetic signals are emitted by the blocking oscillator circuit of the Dutch Vitatron pacemaker, and this unit was originally specifically designed so that the signal was proportional to the battery voltage. This feature is no longer incorporated in the commercial models.[844] A pacemaker monitor developed by van den Berg can be used before or after implantation to check the discharge rate of this or other units.[844]

Valuable information was also obtained by Nickel,[555] who utilized direct connections with the patient's skin instead of a coil receiving electromagnetic signals. He sited pick-up contacts on the skin areas overlying myocardial electrodes and, by displaying the resultant signals on an oscilloscope, was able to determine the time constant of the pacemaker stimuli. The ratio between the voltage 0.5 milliseconds after the beginning of the stimulus to the peak voltage at the beginning of the stimulus is taken as a convenient measure of the time constant, and Nickel quotes ratios of 0.53 for the Elema-Schönander pacemaker and 0.7 for the Medtronic pacemaker. In two patients a decreased quotient was associated with intermittent or absent response to pacemaker stimuli, but after anti-inflammatory treatment the quotient increased and pacing again became regular.

EFFECT OF DRUGS ON STIMULATION THRESHOLD

After the initial postoperative rise, the threshold usually reaches an approximate plateau within a few weeks, but variations about this mean level occur from time to time throughout the day and are particularly likely to be influenced by certain drugs. When patients are awake but resting quietly, the threshold level changes by less than 5 per cent in any one hour, although exercise causes a prompt reduction in threshold energy.[371] This relation of threshold requirements to activity was confirmed by measurements taken when the patients were asleep. These measurements disclosed a considerable rise in the threshold requirements.[371] Small increases in threshold requirements (10%) are produced by procaine amide,[139] and certain other drugs can so increase the threshold requirements that pacing ceases. Morris [530] reported one patient who resumed pacing following withdrawal of diphenylhydantoin (Dilantin®), while Lawrence [424] maintained a patient with external cardiac massage for 20 minutes because the myocardial response to electrical stimulation was blocked by relaxant drugs used during surgery.[484] The effect of administration of potassium depends upon the preceding potassium level; in many cases the threshold is lowered by potassium,[369] and clinical pacing has been restored by its administration.[298, 782] Hayward and Wyman [315] reported that oral (40 mEq) or intravenous (20 mEq/200 ml) potassium caused intermittent return of pacing in patients with pacemaker failure and this intermittent function was associated with coupled beats occurring in the supernormal phase. On the other hand, administration of "polarizing solution" increased the threshold by 27 per cent,[369] and Surawicz [743] reported that when the serum potassium had reached about 7 mEq/liter the stimulation threshold had increased from 0.5 v to 6 v; other reports also indicate that the threshold is increased when potassium levels rise.[304, 695] Sympathomimetic drugs lower the cardiac threshold, and isoproterenol has been shown to restore pacing rapidly when the drug is given by intravenous infusion and to maintain pacing for several hours when it is administered sublingually,[315] while epinephrine and ephedrine, as well as isoproterenol, have all been shown by the General Electric threshold analyzer to lower myocardial threshold.[371]

Steroids have been investigated extensively as a clinical method of treatment in patients with exit block, and it has been shown [371] that glucocorticoids such as prednisone, methylprednisone and dexamethazone lower the threshold significantly, although hydrocortisone apparently does not share this effect. Administration of aldosterone increased the threshold by 28 per cent in one patient,[369] and in another patient 9-alpha fluorohydrocortisone caused an abrupt increase in threshold.[371] Judge found 18 patients with exit block in a series of 128 pacemaker implantations and noted that the serum electrolytes were normal in all 18 cases. Fourteen of these patients were treated with glucocorticoids, and 12 returned to normal pacing within 72 hours during treatment with prednisone 40 to 60 mg daily, seven patients being maintained subsequently with doses of 10 mg daily. These workers have developed a technique of adjusting the steroid dosage to a level which maintains a safety factor of 3:1 of stimulus energy over myocardial threshold.

CAUSES OF A RISE IN THRESHOLD

An increase in threshold requirements in the immediate postoperative period has been found to be almost invariable following direct attachments of electrodes to the heart,[168, 187, 386, 681, 687, 730, 732, 828] although the threshold falls again after this initial rise.[135, 701, 713] A fall in threshold during the first day of pacing was reported by Zucker [840] in patients with congestive heart failure who were paced with bipolar right ventricular endocardial electrodes; he attributed this to a decrease in heart size with closer approximation of the electrode to the endocardium, but did not present data in support of this conclusion. The period over which the threshold continues to rise before falling again varies with the type of electrodes in use, but it is commonly about two weeks,[371] although it may be considerably longer. Provided satisfactory electrodes are used and infection at the implantation site does not occur, the threshold stabilizes in the great majority of patients and reaches stable values within a few weeks,[139, 168, 347, 386, 687, 701] although, occasionally, significant changes may occur for up to three months.[602] Provided pacemaker function is satisfactory the threshold rises whether or not the electrodes have been used for stimulation.[135, 713]

In the absence of complications such as infection or pacemaker faults resulting in abnormal polarization, it seems that the most likely cause for the increase in threshold requirements is the development of fibrotic tissue around the electrode. The physical trauma of insertion, and perhaps also the mechanical effects of cardiac contraction, will result in cell damage in the immediate vicinity of the electrodes, with subsequent fibrotic reaction which will increase the separation between the electrode and viable heart muscle; this increases the effective electrode radius and results in a threshold increase.[494] There are many reports detailing the histological findings around myocardial electrodes; [185, 312, 371, 736, 766] the changes vary from dense fibrous tissue to necrotic hemorrhagic areas and may extend as far as 8 mm from the electrode.[766]

In an investigation on dogs reported by Townsend,[766] myocardial damage was found to be considerably greater with needle electrodes than with epicardial electrodes which did not penetrate the heart muscle; damage was related to continuous rather than intermittent pacing, but not to the length of time the electrodes had been in place. No difference was found between animals paced with monophasic or biphasic stimuli, but very severe damage, including charring of the myocardium, was found in dogs in whom a low level continuous current had accidentally been superimposed upon the pacing signals. In clinical practice the tissue changes do not usually progress, and thresholds have been reported to stay constant for periods of four years; [134] this finding is not invariable and late increases in threshold have been reported by some authors.[562] As expected, rather more powerful stimuli are needed when electrodes are applied to fibrotic areas of the heart, but pacing can nevertheless be carried out successfully.[12, 168, 789] An increase in threshold requirements is also seen in the early stages after insertion of a transvenous electrode, the increase in the case of the Chardack electrode being from about 1.5 ma to 3 ma within 24 hours.[222] This increase is also seen when other transvenous electrodes are used,[168] and is probably due in part at least to the development of fibrous tissue which rapidly develops and fixes the electrode in position.[134]

The development of undue fibrotic reaction may be stimulated by the inclusion of foreign material contaminating the electrodes or the pacemaker [828] or by the absorption on the external pacemaker coating of agents used for sterilization.[530]

Several episodes of pacing failure have been reported in which a transvenous right ventricular platinum electrode developed a black coating which was sufficiently nonconductive to prevent an adequate stimulus reaching the heart. The first report was that of Zucker,[840] who described pacing failure after two months due to the development of a black deposit on the negative pole of a bipolar electrode, and similar causes of failure have been noted by Gordon [283] and by Escher.[215] In one of our own patients pacing failed after fifteen months because of a black deposit covering the platinum tip of a C50 unipolar electrode, and examination of the nature of this deposit was carried out in the research laboratories of the International Nickel Co. (Mond) Ltd.[357] Deposits were extracted from the electrode surface using a plastic film which was then coated with carbon; the plastic was dissolved in acetone to give a preparation suitable for examination in the electron microscope; for electron probe microanalysis a conducting layer of aluminum was sputtered on to the carbon films. A wide variation in composition was found between individual particles;

iron and sulphur were detected in almost every case, and many particles were rich in platinum, while a few contained small amounts of chromium and calcium. It seems likely that the corrosion product was mainly sulfide, and since it contained iron and chromium, a possible mechanism of its development was that the inert covering around the lead wires was not completely effective and the stainless steel (18% chromium) lead wires were involved in the process.

The responsiveness of the myocardium itself to electrical stimulation has been emphasized as a significant factor in the development of threshold changes by Judge.[371] He points out that any agent decreasing the resting membrane potential or increasing the cellular threshold should theoretically increase myocardial responsiveness, but he was unable to demonstrate alterations in serum potassium level in any patients with exit block. It seems likely that alterations in the responsiveness of the heart muscle account for small fluctuations in the threshold and can be influenced by drug treatment but will not explain the alteration from low initial threshold to the final plateau level. Our own investigations indicate that the initial threshold, measured in microjoules, increases by a factor of about ten times by the time the stable plateau value has been reached.[168]

One cause of pacing failure due to high threshold with transvenous electrodes is that the electrode has been positioned in the coronary sinus rather than in the cavity of the right ventricle. If the electrode enters an inferior coronary vein, its tip will pass out towards the apex of the cardiac silhouette seen on the fluoroscopic screen and will apparently be well positioned with its tip impacted in the right ventricular apex. Screening in the AP plane or examination of a PA chest x-ray will not detect the malposition, which will only become apparent if lateral views are available; the error can be avoided if the catheter is passed through the pulmonary valve and then withdrawn to the right ventricle before final positioning. In four of our own patients, stimulation was carried out via a C50 electrode in the coronary sinus, and in each case there was a rapid rise in threshold requirements to unacceptable levels so that pacing ceased between one and seven days after insertion. In one of these patients, pacing was erratic even when the stimulus intensity was increased to its maximum of 10 v; ventricular fibrillation occurred at this time, fortunately with a successful result after defibrillation and thoracotomy for direct attachment of epicardial electrodes and pacemaker implantation. A rapid rise in threshold due to electrode malplacement in the coronary sinus has also been reported by Gordon.[283]

CLINICAL IMPLICATIONS

It is apparent that an implanted pacemaker must develop a powerful enough stimulus to drive the heart satisfactorily when the threshold has reached its stable level, and it is desirable for a safety factor of 2:1 or 3:1 to be available. The great differences in final threshold levels attained when different electrode systems are used limit the interchangeability of units and electrodes, so that a Medtronic unit, delivering 10 μj and designed for high efficiency (Chardack-Greatbatch) electrodes, is unsuitable for use with low-efficiency epicardial wires. Similarly it is unwise for a unit designed for low-efficiency wires, and therefore producing fairly high energy impulses, to be attached to high-efficiency myocardial electrodes since the stimulus intensity may so far exceed the threshold for contraction as to reach the threshold for provocation of ventricular fibrillation; the ratio between stimulation and fibrillation thresholds is of the order of 10:1. A late rise in cardiac threshold may indicate pacemaker failure, electrode damage or possibly infection, but in the absence of these complications it is usually possible to continue pacing with a high-output unit; conversely, the identification of a stable threshold which is unusually low may eventually lead to substitution of a low-output unit having prolonged battery life when routine replacement becomes necessary.[371] Pelaška [895, 896] has designed a range of six pacemakers with progressively greater outputs and chooses the appropriate unit on the basis of threshold measurements. Differences in threshold levels between different electrodes have led to modifications in the design of specific units, so that a Medtronic pacemaker intended for use with the Chardack bipolar electrode has a considerably greater output than the superficially identical model intended for use with intramyocardial electrodes; the low thresholds found with some designs of transvenous electrodes [168] have enabled a considerable reduction in size to be achieved with the Devices pacemaker, but as a result the model intended for long-term transvenous stimulation is unsuitable for use with the normal epicardial electrodes. The initial rise of threshold and subsequent fall in the postoperative period may lead to a temporary failure of pacing even when the implanted unit is capable of delivering stimuli which are adequate when the final threshold has been established, and this phenomenon has been observed clinically, both in our own practice and by Judge,[370] who recommends the use of steroids to lower the threshold temporarily during this phase. The higher output of the Vitatron pacemaker in its "prolonged lifetime mode" has also enabled pacing to be maintained during this temporary period.

SUMMARY AND CONCLUSIONS

Both unipolar and bipolar stimulation is satisfactory in practice; the negative electrode must be placed on the heart when a unipolar system is in use.

Following attachment of electrodes the threshold usually increases for about two weeks but then falls slightly to a final value which remains stable for many years. The final value is between three and ten times the initial value, depending upon the electrode system in use and the parameters chosen to express threshold. With most electrodes in current use, final values for the human heart are about 2 to 5 ma, 2 to 6 v and 5 to 20 μj.

Minor variations in thresholds occur during the day, the values being higher during sleep and lower during exercise. The threshold is lowered by sympathomimetic drugs and glucocorticoids; mineralocorticoids, procaine amide and muscle relaxants increase it.

Noble metals are now usually used for electrode material. If stainless steel is used as the positive electrode it may undergo electrolysis, and this is usually, but not invariably, associated with a faulty pacemaker.

A fibrotic reaction occurs around myocardial electrodes in every case; if infection is also present no stable threshold is achieved.

Chapter 10

HEMODYNAMIC CHANGES DURING
ARTIFICIAL PACING

Dᴙɪᴠɪɴɢ ᴛʜᴇ ʜᴇᴀʀᴛ at a constant rate by electrical stimulation
has been, for many years, a standard technique in physiological
investigations on animals, but it is only since the development of
artificial pacemakers that these investigations have been extended
directly to human subjects. Many hemodynamic studies have been
carried out in patients being treated with artificial pacemakers,
and these investigations all fall into one or more of the following
groups:

1. Studies depending upon alteration in ventricular rate;
2. Studies depending upon a fixed ventricular rate;
3. Studies of the atrial transport mechanism.

STUDIES DEPENDING UPON ALTERATION IN
VENTRICULAR RATE

Animal Experiments

In an investigation on open-chested dogs with surgically induced heart block, Berglund [38] altered the ventricular rate from
below 40 beats a minute to over 200 beats a minute and studied
the myocardial oxygen consumption, coronary blood flow and
cardiac work. He found cardiac output reached a maximum at a
rate between 90 to 180 beats a minute, with a decrease at higher
values. Stroke volume decreased progressively as the ventricular
rate was increased, but myocardial oxygen consumption and coronary blood flow increased even at high ventricular rates when
the ventricular work was constant or even decreasing. The aortic
pulse pressure diminished and the mean aortic pressure rose
slightly as the ventricular rate was increased. Ventricular function
curves obtained by plotting the stroke work against the respective

175

mean atrial pressure were always lower when stimulation rates were fast than when they were slow. Although the coronary blood flow increased at high rates the mechanical work performed by the ventricle also increased, so that coronary flow per unit of work increased as the rate increased. Coronary vascular resistance fell considerably at high ventricular rates. When the coronary inflow tubing was constricted by a screw clamp, elevations of the ventricular rate produced an inadequate rise in coronary blood flow, and left ventricular failure developed with a fall in cardiac output and systemic pressure; these signs of coronary insufficiency were simply reversed by reducing the heart rate. Laurent [420] also studied open-chested dogs and showed that the coronary blood flow and myocardial oxygen consumption increased with increasing heart rate but approached a limit at extremely rapid rates on the order of 300 beats a minute. A reduction in cardiac output at the extremes of the rate range during artificial pacing of a dog's heart was also noted by Miller,[515] who found that the stroke volume was fixed and the cardiac output rate-dependent below 60 beats a minute but that above this, cardiac output was independent of pacing rate. At very fast rates he demonstrated by cineangiography that there was reduced diastolic filling of the ventricle and that this accounted for the fall in cardiac output. In a study of the effect of heart rate on left ventricular volume in dogs, Bristow [72] reported that cardiac output rose slightly when the heart rate varied between the range of 80 to 140 per cent of the original rate, and that the left ventricular end-systolic volume altered in the same direction as the stroke volume, but to a lesser extent. The cardiac output was also found to be almost independent of ventricular rate by Warner and Toronto,[787] who studied dogs both at rest and on exercise shortly after production of complete heart block.

It seems clear that in dogs the production of complete heart block results in a low cardiac output with the later development of heart failure,[73] but that the cardiac output can be returned to normal by artificial stimulation of the ventricles. As the stimulation rate increases to high levels the cardiac output falls again, although the coronary blood flow and myocardial oxygen consumption continue to increase. In the presence of impaired coronary filling, acute heart failure can be induced by rapid rates.

Investigations in Man

Changes in cardiac output with alterations in ventricular rate were studied originally by Müller and Bellett [536] and by Escher,[216] while many other reports along similar lines have appeared since then.[34, 42, 43, 107, 217, 260, 311, 372, 418, 487, 648, 675] In these, as in other less exhaustive investigations,[35, 220, 510, 765] it was firmly established that the low cardiac output associated with complete heart block is augmented when the heart rate is increased by an artificial pacemaker. Further increments in rate result in further increases in cardiac output until a maximum level is reached. In patients with good myocardial function further increases in ventricular rate do not then significantly increase the cardiac output.[42, 311, 372, 487, 712] Ross [633] found that in subjects without heart block the cardiac output remained unchanged when the heart rate was increased by pacing the atrium. Similar studies by Stein [729] included slowing of the ventricular rate by paired and coupled pacing of the atrium (see p. 201); cardiac index was not significantly changed when heart rate was decreased by as much as 50 per cent below, or increased by as much as 100 per cent above the sinus rate, either at rest or during exercise. It seems clear therefore, that in normal subjects and in pacemaker patients with good myocardial function the cardiac output is not dependent upon pacing rate but is adjusted largely by alteration in the stroke volume. In the presence of heart failure,[368] or when ventricular function is impaired,[34, 190, 487, 712] the stroke volume is relatively fixed and so the output is rate-dependent; under these circumstances the cardiac output will not become independent of ventricular rate but will continue to increase as the pacemaker rate increases.

As the heart rate is increased a point is reached in all patients at which the fall in stroke volume is greater than that which would be appropriate to maintain a steady cardiac output.[31, 487, 497, 712] The situation in resting patients is thus very similar to that previously described in experimental animals with complete heart block, the cardiac output increasing initially but decreasing later as the pacemaker rate becomes rapid. The most likely explanation for this fall-off in flow at rapid rates is that a long diastolic period is necessary for adequate ventricular filling in the absence of an effectively placed atrial systole.[487, 712] The effect occurs at lower rates in patients with poor myocardial function because the atrial transport mechanism is of increased importance when the left ventricle is diseased.[66] Other factors which may be involved are the development of atrioventricular valve regurgitation at high rates and the relative inefficiency of beats stimulated from the ventricle.[275] This inefficiency of paced beats is illustrated by the results of an investigation of one of our patients with aortic stenosis and heart block [307] in whom the findings during idioventricular rhythm at 41 beats a minute were compared with those during paced rhythm at 42 beats a minute. Although the cardiac output remained unchanged, the left ventricular peak systolic pressure increased from 175 mmHg to 190 mmHg, and the gradient across the aortic valve increased from 70 mmHg to 90 mmHg during pacing; at the same time the PC wedge pressure rose from 20 mmHg to 25 mmHg. Pacing increased the mean left atrial pressure and left ventricular work without any appreciable alteration in heart rate or increase in cardiac output. It has also been suggested [31] that a reduction in coronary flow at rapid rates may result in ventricular ischemia, producing a decreased cardiac output, but this seems unlikely in view of animal work showing that coronary flow increases at rapid rates, even when the cardiac output falls.

Optimal Rate

The lowest pacemaker rate at which the maximal resting cardiac output is reached is associated with the minimum level of left ventricular work since the aortic pressure does not vary significantly with alterations in pacemaker rate over this range. It is therefore reasonable to assume that the optimal rate during pacing is that corresponding to maximal cardiac output. Little information is available as to whether the optimal rate is a constant finding for each patient, although it seems likely that in short-term investigations at least the optimal rate remains fairly constant. McGregor and Klassen [487] found the response to be highly repeatable in one patient, and a similar observation was made by Benchimol.[31] Observations made in our own laboratory show that repeated determinations of the optimal rates over a few weeks produce similar values. The optimal rate probably varies with the state of ventricular function; McGregor and Klassen investigated patients in heart failure and found that under these circumstances the cardiac output was highly rate-dependent until the heart failure had been successfully treated, when cardiac output became almost independent of rate in the usual manner. In investigations covering a longer period of time, Bishop [47] studied the same patient after an interval of a year and found that the response to increased ventricular rate was identical. We have investigated one patient after one year and after two years of continual artificial pacing and found that the optimal rate had not altered but that the cardiac output was considerably less dependent upon pacemaker rate than initially, a finding which probably indicates an improvement in myocardial function with long-term pacing (Fig. 14).

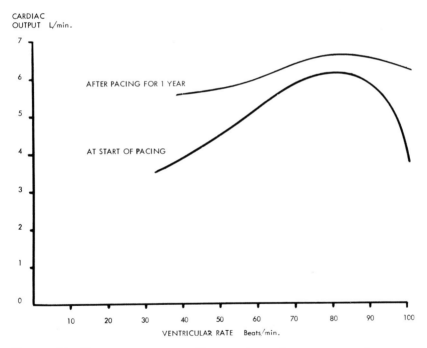

FIGURE 14. Rate-output curves. Changes in cardiac output with pacing rate in a 37-year-old patient with heart block and cardiomyopathy. The output was less dependent upon ventricular rate after continuous fixed-rate pacing for one year.

The six patients originally reported by Müller and Bellett in 1961 had maximal outputs at rates of between 50 and 65 beats per minute, while Escher found highly specific optimal rates within the range of 60 to 100 beats a minute in her ten patients.[216] Segel [675] reported optimal rates in 12 patients to lie between 70 and 80 beats a minute with a mean of 73 beats a minute, while we [712] found a mean rate of 72 beats per minute gave maximum output in a group of 14 patients of this type. Piemme found optimal rates to range from 84 to 100 beats a minute and to be highly specific for each patient.[595] Carleton [107] investigated 12 patients and found optimal rates of approximately 70 beats a minute. Benchimol [34] found an optimal rate of 76 beats a minute in one patient and Samet [648] reported optimal rates between 80 and 105 beats a minute in his "Group 2," which was made up of six patients. Escher [217] reported that the optimal rates for most of her patients were in the seventies and correlated with the level at which the greatest percentage increase of cardiac output in relation to rate was reached. The patient reported by Gaal, Goldberg and Linde [260] had an optimal rate of 75 beats a minute at rest, and this was unchanged during exercise; our own investigations [712] have shown that the optimal rate during exercise is often very similar to the resting value, and Carleton [107] came to a similar conclusion.

Changes in Atrial Rate at Rest

As the ventricular rate is altered with an artificial pacemaker there is often, although not invariably,[217] an alteration in the atrial rate also. The atrial rate is often rapid during complete heart block with a slow idioventricular rate, but as the ventricular rate is increased by artificial pacing the atrial rate initially falls.[42] If the pacemaker rate becomes fast there is often a secondary increase in the atrial rate also, so that a graph of atrial rate against pacemaker rate shows a minimum value (Fig. 15). The pacemaker rate at which the atrial rate reaches its minimum corresponds to the rate at which cardiac output is a maximum, and attempts have been made to determine the optimal pacemaker rate from a study of the atrial rate changes.[712, 846] This test is difficult to apply in practice, owing to alterations in the atrial response produced by

ATRIAL RATE

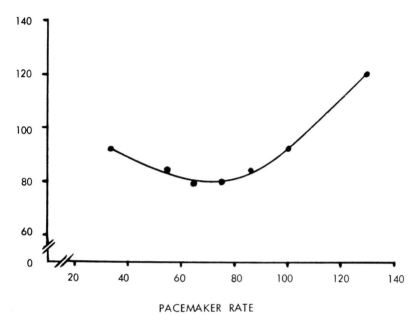

PACEMAKER RATE

FIGURE 15. Atrial-ventricular rate. Relation between ventricular rate (pacing rate) and atrial rate at rest in a 40-year-old woman with complete heart block and poor myocardial function.

changes in sympathetic tone, the effects of drugs and reflex changes induced by respiration or alterations in body position, as well as by the Erlanger-Blackman phenomenon (see p. 31). The alterations in atrial rate consequent upon alterations in pacemaker rate are probably of reflex origin since the response can be abolished by atropine or drugs with an atropine-like action such as chlorpromazine.[712]

Changes in Stroke Volume

At slow idioventricular rates the ventricular stroke volume is large, and values up to 230 ml have been reported.[744] As the ventricular rate is increased the stroke volume falls progressively [43, 107, 372, 675, 712] unless the patient has very poor myocardial function, when the stroke volume may remain fixed.[34, 487, 712] We have noticed in several of our patients who had exceptionally slow idioventricular rates (20 beats/min or less) that at very slow rates there was a reduction in stroke volume, and it seems likely that this was due to diminished ventricular performance secondary to inadequate coronary flow.

Changes in Venous Pressure

The right atrial pressure is usually high in complete heart block [43, 713] but falls as the ventricular rate is increased. If the pacemaker rate is very fast there may be a secondary rise in venous pressure [712] so that the minimum value is reached at a pacemaker rate within the resting physiological range.[217] This pacemaker rate is associated with maximal resting cardiac output.[712]

The left atrial pressure measured indirectly as PC wedge pressure is frequently also high in pacemaker patients but remains fairly constant as ventricular rate is increased.[675] At high pacemaker rates there is often a sharp increase in the PC wedge pressure, and this effect may occur above about 100 beats a minute.[43, 712]

These changes in right and left atrial pressure are of course quite separate from the fall in venous pressures which occurs when a patient in heart failure improves during treatment with an artificial pacemaker.

Pulmonary Arterial Pressure

During a slow idioventricular rhythm the pulmonary artery mean pressure is usually normal or slightly elevated,[43, 217] and the pulse pressure is wide with a high systolic level. As the ventricular rate increases the usual response is for the systolic pressure to fall and the diastolic to rise so that the pulse pressure diminishes while the mean pressure remains relatively stable,[43, 217, 716] although Segal found that an increase in ventricular rate in his patients was associated with increasing mean and diastolic pressures and little change in the average systolic level.

Systemic Arterial Pressure

The systemic pressure behaves similarly to the pulmonary arterial pressure, with the exception that at very slow ventricular rates the mean pressure is often low,[43, 217] although, as a consequence of the large stroke volume, the pulse pressure and the systolic level are high.[715] A sudden increase in pacing rate from normal to high levels results in a rapid drop in aortic pressure, presumably because the very short diastole does not allow normal ventricular filling. This pressure drop is transient and restoration to control levels occurs in about 20 seconds.[43]

When the ventricular rate is increased from the idioventricular rate there is an initial increase in the systemic mean arterial pressure,[42, 43] but at higher rates the mean pressure remains approximately constant, although the pulse pressure diminishes in the same way as in the pulmonary artery.[714] In a study of 13 patients, Benchimol [31] found that the systemic mean arterial pressure continued to increase as the pacemaker rate increased, even when the optimal rate had been passed and the cardiac output was falling; Segal also reported that the systemic mean pressure continued to rise at an increasing heart rate, although he found that the average systolic pressure remained unchanged.

An unusual response of the systemic arterial pressure to artificial pacing was reported in 1960 by Tsuboi and Ebina,[769] who found that in dogs and in one patient the systemic blood pressure was affected not only by the heart rate but also by the stimulating voltage. They quote values for a 35-year-old man of 70 mmHg at 2 v, rising to 120 mmHg at 6 v and found a maximum blood pressure level at 5.5 v. We have been unable to confirm this observation, and in our studies the arterial pressure has been independent of stimulating voltage.

Oxygen Consumption

The oxygen consumption of a patient in complete heart block is usually normal, but Segal [675] found that as the heart rate was increased by pacing there was a concomitant increase in oxygen consumption. He argues that this was due to an increase in the myocardial oxygen uptake since the requirements for the rest of the body probably are not affected by a change in pacemaker rate. His figures indicate that a twofold increase in heart rate doubled the myocardial oxygen uptake, and this is consistent with the results of animal experiments previously described.[38] These results could not be confirmed by Bevegård,[43] who found no significant changes in oxygen consumption in 22 patients when the pacing rate was increased. During steady state exercise the oxygen uptake is higher for any given ventricular rate than at rest. If the ventricular rate is increased during steady state exercise the oxygen uptake alters in the same manner as when the subject is at rest.[377]

Arterial-Venous Oxygen Difference

Arterial-venous oxygen difference is wide in patients with slow idioventricular rates, but narrows as ventricular rate is increased,[43, 675] and this is so whether the patient is at rest or performing steady state exercise. The AV oxygen difference is higher during exercise than at rest with identical ventricular rates, and if the exercise is submaximal an increase in pacemaker rate will reduce the AV difference.[377] If the patient is exercising at his maximum level, an increase in rate does not affect the arterial-venous oxygen difference, which remains fixed at the upper limit obtainable by that subject.[377]

Other Parameters

When the heart rate is increased from its slow idioventricular rate to the optimal level, Benchimol [31] found that the left ventricular work increased while the peripheral resistance, circulation time and left ventricular ejection time decreased. Bevegård [43] found no alteration in peripheral vascular resistance when the ventricular rate was altered, and also reported that the central blood volume did not alter systematically with change in rate in five patients. The effect of inflation of antigravity suits in four patients did not produce significant changes. There is a tendency for the right ventricular end-diastolic pressure and the ventricular filling pressure to fall as the heart rate is increased.[31] If the pacemaker rate is considerably faster than the optimum the left ventricular work, cardiac index and ejection time continue to decrease, but the peripheral resistance and circulation time increase again.[31]

STUDIES DEPENDING UPON A FIXED VENTRICULAR RATE

Postural Changes

When normal subjects change from the supine to the erect posture there is a fall in cardiac output of about 20 per cent, and this is mediated both by alterations in heart rate and in stroke volume.[41] Since the physiological control of rate has been lost in patients with fixed-rate pacemakers, any adjustment in cardiac output with posture must be dependent entirely upon alterations in stroke volume. A comparison between five normal subjects and five patients with fixed-rate artificial pacemakers is illustrated in Figure 16. The normal subjects showed a drop of 25 per cent in cardiac output accompanying the alteration from supine to the sitting posture, and the mean fall in cardiac output in the pacemaker group was almost identical with that of the normals. In the investigation reported by McGregor and Klassen,[377] one subject was paced at substantially the same rate sitting and supine dur-

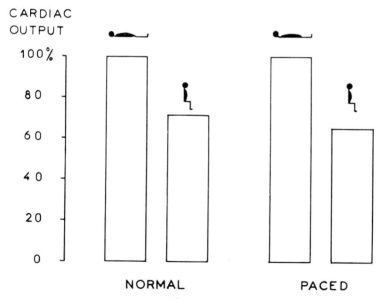

FIGURE 16. Postural effects. Mean changes in cardiac output with changes of posture in five normal subjects and five patients with fixed-rate artificial pacemakers. The fall in both groups is very similar.

ing two separate studies. The cardiac output was lower in the sitting position by just over 20 per cent. Similar measurements were made by Gaal [260] on one patient who was investigated in the supine and sitting position. There was a fall of 23 per cent in cardiac output with the change to the sitting position.

Effect of Exercise at Fixed Heart Rate

In the normal subject the stroke volume initially increases at the onset of exercise by about 10 per cent when the subject is supine, but by considerably more when erect.[41] After this initial increase the stroke volume remains relatively fixed, and the increase in cardiac output is directly proportional to the increase in heart rate.[337] This normal response is completely absent in patients with fixed-rate artificial pacemakers, and several investigators have studied the effect of exercise under these conditions. One of the earliest reports was that of Bevegård,[42] who reported fully on two patients, with a footnote mentioning three others. His patients were able to increase their stroke volume and therefore their cardiac output on exercise despite a fixed heart rate; they obtained only a negligible increment in cardiac output at higher ventricular rates, and these findings were later confirmed by a comprehensive study of 22 patients from the same laboratory.[43] This increase of stroke volume with exercise is characteristic of pacemaker patients with good myocardial function, and in this group the cardiac output is to a great extent independent of heart rate and is affected only by the level of exercise, so that the cardiac output increases linearly with work load in the normal manner.[43, 487, 712] Stroke volume in these patients may reach high levels, and values during exercise of 200 ml [712] and 320 ml [744] have been reported. During submaximal exercise patients with good myocardial function rarely benefit from an increase in pacemaker rate above about 90 beats a minute.[43, 107, 712]

The inability of patients with poor myocardial function to increase their stroke volume is characteristic and has been used as a screening test in a wide variety of clinical conditions.[758] When this situation is present in patients with artificial pacemakers it follows that their cardiac output must be entirely rate-dependent even on exercise, and this conclusion has been confirmed in several investigations.[34, 260, 487, 712] One patient studied by McGregor was initially in heart failure, but after treatment for three days with a pacemaker and diuretics subsequently showed a normal response to exercise, with an increase in stroke volume and cardiac output despite the fixed heart rate. Escher [217] reported the results during exercise on four patients with fixed-rate pacemakers who showed only minimal increases in cardiac output despite large increases in the oxygen consumption, and in one patient reported by Benchimol [34] and two of the six subjects studied by McGregor [487] there was no increase in the cardiac output with exercise. The most striking feature during effort in these patients with poor myocardial function was the large difference between the arterial and venous oxygen saturations.

Maximal Exercise

Most exercise studies carried out on pacemaker patients are designed to study submaximal exercise levels, but one report from Stockholm is concerned solely with maximal levels of exercise.[377, 718] In this study ten patients were exercised up to maximal levels on a bicycle ergometer, and the influence of different fixed pacemaker rates on their performance was studied. The maximal oxygen uptake was shown to be related to the heart rate provided that this was fairly slow, but once the pacemaker rate had reached 80 to 90 beats a minute, the maximal oxygen uptake and maximal exercise level were not increased by further increments of pacemaker rate in eight out of the ten patients. Of the 22 patients reported by Bevegård,[43] eight were exercised at levels close to their maximal capacity; at paced rates up to 110 beats a minute the stroke volume increased approximately to the maximal obtainable in six cases. The remaining two patients were unable to reach their maximal stroke volume with ventricular rates of 72 beats a minute and 106 beats a minute respectively, while when the ventricular rates were increased to 120-150 beats a minute three further patients were unable to attain their maximal stroke volumes. In all eight patients the maximal cardiac output during exercise was reached with relatively slow ventricular rates, and in no case was there an increase when the ventricular rate was faster than 110 beats a minute. An increase in cardiac output during exercise when the pacemaker rate was increased was reported by Landergren,[412] who also showed that the exercise capacity was increased with a rapid ventricular rate. The maximal rates used in this investigation were of the order of 105 to 110 beats a minute, and it seems likely that the same factors operate during exercise as at rest in restricting the maximal beneficial pacemaker rate. It seems clear that little, if any, benefit will be obtained by increasing the pacemaker rate above about 100 beats a minute during exercise even in patients with good myocardial function; when atrial-triggered pacemakers are used the situation may be completely different since a properly timed atrial systole should become increasingly important at high exercise levels.

STUDIES OF THE ATRIAL TRANSPORT MECHANISM

The varying relationship between atrial and ventricular systole in patients with A-V dissociation leads to fluctuations in ventricular performance depending upon the presence or absence of a correctly placed preceding atrial contraction. When atrial systole precedes ventricular contraction by a physiological interval, ventricular filling is augmented,[547] and the respective ventricular end-diastolic pressure increases,[66] as compared to ventricular beats in which there is no preceding effective atrial systole. As a result of these changes during diastole the ventricular contraction produces a higher systolic pressure, and this effect has been shown to occur on both the right and left sides of the heart.[30, 66, 372, 497, 510, 546, 650, 715, 716, 744, 813] From observations of this type it is possible to compare the delay between atrial and ventricular systole with the corresponding pulse pressure, and when this is done a curve of the shape shown in Figure 17 is obtained. Similar figures have been published by Johansson,[267] Carleton [107] and us, showing considerable augmentation of the systolic pressure when the PR interval falls within the physiological range. The acute effects of atrial systole upon ventricular performance are dependent upon the pacing rate of the ventricle, and Benchimol [30] reported that a properly timed atrial contraction was most effective for ventricular rates between 50 and 80 beats a minute; in other studies the effect of atrial systole upon systemic arterial pressure has become increasingly noticeable as the ventricular rate was in-

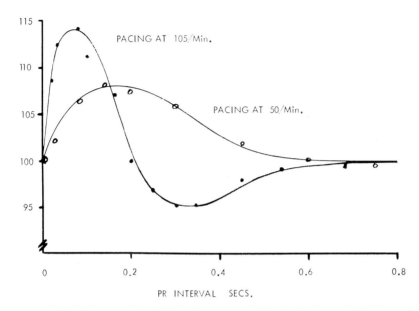

AORTIC PULSE
PRESSURE %

PACING AT 105/Min.

PACING AT 50/Min.

PR INTERVAL   SECS.

FIGURE 17. PR interval and blood pressure. Relation between PR interval and aortic pulse pressure of the corresponding beat for a patient in complete heart block with fixed-rate ventricular pacing. The relative importance of atrial systole is greater at 105 beats per minute than at 50 beats per minute. Maximum augmentation of pulse pressure occurs with physiological PR intervals; at 105 beats per minute, an atrial contraction falling late *diminishes* the aortic pulse pressure below control levels.

creased.[86, 104, 107] It has been noted by Jonsson [43] and in our own laboratory also that when atrial systole occurs at a critical time before ventricular systole the pulse pressure in the subsequent beat may be considerably lower than that of the control value with ineffective atrial systole, and this effect is attributed to diminished ventricular filling produced by emptying of the venous reservoir by the contraction of the atrium. The exact timing of atrial systole for this effect to be produced varies with heart rate and from patient to patient, but the PR interval is always longer than the physiological range. It is to be noted that these investigations on augmentation of ventricular systolic pressure are all based on beat-to-beat studies in which no compensating mechanism can act, and so they provide no evidence for the superiority of atrial-triggered pacing on a long-term basis. Chardack [125] has published tracings of investigations on dogs' hearts demonstrating that the mean systolic pressure level was not affected by recurrent synchronization of atrial and ventricular contractions, although the systolic pressure fluctuated above and below the level attained during synchronized pacing.

Atrial-Triggered Pacing

The effects of atrial systole have been investigated many times during animal experiments.[73, 459, 517] Snyder and Wood [708] found that an ineffective atrial systole resulted in a 10 per cent decrease in cardiac output and that this effect was constant over a wide range of heart rates, but Mitchell,[518] using an open-chested dog supported by right heart bypass, found that the influence of atrial systole in determining ventricular stroke volume was greater at higher heart rates. Sellers,[678] studying dogs with denervated hearts, showed 15 per cent decrease in cardiac output during ineffective atrial systole, and Skinner [703] found an absent atrial systole to be associated with a reduction of approximately 30 per cent in aortic blood flow. Stephenson and Brockman [731] found higher aortic pressures and stroke volumes in dogs during atrial-triggered pacing than during direct ventricular pacing.

Similar studies carried out in man by Martin [498] showed that stroke volume and cardiac output were lower when pacing was carried out without physiological placing of atrial systole compared to the values obtained during atrial synchronized pacing. The acute effects of alteration in the timing of atrial systole in man were studied in one of our patients by a technique of pacing both atrium and ventricle via two transvenous endocardial electrodes with a stimulator giving an adjustable delay between two pulses.[716] When the atrium and ventricle were made to contract at the same time atrial systole was ineffective and there was a sudden drop in cardiac output of 30 per cent. This fall in output was an immediate change, and after a few minutes the cardiac output had increased to the control value, despite the continued absence of effective atrial systole, showing that an increase in ventricular stroke volume had occurred.

A sustained improvement in hemodynamic function when atrial-triggered pacemakers are used as compared to fixed-rate ventricular pacing has been shown by Escher,[217] who demonstrated in three patients that the cardiac index at rest was higher when the PR interval was at the upper limit of normal (0.23 sec) than when it was short (0.1 sec). One patient was studied both at rest and on exercise during atrial-triggered and fixed-rate ventricular pacing; during atrial-triggered pacing the cardiac index increased and the AV oxygen difference decreased. An excellently controlled investigation into the atrial contribution to cardiac output has been reported by Samet, Bernstein, Nathan and Lopez,[649] who compared hemodynamic findings in six patients with complete heart block during different types of pacing at identical ventricular rates. Both atrium and ventricle could be independently paced via bipolar endocardial electrodes, and, in addition, ventricular pacing could be triggered from the atrium with a physiological PR interval. The results, which were obtained at rest only, indicate a mean increase of 10 per cent in the cardiac output when ventricular contraction was preceded by an atrial systole. There was considerable variation between the six patients studied, and in some cases atrial-triggered pacing produced no increment in stroke volume. Throughout the series there was a tendency for the effect of the atrial transport mechanism to become more marked as the ventricular rate was increased, and in one patient the cardiac output reached a maximal level with a PR interval of 1.08 seconds. Similar studies during exercise have been carried out by Nathan [543] and by Karlöf [387] and clearly demonstrate that the cardiac output is greater for any given level of exercise during atrial-triggered pacing than during fixed-rate ventricular pacing.

The pressure changes during atrial-triggered pacing are broadly similar to those already described for direct ventricular pacing, although, of course, the cyclical pressure variations due to transient synchronization of atrial and ventricular systoles are not present. Investigations of the effects of sudden alterations from complete heart block with slow idioventricular rates to atrial-triggered pacing [43, 387] have demonstrated an immediate increase in systemic arterial pressure, a fall in right atrial pressure, and an increase in cardiac output at the onset of pacing. These changes stabilize at new steady levels very shortly after the onset of pacing, and these levels show considerable improvement over the values in complete heart block.

Pacing in Sinus Rhythm

Although it is by no means unusual for A-V conduction to return in paced patients (see p. 96), there appear to have been very few hemodynamic investigations in such subjects. One patient with obstructive cardiomyopathy was paced via electrodes in the ventricles for diagnostic reasons by Lockhart,[472] who found that alternate sequences of fusion beats and paced beats occurred at identical rates. The right ventricular systolic pressure and the outflow gradient were lower during the paced beats; presumably this effect was due, in part at least, to loss of the normal relationship between atrial and ventricular systole. A similar observation was reported by Slama,[763] who noted in patients with sinus rhythm and artificial pacemakers that the heart beat was less effective, as judged from carotid pulse tracings, whenever fusion beats occurred. An investigation of three of our patients with parasystole due to sinus rhythm and fixed-rate artificial pacemakers [716] demonstrated that at rest it was not possible by means of alterations in the pacing rate to raise the cardiac output above that produced by sinus rhythm. During steady state exercise on a bicycle ergometer the cardiac output fell when the pacemaker rate was increased, and this effect was due, in part at least, to the increasing loss of the atrial transport mechanism as the pacemaker-induced beats became more frequent. In the same investigation one patient was exercised at increasing work loads at each of two fixed pacemaker rates; cardiac output increased linearly with work load in the normal manner, and the patient's performance was virtually identical at the two pacemaker settings.

Spontaneous Synchronization

Segers [676] noted that atrial and ventricular beats might synchronize at the same rate in patients in complete heart block, and the phenomenon has been described in patients with fixed rate artificial pacemakers.[85, 218] This synchronization usually depends upon an increase of the slower rate towards the faster rate and is more likely to occur when the two rates are fairly similar. In the patient reported by Ettinger,[218] the atrial rate increased from its intrinsic level of 60 beats a minute to synchronize with the paced ventricular rate, provided this was not faster than 75 beats per minute. The clinical importance of this type of synchronization is negligible, since the atrial rate will diverge from the paced ventricular rate as soon as the patient increases his activity.

Limits of Atrial-Triggered Pacing

If an atrial tachycardia develops it is obviously undesirable for the ventricle to follow the atrial rate with a 1:1 response. Cordis and Elema-Schönander pacemakers deal with this problem by the introduction of a 2:1 block between atrium and ventricle, when the atrial rate reaches a certain preset value; if necessary, 3:1 and 4:1 blocks are introduced as the atrial rate increases. This approach has proved successful in practice, but its disadvantage is that when the patient exercises the ventricular rate is halved when the atrial rate reaches the limiting value. This results in a fall in cardiac output at a time when an increase would be more appropriate.[116] The upper limit for synchronous pacing with the Elema-Schönander pacemaker is usually set at 150 beats per minute. When the atrial rate exceeds this limit ventricular beats are dropped with increasing frequency, so that the 2:1 block has been slowly introduced by the time the atrial rate has risen by 10 per cent over the limit. Although it is theoretically possible for the ventricular rate to be held at a constant level by dropping ventricular beats as necessary without the introduction of a 2:1 block, the disadvantage of this method is that the ventricular diastolic filling time is not constant, and the maximal rate of ventricular response is achieved by means of a few very rapid ventricular beats followed by a longer pause when the ventricular beat is dropped.

If atrial fibrillation develops, atrial potentials sufficient to trigger the pacemaker occur randomly, and the resultant ventricular rhythm is irregular and complicated by periods of fixed-rate pacing and perhaps also by rapidly changing pacemaker block; atrial-triggered pacemakers are probably contraindicated during atrial fibrillation.[115] In at least one patient treated with an Elema-Schönander pacemaker, stimulation continued at the basic fixed rate when atrial fibrillation developed, but a 2:1 block appeared when the rhythm altered to atrial flutter.[760]

If the atrial potential is inadequate to trigger the pacemaker, or if atrial asystole occurs, all commercially available units automatically stimulate at a fixed rate so that the situation is identical with that produced by fixed-rate ventricular pacing. A somewhat similar situation has been reported to occur temporarily after the insertion of an atrial-triggered pacemaker in which a conduction delay occurred transiently between the atrium and the pick-up electrode ("atrial-pacemaker block").[540] This resulted in an unduly prolonged PR interval for a short time postoperatively and was associated also with complete failure of atrial-triggering for a short time during which the pacemaker stimulated at its fixed preset rate.

Choice of Rate for Fixed-Rate Pacing

The choice of an optimal rate for a fixed-rate direct ventricular pacemaker depends upon the definition of the term "optimal," and there are many criteria which may be used in this respect. Furthermore, the optimal rate is not constant for any given patient but varies with the state of ventricular function and possibly also with the degree of exercise. The choice of rate will often be influenced by factors apart from the hemodynamic response, such as the need for a rapid rate to suppress arrhythmias.[196, 216, 381, 714, 806] In patients with good myocardial function the resting cardiac output is likely to be independent of pacemaker rate, and under these circumstances the slowest ventricular rate at which an adequate output and systemic arterial pressure can be maintained is the most satisfactory choice; it is on these grounds that a subnormal rate is so strongly advocated by Chardack,[125] who considers a rate of 60 beats a minute to be the most satisfactory. Most patients, however, attain their maximal resting cardiac output with pacemaker rates between 70 and 80 beats a minute, and since rates of this order allow moderate levels of exercise, most commercially available units provide stimulation rates within this range.

If the optimal ventricular rate is judged on the basis of changes in the right atrial pressure or on the basis of alterations in the atrial rate, the resulting pacemaker rate will be approximately the same as if the choice had been made on the basis of maximal cardiac output.[712, 846]

There is a case for the increase of pacemaker rate during exercise, but there are very few patients in whom a rate of above 100 beats a minute provides any benefit, and as pacemaker patients are usually in the older age group there seems little point in providing a pacemaker which is designed to allow high levels of exertion.

The choice of pacemaker rate is very rarely influenced by subjective symptoms on the part of the patient, since in general pacemaker patients are unaware of their rate unless the pacemaker is stimulating at the extremes of rate, or unless competition is present between natural and artificial pacemakers. Our experience is in accord with that of Elmqvist,[207] in that most patients cannot decide at which rate to set an adjustable pacemaker. In a few instances patients may prefer a particular pacemaker rate, although in general patients express dislike only of unduly slow or unduly fast rates.

Another method of determining the optimal heart rate is based upon the work of Sjöstrand,[336] who demonstrated that in normal subjects the resting pulse rate in the upright position is related to the total body hemoglobin and to the height of the patient. From a knowledge of these parameters, a theoretical value for the pacemaker rate can be obtained from the normal regression line (Fig. 18), and values calculated by this method are usually of the order of 80 to 90 beats a minute.

Effect on Intracardiac Shunts

We have been unable to trace any reports of hemodynamic investigations in patients with complete heart block and intracardiac shunts treated by artificial pacemakers. In two patients with ventricular septal defects investigated in our laboratory the degree of left to right shunting was unaffected by a change in pacemaker rate over a wide range, while the alterations in sys-

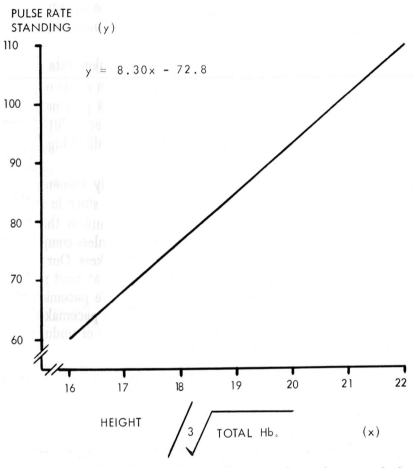

FIGURE 18. Sjöstrand's regression line relating standing pulse rate to body height (cm) and total body hemoglobin (gm) for normal subjects. Based on data published by Sjöstrand.[336] From a knowledge of the height and hemoglobin values a pulse rate value can be deduced which is theoretically optimal for normal subjects.

temic cardiac output and arterial pressures were similar to those already discussed for patients with ventricular pacing.

SUMMARY AND CONCLUSIONS

In patients with complete heart block the cardiac output is low but can be increased to normal by artificial pacing. In patients with good myocardial function, or in normal subjects without heart block, cardiac output is independent of ventricular rate, both at rest and on exercise, apart from a reduction in flow at the extremes of rate. In patients with poor myocardial function the output is rate-dependent, and increases as the pacemaker rate increases. At rapid ventricular rates there is a fall-off in flow in all subjects; this is largely due to the reduction in diastolic filling time, particularly in the absence of a suitably timed atrial systole.

Myocardial oxygen uptake and coronary blood flow increase with ventricular rate even when cardiac output has begun to fall. Angina and acute heart failure can be produced by rapid pacemaker rates when coronary vessels are stenosed.

Systemic and pulmonary artery mean pressures change little when pacing rates are altered within the physiological range; systolic and pulse pressures fall as the ventricular rate is increased. Pressure changes are rapid, and a new steady state is usually achieved within 30 seconds of a change in rate.

Various methods of determining the optimal rate for a fixed-rate pacemaker are discussed, and a new method is described, based on physiological data published in Scandinavia. On exercise patients with fixed ventricular rates can increase their stroke volumes unless myocardial function is very poor. Fixed-rate pacemakers allow moderate activity, and very few patients would benefit from rates over 100 beats per minute.

Atrial-triggered pacing produces both acute and sustained improvements in hemodynamic function at rest and on exercise when compared to fixed-rate pacing.

Chapter 11

SPECIAL CONSIDERATIONS

PACING IN ACUTE MYOCARDIAL INFARCTION

COMPLETE HEART BLOCK developing during an acute myocardial infarction greatly increases mortality, which reaches at least 50 per cent,[186] although in 90 per cent of the survivors the heart block is transient and sinus rhythm returns within two weeks.[186, 413, 658] The long-term mortality among patients who return to sinus rhythm is comparable with that of patients who did not develop complete heart block during their cardiac infarction.[142] All three techniques of short-term pacing described in Chapter 5 have been used successfully in complete heart block associated with cardiac infarction. An external pacemaker with skin electrodes has been recommended by Zoll,[835] and we have also used this method with success on several occasions. The disadvantages of prolonged use of skin electrodes for pacing restrict the use of the method to emergency procedures, but it can well maintain a patient for the period while transvenous endocardial pacing is being set up. Albert [13] particularly recommends the use of percutaneous wires, the second method described on page 53. The third method, pacing endocardially, is particularly well suited should Stokes-Adams attacks develop; [177] a small bipolar endocardial electrode such as the C51 size 5F (U.S.C.I.) is usually chosen for this application, and may be rapidly passed to the apex of the right ventricle from an arm or leg vein. The electrode should be passed under fluoroscopic control (see p. 56), which usually entails that the patient be moved to a catheterization laboratory, but this has caused little difficulty either in our own practice or in that of others.[177, 306, 709] It is possible for electrodes of this type to be passed blind in the ward,[714] but we consider the risks of this technique too high for it to be recomended, particularly in the case of a patient with a recent cardiac infarction. The blind

198

passage of fine insulated wires [308] may be more satisfactory, although the risk of provocation of dangerous arrhythmias as the wire crosses the tricuspid valve may limit the use of this technique also. When the electrode is in position, stimulation is carried out at about 70 beats a minute or at the rate which will suppress multiple ventricular ectopic beats, whichever is the slower, and the patient is returned to the ward for continuous electrocardiographic monitoring. The use of myocardial depressant drugs such as procaine amide may be continued with less risk of severe hypotension than during idioventricular rhythm, and Chardack [125, 128] found procaine amide effective in suppressing ectopic activity after an acute myocardial infarction, although pacing at rates up to 100 beats a minute had not been effective. In the case of the patient reported by Dellman,[177] the institution of right ventricular endocardial pacing was accompanied by an increase in the blood pressure, so that over the next few days it was possible to withdraw vasopressors.

After a variable period of time A-V conduction will return in the majority of cases, and this will usually result in interference between the competing rhythms. This allows the pacemaker stimulus to fall in the vulnerable period of the cardiac cycle, and as the threshold for the provocation of ventricular fibrillation is exceptionally low in the presence of myocardial ischemia (see p. 105) the risk of pacemaker-induced arrhythmias is very high. In two of our own patients, not previously reported, being treated with artificial pacing after acute myocardial infarction, sudden ventricular fibrillation developed shortly after the appearance of competing rhythms, and the same phenomenon has been noted by others.[306, 374] To avoid this risk we now routinely use a pacemaker which stimulates only when no spontaneous ventricular activity has occurred during a preceding adjustable time interval,[426] and similar "on demand" pacemakers have been described from other centers (see p. 96).

There is usually a dramatic improvement in the condition of shocked patients when their slow idioventricular rate is controlled by artificial pacing, and many successful clinical results have been reported.[177, 712, 854] Paulk and Hurst [586] analyzed the records of 1,400 patients who were admitted to hospital with cardiac infarction and found 47 (3.3%) who developed complete heart block. Forty-one of these 47 patients were paced with bipolar electrodes, and 22 survived. Sinus rhythm returned in 17 of these 22 survivors, and an implanted pacemaker was later inserted in three of the five survivors with persistent complete heart block. Nineteen of the 41 patients had a cardiac arrest with resuscitation before pacing started and in this group the mortality was 63 per cent; 22 of the 41 patients had complete block but no major cardiac arrest, and the mortality among these patients was only 31 per cent. These figures compare with those of Cosby,[147] who reported no improvement in mortality figures when patients with acute ischemic block were paced; they found a mortality of 60 per cent in unpaced patients and 62 per cent in 17 paced patients.

In a review of 18 cases Courter [152] found that pacing had been of no benefit; six (39%) of these patients died within 34 days and of nine shocked patients, six (67%) died. More encouraging results were reported by Bruce,[79] who listed 23 patients, with two more in a footnote, who had been treated with artificial pacing for heart block developing during acute myocardial infarction. Twelve of the 25 patients (48%) recovered with sinus rhythm, and a further two recovered but had persistent heart block. Six patients died (23%) and four (16%) required an implanted pacemaker. The authors note that of their own nine patients the overall mortality with pacing was 11 per cent compared with 62 per cent in eight previously reported cases, but the figures are probably too small for statistical significance to be reached. In one case, ventricular fibrillation was provoked during insertion of the electrode.

Harris and Bluestone [305] reported 19 patients who developed complete heart block and one with a very slow nodal rhythm following acute myocardial infarction, who were paced with a transvenous electrode. Nineteen patients returned to sinus rhythm within ten days, and the remaining patient was eventually treated with an implantable pacemaker. Seven patients died; five of these developed intractable heart failure, and at necropsy large areas of infarcted myocardium were found. The last two patients who died had initially returned to sinus rhythm during pacing, but later reverted to complete heart block at 19 and 21 days.

In a review of the literature covering 125 cases paced for cardiac infarction and acute heart block,[868] we found that 60 per cent recovered but 9 per cent remained in block. Artificial pacing probably halves the mortality in patients who do not have a major episode of cardiac arrest.

Our current practice is to rely upon the "on demand" pacemaker after A-V conduction has returned and to leave the electrode *in situ* for a total of at least 21 days. If uninterrupted A-V conduction has then remained stable and the PR interval is within normal limits we remove the electrode, although others [177] have recommended that it remain in the heart for longer.

The position regarding pacing of patients who do not develop block is not yet clear. Results have been very disappointing when bradycardia or asystole occur,[868] but pacing for suppression of arrhythmias may occasionally be indicated [402] (see p. 62).

PAIRED PACING

The technique of paired pacing or paired electrical stimulation of the heart was initially reported in 1963 by Lopez, Edelist and Katz,[476] who showed that the "make" and "break" at each end of a long impulse caused electrical depolarization of the heart of dogs. When the impulse was of critical length the second depolarization occurred at a time when the heart was incapable of contracting mechanically although it could still respond electrically, and as a result the refractory period was prolonged and the effective ventricular rate reduced. The effect can equally well be produced by pairs of short electrical impulses separated by a critical interval. This interval varies according to the heart rate and the level of sympathetic tone, but is of the order of 150-200 milliseconds in dogs and about 300 milliseconds in human subjects. The most satisfactory way in which the interval between the two pulses can be determined is by continual monitoring of ventricular pressure; if the interval is too long both stimuli will result in ventricular contractions, while if the interval is too short the second stimulus will be applied during the absolute refractory period and will have no effect. When the interval is approximately correct, the down slope of the ventricular pressure trace is distorted by the extremely premature beat induced by the second stimulus, and adjustment of the delay between the two stimuli will result in the almost total disappearance of this second pressure response. Complete disappearance of the second pressure response is usually referred to as "fusion" and is considerably easier to achieve in the dog than in human subjects. When fusion or near-fusion has been attained an electrocardiogram will show two electrical depolarizations for each systolic pressure peak so that there are two electrical events occurring for each mechanical event (Fig. 19). Once fusion has been achieved the heart is controlled by the paired stimulator and the rate may be increased or decreased at will within wide limits, although the interval

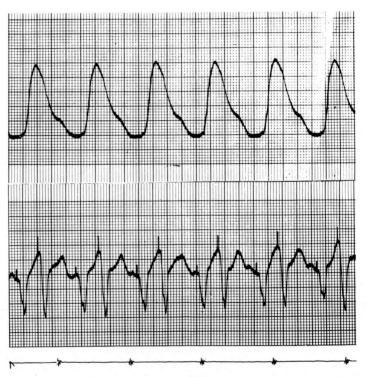

FIGURE 19. Paired pacing in a woman of 53 with mitral valve disease and intractable heart failure.

Upper record: right ventricular pressure; rate 73 beats per minute. Note the small pressure event distorting the downslope.

Lower record: ECG showing two stimuli and two depolarizations for each mechanical contraction.

between the two pulses may need to be adjusted to maintain fusion at different rates. Paired stimulation has two independent effects, the effect on heart rate and a potentiation effect on muscle contraction.

Effect on Rate

Provided the delay between the two stimuli is correct, the heart rate can be slowed below its spontaneous rhythm by paired pacing of the ventricle so that many arrhythmias can be controlled; the effects of this technique are discussed later (see p. 213).

Potentiation

During paired stimulation of the ventricles the effective ventricular contraction is augmented by comparison with ventricular contraction during single pacing and usually also by comparison with spontaneously occurring beats. This effect is independent of the stimulating rate and is clearly related to the well-known postextrasystolic potentiation [67, 69, 131] in which the first contraction following an extrasystole takes place at an increased rate and develops an increased maximal tension; the effect decays over the next few contractions until the control levels are reached. The extent of the potentiation is related to the prematurity of the extrasystole.[325, 326] Postextrasystolic potentiation can also be demonstrated in the isovolumic ventricle [694] and in isolated papillary muscle.[867] During maintained paired stimulation of the ventricles every effective contraction is a postextrasystolic beat, since it follows the premature ineffective depolarization induced by the second stimulus of the preceding pair; the resulting maintained potentiation has been called "electro-augmentation" by Ross and his co-workers at Bethesda.[634] The potentiation produced by repetitive extrasystoles occurring in each cardiac cycle, as in paired pacing, is considerably greater than that following a single extrasystole, and when stimulation is interrupted the potentiation does not disappear immediately but declines during the next few beats.[325] A further factor of importance in determining the degree of potentiation is the preceding state of myocardial contractility; postextrasystolic potentiation is more marked when myocardial

function is poor.[702] Although the effects of electro-augmentation
and of changes in rate can be clearly distinguished they may
occur together during experimental and clinical application of
paired pacing so that the actual effect on ventricular performance
is influenced by potentiation and by alteration in the diastolic
filling time. Electro-augmentation is not increased when a third
electrical stimulus is added.[250, 506]

Coupled Pacing

During paired pacing, the first impulse causes a ventricular
contraction and the second impulse results in the premature electrical depolarization. Application of a single electrical stimulus
at the correct interval following the R wave of a spontaneous
ventricular contraction will result in a similar electrical depolarization without mechanical contraction, and this technique is
referred to as "coupled pacing."[69, 133] During coupled pacing the
two depolarizations result in prolongation of the refractory period
of the ventricle so that the next atrial impulse arrives during the
refractory phase and does not result in a ventricular contraction;
there is thus an immediate halving of the ventricular rate as
coupled pacing becomes effective. The major differences between
paired and coupled pacing are that with the latter technique
the heart rate is not under the control of the stimulator and that
the normal time relationships between atrial and ventricular contractions are maintained. Frommer [250] has noted that there is a
surprising lack of reflex change in heart rate following the onset
of coupled pacing so that the reduction in ventricular rate is
maintained. Since each ventricular contraction is a postextrasystolic beat during coupled pacing, electro-augmentation occurs in
the same manner as during paired pacing.

Paired Pacing of the Atrium

During paired or coupled pacing the electrical impulses are
usually applied to the ventricle, but in the presence of normal
A-V conduction the techniques can also be applied to stimulation
of the atrium. Under these circumstances the effects on the
atrium are of less importance than the resulting ventricular consequences. The atrial rate can be slowed with a resulting slowing

of the ventricular rate but the second of each pair of atrial depolarizations fails to pass through the A-V node since this is still
refractory from the first impulse. As a result the slowing of the
ventricular rate is unaccompanied by electro-augmentation. This
mechanism of an electrical 2:1 A-V block can be demonstrated
both in animals and in human subjects.[172, 388, 470] The atrial contribution to ventricular filling is maintained during paired pacing
of the atrium.

Risk of Ventricular Fibrillation

The second stimulus of each pair must be applied at or close
to the vulnerable period in the cardiac cycle so that the risk of
provocation of ventricular fibrillation in a patient whose fibrillation threshold is low must always be present. The safety factor
between the threshold currents needed for coupled pacing and
for the provocation of ventricular fibrillation in dogs was studied
by Frommer,[250] who found that the lowest current producing
ventricular fibrillation was at least 30 times the threshold for pacing and similar factors were obtained on patients also. In a comparison between coupled pacing and paired pacing he found
that in three dogs there was no difference, but in four other dogs
coupled pacing was significantly safer than paired pacing. He
noted that paired stimulation produced brief runs of ventricular
arrhythmias much more frequently than coupled pacing, especially when there was an incomplete atrioventricular block. As
Frommer points out, the safety factor may be considerably
influenced by hypoxia, electrolyte disorders, drugs and other
factors; and other workers in this field have also emphasized the
inherent dangers of paired stimulation.[70] The actual development
of ventricular fibrillation during paired pacing in anesthetized
dogs has been reported by Castle and Briggs,[114] and the development of this arrhythmia in patients has been noted both in our
own experience [614] and that of others.[388]

The period of takeover of the ventricular rhythm by the paired
stimulator is associated with an unusually high risk of ventricular
fibrillation, since the threshold stimulus intensity and the correct
interval between the impulses is initially unknown. For normal
pacing with single impulses the stimulator rate must be faster

than the heart rate, but if the rate of a paired pulse stimulator is increased to above the spontaneous ventricular rate and takeover is then attempted, it is possible that the interval between the paired impulses will be too long so that the ventricle responds individually to each of the stimuli. As a result, the ventricle will be driven at more than twice its preceding rate. The heart may then develop ventricular fibrillation before the interval between the impulses can be shortened for fusion to occur, and we are aware of at least one patient in whom ventricular fibrillation was provoked by this mechanism. This risk is avoided by a method of takeover which is widely used by most groups working with this technique, including our own, in which the paired stimulator rate is set to slightly above half the heart's spontaneous rate and the interval between the two pulses is deliberately made too long for fusion to occur. The stimulus strength is then slowly increased until the heart responds to every stimulus at which point it will be overdriven at slightly above its preceding spontaneous rate. The interval between the two stimuli is then progressively reduced until fusion occurs, at which point the mechanical heart rate will suddenly halve and electro-augmentation will be produced. The development of fusion can best be monitored from the continuous display of a ventricular pressure trace, and initial reports of paired pacing stress the importance of complete fusion, but Chardack [132] has pointed out that accurate timing of the ineffective extrasystole is not as critical as had been thought previously. He showed that most of the benefits of paired stimulation could be obtained when the second impulse of each pair was delayed by as much as 100 milliseconds from its optimal position and that monitoring of the ventricular pressure, although desirable, was not essential. For this technique to be used the interval between the two stimuli is decreased to the minimum which still results in two electrical depolarizations as judged from the ECG, and the interval is then increased by about 30 milliseconds.[129]

Results of Animal Investigations

Since the initial reports of Lopez,[476] many other reports have demonstrated that in dogs the heart rate could be slowed by paired pacing to beneath its spontaneous rate whether the dog was in sinus rhythm or an abnormal rhythm was present. Control of ventricular rate could be achieved during spontaneous or artificially induced tachycardia whether of ventricular or supraventricular origin,[67, 131, 477] and even ventricular arrhythmias induced by toxic doses of Ouabaine can be controlled by paired electrical stimulation;[251] our own observations are in keeping with these findings,[614] and in common with other groups we found that the maximum slowing of effective ventricular rate which can be achieved with this technique is about 45 per cent.

Electro-augmentation has been demonstrated by an increase in the contractile force of the myocardium,[67, 131] by an increase in peak systolic blood pressure[67, 131, 388, 614] and by an increase in the rate of contraction of the ventricular muscle with a resulting increase in the rate of rise of intraventricular pressure (dp/dt).[131, 614, 634] The potentiation effect continues for as long as paired stimulation is maintained, apparently without producing permanent damage to the ventricular muscle.

This potentiation is accompanied by an increase in the myocardial oxygen consumption. Sarnoff[651] found a mean increase of 40 per cent in myocardial oxygen uptake during coupled pacing when the effective ventricular rate, mean aortic pressure and stroke volume were held constant, and Ross[634] found paired stimulation produced an average increase of 35 per cent under similar conditions. Chardack[132] found an increase of about 70 per cent in myocardial oxygen consumption during paired pacing at an identical rate to the control value and showed that there was little difference in the extra energy consumption whether fusion of the premature extrasystole was achieved or not. Although the oxygen uptake of the heart is increased per beat by paired pacing, the oxygen uptake per minute can be maintained at control values if the heart rate is slowed to about 60 per cent of its original value.[132] If a third stimulus is added so that three electrical depolarizations occur for every ventricular contraction, the myocardial oxygen uptake is increased even more than during paired stimulation.[506]

The coronary blood flow increases during paired stimulation at the control rate, but the percentage increase in flow is less than the increase in myocardial oxygen uptake.[132, 172, 634] Katz[388] found that the alterations in coronary flow roughly paralleled the oxygen consumption of the heart.

The effect of paired stimulation on dogs following ligation of the major branch of the left coronary artery have been studied by Singer,[702] who found that ventricular tachycardia and fibrillation developed when the technique was undertaken soon after ligation. Ninety minutes after coronary artery ligation, paired pacing did not initiate ventricular fibrillation, and animals studied a week later responded in a manner very similar to that of normals. The authors noted that abrupt cessation of paired stimulation in dogs following coronary artery ligation sometimes produced a marked fall in systemic blood pressure, and although this effect occurs occasionally in normal animals, recovery was delayed well beyond normal in the animals with ischemic myocardium; in one instance only they noted that there was also a sudden fall in cardiac output at cessation of paired pacing and they recommend that gradual weaning of the animal from the paired stimulator should be carried out. This may be achieved if necessary by a technique described by Hoffman[325] in which the second impulse of the pair is dropped initially from every other cycle and subsequently more frequently until a slow reduction of potentiation has occurred and the heart is being driven by single pacing only.

The marked potentiation effect produced by paired stimulation suggests that the technique might be valuable in the treatment of heart failure, and this field has been investigated in dogs by several workers. Hoffman[325] induced acute failure in dogs by partial constriction of the pulmonary artery and administration of beta-adrenergic blocking drugs. The resulting changes were of sufficient magnitude to lead to death in all control animals, but paired stimulation led to a dramatic improvement in that the heart size decreased, the end-diastolic pressure fell, and both right and left ventricular systolic pressures increased; these improvements were maintained for the duration of the period of paired stimulation, and if the pulmonary artery constriction was removed and no further beta-adrenergic blockade performed, the circulation could be maintained long enough for the animal to survive. They also noted that pulmonary edema rapidly disappeared after the onset of paired stimulation and that the circulation could be maintained in animals who had been successfully defibrillated after ventricular fibrillation but in whom there was little mechanical function of the heart. Heart failure in dogs was also produced experimentally by Kerth and Kelly,[396] whose technique combined constriction of the aorta with the administration of beta-adrenergic blocking drugs. They were able to demonstrate that paired pacing led to an increase in left ventricular systolic and aortic pressures but decreased the left ventricular end-diastolic pressure and that these effects were continued throughout the period of paired pacing. Similar observations were made by Tatooles and Braunwald,[754] who studied dogs with complete heart block with and without myocardial failure induced by partial excision of the tricuspid valve; they demonstrated that paired stimulation increased myocardial contractile force, peak left ventricular pressure, dp/dt and peak aortic flow, and that these changes were greater in animals with cardiac failure. The improvement in left ventricular performance produced by paired pacing during acute cardiac failure has also been documented by Cranefield [154] and in our own investigations.[614]

The cardiac output remains almost unchanged during paired pacing unless it was low initially, in which case there is often a dramatic increase. This increase in flow occurs whether the technique is being untilized to slow a tachycardia [131, 614] or to treat acute heart failure.[396] The unchanged cardiac output during paired stimulation of relatively normal dogs' hearts was confirmed by Lister,[471] who demonstrated the effect both during short-term experiments and over a period of five days in a dog with an implanted stimulator. The special Medtronic unit which was implanted in this dog maintained paired stimulation continuously over the five-day period with a mechanical ventricular rate of 84 a minute; hemodynamic measurements during this time showed a fall in the right ventricular pressure and the systolic aortic pressure, although the mean aortic pressure remained unchanged and the right ventricular end-diastolic pressure increased. After the period of paired pacing, the pacemaker was removed at a second thoracotomy and the animal allowed to recover.

The effect of paired pacing on potassium ion loss from the myocardium has ben studied on the cat heart by Mansfield and McDonald,[495] who showed that paired pacing resulted in rather more potassium loss and a higher myocardial oxygen uptake than single pacing at twice the control rate. Potassium loss during coupled pacing was also reported by Sarnoff,[651] who found that the amount of potassium lost was comparable to the loss following a strongly inotropic dose of acetyl strophanthidin. Meijler and Durrer,[506] working with the perfused isolated rat heart, investigated the role of calcium and were able to show that potentiation phenomena were entirely abolished during high calcium perfusion, possibly because the calcium itself had already resulted in maximum possible potentiation.

Cessation of paired or coupled pacing occasionally results in an acute fall of the systolic ventricular and arterial pressures. Ross [634] found this period of reduced ventricular performance occurred fairly frequently and was characterized by elevation of the left ventricular end-diastolic pressure and a reduction in ventricular dp/dt, ejection rate and stroke power. The depression could be produced by periods of paired stimulation as short as 30 seconds, and its duration and severity increased following longer periods of paired stimulation; in addition, the depression was more marked when myocardial performance had initially been poor before paired pacing. These findings were emphasized by Singer, Galst and Wagner,[702] who found transient falls of about 50 per cent in systemic blood pressure at the termination of paired stimulation in two experiments, and minor elevations in right ventricular end-diastolic pressure occurred in seven investigations with relatively normal dog hearts. Cessation of paired pacing in their dogs with coronary artery ligation resulted in more dramatic and sustained falls in systemic blood pressure, the most pronounced of which was from 125/84 to 60/40 with restoration to a systolic level of 100 mmHg taking seven minutes.

Investigations on Human Subjects

Preliminary reports by Chardack [131] and by Braunwald [67] indicated that similar results to those found in animal experiments might be expected in human subjects, although it soon became apparent that fusion of the premature extrasystole with the main ventricular contraction was very much more difficult to achieve in man. Thirteen patients were studied during the course of cardiac catheterization by Braunwald,[69, 70] who was able to show that electro-augmentation occurred in man and could be maintained for periods of several hours, but that despite the increase in several parameters of ventricular performance, there was little hemodynamic benefit; these results are similar to the findings in dogs in whom the cardiac output was not compromised before the onset of paired stimulation. The same authors studied other patients one to three days following cardiac operations with similar results to those found during catheterization. During these investigations there were no episodes of persistent arrhythmias, and upon discontinuation of the paired stimuli there was no evidence of depression of myocardial contractility. Little change occurred in the cardiac output of any of these patients, including four who were in heart failure at the time of the study, although ventricular end-diastolic pressures fell, particularly when they had previously been elevated. Paired pacing in one patient at open-heart surgery for rheumatic mitral heart valve disease was reported by Lister;[471] the patient was in severe congestive heart failure and on long-term digitalis therapy. Poor fusion was obtained, and only slight augmentation of right ventricular and aortic pressures could be demonstrated. Paired stimulation has also been used clinically by a modification of the radio frequency pacemaker used by Glenn;[19] ventricular rate was slowed and electro-augmentation demonstrated. No ventricular arrhythmias were provoked. Meijler and Durrer[506] used paired stimulation via a right ventricular endocardial electrode in one patient with mitral incompetence. The electro-augmentation diminished the intensity of the pansystolic murmur, and they concluded that regurgitation might have been due to inefficiently contracting papillary muscle. In one patient with rheumatic heart disease studied in our laboratory (not previously reported), paired pacing via a right ventricular endocardial electrode led to considerable deterioration in the hemodynamic state, with a fall in cardiac output and an increase in PC wedge pressure. There was evidence of increased mitral regurgitation during the period of paired stimulation.

Clinical Application

Paired stimulation has also been applied as a therapeutic measure to other patients in whom conventional therapy has failed.
Katz [388] reported the use of paired stimulation of the ventricle in
one patient with severe congestive cardiac failure. The cardiac
output increased from 1.3 liters/min to 2.3 liters/min as the effective ventricular rate was slowed from 100 beats per minute to
70 beats per minute; this represents an increase in stroke volume
of approximately two and one-half times. Ventricular fibrillation
developed as a complication but was successfully treated by countershock. Braunwald [65] has been able to maintain adequate circulation in patients in whom great difficulty was being experienced in terminating cardiopulmonary bypass following surgery,
and has found that paired stimulation for several hours has occasionally resulted in considerable improvement in myocardial
performance. Meijler and Durrer [506] report an attempt to improve
severe congestive failure in one patient by paired pacing which
was continued without significant benefit for 12 days; although
both right and left ventricular dp/dt increased, the authors felt
that this resulted in deterioration of tricuspid and possibly also
of mitral incompetence. Langendorf and Pick [415] report the case
of an 80-year-old female patient with recent myocardial infarction causing complete A-V dissociation and Stokes-Adams attacks;
pacing with single stimuli through an endocardial electrode was
unsatisfactory because of a low blood pressure, and although
paired pacing resulted in satisfactory ventricular capture there
was no improvement in the clinical state and the patient died.
Six human cases were reported by Kerth and Kelly.[396] They found
no change in the normal cardiac output of one patient with complete heart block during single or paired pacing, although the
right ventricular end-diastolic pressure dropped from 10 mmHg
to 5 mmHg during paired stimulation. A second patient, also with
complete heart block, responded to every impulse from the paired
stimulator, and the resulting ventricular tachycardia had to be
controlled by countershock. When fusion was poor, the small ventricular contraction provoked by the second stimulus prevented
adequate filling, and the patient experienced angina. Of the remaining four patients two were moribund following cardiac arrest,

and paired stimulation did not produce enough improvement for prolonged survival, and two were successfully paced for short periods in the operating room before institution of cardiopulmonary bypass.

Our own experience of paired pacing as a therapeutic measure includes four patients in whom conventional therapy had failed to control dangerous arrhythmias.[614] In one patient, ventricular fibrillation rapidly followed the onset of attempted paired stimulation and was successfully reverted by countershock; in another patient with a recent myocardial infarction, paired pacing resulted in repetitive ventricular responses and was abandoned. In the remaining two patients, satisfactory ventricular control was achieved and paired pacing was continued without incident for a considerable time. In one patient in intractable heart failure associated with an acute septal perforation following myocardial infarction, paired pacing was maintained for 24 hours. The degree of left to right shunt was unaltered by paired pacing, and we were unable to demonstrate electro-augmentation, while there were no beneficial effects on the systemic arteriovenous oxygen difference nor on the pulmonary or aortic arterial pressures; single pacing of the ventricle at a faster rate than the spontaneous rhythm produced deterioration although the degree of left to right shunt did not change. Fusion was extremely difficult to achieve in this patient, and occasionally each stimulus of the pair produced sufficient ventricular contraction for the VSD murmur to become audible. As there was no clinical or hemodynamic evidence of benefit the technique was abandoned. The last patient developed a rapid ventricular rate following aortic valve surgery under cardiopulmonary bypass, and the arrhythmia was complicated by sinus tachycardia, atrial fibrillation, ventricular tachycardia and intermittent A-V dissociation; paired stimulation through wires attached to the ventricle during his operation was carried out continuously for 48 hours with both clinical and hemodynamic benefit. The pulmonary artery oxygen saturation increased from 34 per cent to 56 per cent, and the effective ventricular rate was slowed by over 30 per cent. In the last two patients, there was no evidence of ventricular arrhythmias produced by paired pacing.

Paired stimulation has also been applied safely for a period of three hours by Stock [735] to a patient who experienced an acute myocardial infarction with intractable shock five days previously. No ventricular arrhythmias developed in this patient, and there was no fall in blood pressure upon cessation of paired pacing, but no details of clinical results are given. In view of the findings in animal experiments that the myocardial oxygen uptake is increased out of proportion to the increase in coronary flow and to an extent greatly surpassing gain in contractility,[506] and the known risk of provocation of ventricular fibrillation, particularly in the presence of myocardial anoxia (see p. 107) it seems that paired pacing should not be applied in patients with ischemic heart disease unless all conventional therapy has failed.

A successful clinical extension of the technique of paired pacing has been reported by Bayley.[26] A 43-year-old man who presented with chest pain developed runs of ventricular tachycardia at 200 beats per minute, which could not be controlled by drugs. Paired stimulation of the ventricle with an endocardial electrode enabled a ventricular rate of 106 beats per minute to be maintained for 24 days, during which the patient carried a pocket-sized paired stimulator. Control of the ventricular rate was maintained with difficulty, and the patient needed medical treatment for congestive failure so the stimulator was modified to provide triple pulses, and this enabled the ventricular rate to be controlled at 70 beats per minute for three days. He then reverted to sinus rhythm and the pacemaking electrode was removed 14 days later. Although his electrocardiogram was compatible with an anterior myocardial infarction, no adverse effects were noted in this patient during paired or triple stimulation. It seems possible that further pulses could be added as necessary to cause recurrent electrical depolarization without mechanical contraction.

The possibility of control of sinus tachycardia in human subjects by coupled or paired stimulation of the atrium was suggested by Langendorf and Pick,[415] who were able to apply the method successfully in a 24-year-old patient with mitral stenosis. By pacing the right atrium with an endocardial electrode, they slowed the ventricular rate from its control value of 68 beats per minute to 43 beats per minute, and they point out that this method of ventricular slowing would avoid the increased oxygen consumption of the ventricular myocardium associated with paired pacing of the ventricle. Paired stimulation of the atrium was also used by Lister [470] to control the ventricular rate in seven patients who were all being treated with digitalis and quinidine. The stimuli were applied by means of endocardial electrodes, and when the delay between the pairs of stimuli was 295 to 315 milliseconds, every second atrial depolarization was blocked at the A-V node and ventricular slowing by 20 to 45 per cent was achieved. No arrhythmias were provoked by this maneuver, and there were no significant changes in cardiac index or mean arterial pressures.

Present Position of Paired Stimulation

Paired stimulation provides probably the most potent inotropic intervention known. In laboratory animals the technique can be used to slow tachycardias, whatever their etiology, and to reverse acute heart failure; when the cardiac output is initially compromised, paired stimulation results in an increase, but if the cardiac output is relatively normal, there is no change. Myocardial contractility increases greatly, and there is an increase in coronary blood flow. The increase in myocardial oxygen consumption is proportionally greater than the increase in coronary flow or the improvement in contractility.

The clinical application of paired stimulation is still in the early stages. It seems reasonable for the technique to be used in an attempt to control intractable arrhythmias, and in many instances the method of choice appears to be paired stimulation of the atrium by means of a bipolar electrode; if the arrhythmia is of ventricular origin or if atrial fibrillation is present, the electrode should be positioned within the right ventricle. The inotropic effect of paired ventricular stimulation, may be useful in the short-term management of patients with normal coronary arteries but with myocardial function which is temporarily depressed, as for example following prolonged bypass for cardiac surgery. The increased myocardial oxygen uptake during paired stimulation indicates that ischemic heart disease is a relative contraindication; the technique should be used only when conventional therapy has failed to control a deteriorating situation. Even when paired stimulation is being applied for its inotropic effect the opportunity should be taken to slow the ventricular rate as much as possible, with the object of preventing the myocardial oxygen uptake per minute from exceeding the capabilities of the coronary blood flow to supply oxygen. Paired stimulation of the ventricle is particularly hazardous in the type of patients in whom the indications for its use are strongest, and the risks of ventricular fibrillation must be weighed carefully against any possible benefit. Although coupled pacing is probably slightly safer, it seems doubtful if the difference will be clinically significant.

BIOLOGIC ENERGY FOR PACING

The possibility of deriving electric power for an artificial pacemaker directly from the body itself is extremely attractive, and has been approached in several ways. One possibility is to use the beating of the heart itself as a power source, and Long [474] states that the power output of a beating heart is about 8 w for a man, 12 w for a cow and 0.6 w for a dog. It is theoretically possible for the mechanical action of the heart to be converted to electrical power in a variety of ways. A small magnet could be attached to the heart in such a manner that its movement induced an electric current in a suitably placed coil, or a piezoelectric crystal could be distorted by each heart beat. Such systems could theoretically deliver several milliwatts and an accelerometer made experimentally by Long actually produced 1 mw.

Piezoelectric Methods

The production of electrical power by distortion of piezoelectric crystals forms the basis of experiments carried out at several centers. Workers from the group at Newark Beth Israel Hospital in New Jersey [538, 578, 842] have described two distinct applications of this method. The first technique makes use of the respiratory movements of the diaphragm to wind a watch-like mechanism which produces rhythmic striking of a set of piezoelectric crystals. This apparatus, developed by Van Haaften of the Bulova Watch Company, has already paced a dog's heart satisfactorily when hand wound, but still requires considerable further development before implantation and satisfactory operation by the diaphragm. The impulse produced was 1.6 milliseconds duration and had an amplitude of 0.7 to 1.0 v; the apparatus drove the dog's heart at 80 beats per minute via an intracardiac bipolar electrode. The advantages of this approach are that irregularity of diaphragmatic movement will not affect pacing, and that the electrical output from the stimulus is sufficient to stimulate the heart with only an extremely simple electronic circuit intervening. The authors recognize that diaphragmatic movement may not be sufficient to maintain the mainspring fully wound during sleep and that patients with pulmonary emphysema or pleurisy may also have inadequate diaphragmatic movement; they suggest that the winding lever could perhaps be adapted to use the movement of the heart itself. The second technique investigated by this group involves the arrangement of about ten thin crystals around the aorta in such a way that the arterial pulsation produced movement of all the crystals; the resulting electrical output was usually about 12 v and was used to drive an artificial pacemaker. This pacemaker produced an impulse of 1.6 milliseconds duration with an amplitude of 0.75 to 1.0 v, and in experimental tests on dogs successful pacing was achieved when the crystals were placed around either a simulated or an actual aorta.[79]

Considerable success with an implantable pacemaker driven by the heart has been achieved by Enger, Kennedy and Michel at Cleveland,[209] who have used their most recent unit in five dogs. This pacemaker is in the form of a disc 4.3 cm in diameter. The disc weighs 10 gm. Piezoelectric crystals are distorted by left ventricular contractions, and the resulting electrical energy is stored in a tantalum capacitor; pacing impulses from a pulse generator fed from this capacitor are delivered to the ventricle via bipolar implanted electrodes. Idioventricular contractions have proved sufficient to drive this pacemaker which then slowly increased the ventricular rate to a final preset level of 120 beats a minute. The storage capacity of the unit is adequate to drive the heart for several beats, and the pacemaker can be retriggered by external massage of the chest if pacing ceases.

Temperature Methods

Another approach to the problem of obtaining electrical energy from the body is to use thermocouples situated in hot and cold areas. This possibility has been examined in several centers,[94] but no satisfactory unit has yet been produced. Parsonnet[572] was unable to find consistent hot and cold spots in the body and found the method impracticable.

Direct Electrical Methods

Since the tissue fluids behave as an electrolyte, there will be a potential difference between two dissimilar metals implanted in the body, or between one metal electrode and an inert electrode. Experiments carried out in Canada by the National Research Council[341] have resulted in the development of small stimulators powered from dissimilar electrodes on moist skin; early models of these units delivered 2.5 μj. The technique has also been studied elsewhere, and a preliminary report by Satinsky[652] describes the successful application of this method in ten dogs and two patients. A potential difference of 0.5 to 0.6 v between implanted electrodes of platinum black and stainless steel was converted to a stimulus of 1.5 v applied directly to the heart. The impulse duration was two milliseconds and the energy ten μj.

(PACING TO CONTROL BLOOD PRESSURE DURING CEREBRAL SURGERY)

Small[706] of Birmingham, England, has in twelve patients used rapid endocardial pacing to reduce bleeding for a few crucial minutes during brain surgery, particularly for aneurysms. By pacing at rates up to 200 impulses a minute the systolic pressure may be temporarily held at about 25 mmHg. In nine patients, ventricular fibrillation occurred, but sinus rhythm was readily established by DC defibrillation. The operations were carried out at 31 to 32 C. No morbidity or mortality resulted from the maneuver, which greatly facilitated surgical hemostasis by temporarily reducing bleeding.

EXPERIMENTAL WORK ON THE RELIEF OF BLOCK WITHOUT ELECTRICAL PACEMAKERS

Rylant[643] showed that a sino-atrial node, transplanted as a free graft to the right atrium of the same animal, could control the heart rhythm and that such a transplant to the atrium of another animal of the same or different species controlled the rhythm for 10 to 30 days before it was absorbed. The graft took over from the atrioventricular node six hours to five days after grafting. Most of the work was done in dogs, but the graft functioned for a longer period in goats, perhaps because these animals were more closely related; it functioned indefinitely in animals of the same litter. Ernst,[213, 214] working with dogs, transplanted the sino-auricular node to the ventricle, preserving the nutrient artery in the form of a pedicle. He found that the transplanted node would not control the ventricle until a period of more than a month had elapsed, but after two months he obtained equivocal ECG evidence and some histological evidence of viability of the node. In one group of dogs he did not create block until a second operation two months after the transplant; these dogs then showed a nodal rhythm, and this ceased on excising the transplanted node. A second group in which he created block at the time of transplant, using an implanted artificial pacemaker to control the heart rate prior to a second operation was disappointing. Of the five dogs surviving to the second operation the three that were in sinus rhythm continued in this rhythm after destruction of the transplanted node.

Starzl [728] attempted a more critical experiment in dogs, using Ernst's transplantation technique. Since it is well known that surgically created block is often transitory, he created block at an initial operation and transplanted the node only in those dogs in which the block persisted for two to nine weeks. The nine dogs who survived the transplant operation were observed for 11 to 97 days (average 65 days); in none of them was there at any time ECG evidence of the transplanted node controlling the ventricle. Albert [881] had similar results with pedicled graft experiments. Papadopoulos [567] has attempted to bridge the atrium to the ventricle with a portion of the phrenic nerve split longitudinally. At an initial operation the nerve was threaded through the atrium and then into the ventricular wall, block being created at the same operation. He claims that in the 12 dogs in which this operation was performed, normal conduction returned on the 14th to 18th postoperative day. No explanation is given as to how the phrenic nerve produced a delay of an apparently normal PR interval.

Fifteen days after the return of normal conduction the bridging nerve was cut, and the authors claim that block resulted immediately in each case.

Folkman [231, 232, 233] has approached the problem in an entirely different manner. He showed that in dogs with surgically established block of at least a month's duration it was possible to speed the heart by transplanting a pedicle graft of thyroid to the ventricle, thus creating a localized area of hyperthyroid myocardium. This resulted in an increased heart rate starting 8 to 12 hours after operation and lasting up to ten days, at which stage he showed that the transplanted thyroid tissue was still viable. He then showed that the introduction of tablets of tri-idiothyronine into the myocardium had the same effect starting in 8 to 12 hours, but the hormone was expended in 30 hours. His next stage was to use slow-release pellets of his own design, consisting of small silicone rubber containers with the hormone enclosed. These were consistently effective for four or five days and thereafter only intermittently so. This intermittent effect, which lasted several months, eventually gave way to the idioventricular rhythm. The pellet, if moved to a new area of myocardium, became active again, so demonstrating that it continued to release hormone. He produced some experimental evidence suggesting that the failure to sustain its pacemaker action was not the fibrotic reaction around the pellet but rather that new blood vessels in the vicinity carried the drug away, preventing a sufficient concentration being built up. The period of effective action could be prolonged by an iontophoretic technique driving the hormone into the myocardium electrically. Among the many substances which he tried in place of tri-idiothyronine, the only active compounds were isoproterenol, ethylene diamine tetra-acetic acid, and digotoxin.

SUMMARY AND CONCLUSIONS

Patients who develop complete heart block during the course of a myocardial infarction have a poor prognosis and should be treated by artificial pacing; the mortality is probably halved, except in the group who develop major cardiac arrest, when pacing does not improve the prognosis. The position with regard to patients who do not develop block is not yet clear, but it is possible that pacing may be indicated occasionally to suppress arrhythmias.

Paired pacing has proved a useful laboratory technique but is disappointing clinically. Tachycardias of many different etiologies can be controlled, but there is considerable risk of provocation of ventricular fibrillation. When cardiac output is low it can be increased by paired pacing, but in most instances there is little evidence of hemodynamic improvement.

The application of biologic energy for pacing is still in the experimental stage, but several successful pacemakers have been used in dogs. Most such units depend upon distortion of piezoelectric crystals, but the direct use of the tissue fluid as a battery electrolyte with the development of a potential different between two dissimilar metals is also being investigated.

Attempts to transplant the sino-atrial node to the ventricle, or to produce a neural A-V bridge have not yet progressed to the stage of clinical application.

REFERENCES

1. ABELSON, D. S., SAMET, P., RAND, G., MORACA, J. (1961): Endocardial pacemaking and insertion of a permanent internal cardiac pacemaker. *New Eng. J. Med.*, **265**:792.
2. ABER, C. P., JONES, E. W. (1960): Complete heart block treated with corticotrophin and corticosteroid. *Brit. Heart J.*, **22**:723.
3. ABER, C. P., JONES, E. W. (1965): Corticotrophin and corticosteroids in the management of acute and chronic heart block. *Brit. Heart J.*, **27**:916.
4. ABLAZA, S. G. G., BLANCO, G., MARANHAO, V., GOLDBERG, H. (1965): Total replacement of aortic valve in a patient with internal pacemaker. *Arch. Surg. (Chicago)*, **90**:694.
5. ABRAMS, L. D. (1965): Experience with the inductively-coupled cardiac pacemakers. *Resuscitation & Cardiac Pacing* (Proc. of Conference, Glasgow, March, 1964). London, Cassell, p. 202.
6. ABRAMS, L. D. (1965): Problems associated with emergencies arising in cardiac action during and after cardiac surgery. *Resuscitation & Cardiac Pacing* (Proc. of Conference, Glasgow, March, 1964). London, Cassell, p. 250.
7. ABRAMS, L. D. (1965): *Communication to British Cardiac Society* (April, 1965).
8. ABRAMS, L. D., HUDSON, W. A., LIGHTWOOD, R. (1960): A surgical approach to the management of heart block using an inductive coupled artificial cardiac pacemaker. *Lancet*, 1:1372.
9. ABRAMS, L. D., NORMAN, J. C. (1964): Experience with inductive coupled cardiac pacemakers. *Ann. N. Y. Acad. Sci.*, **111**:1030.
10. ADAMS, R. (1827): Cases of diseases of the heart. *Dublin Hosp. Rep.*, 4:353.
11. A.G.R.E.E. *Report* (June, 1957). Reliability of military electronic equipment. Washington, U.S. Government Printing Office.
12. ALBERT, H. M., GLASS, B. A., ANDONIE, J. A., CRANOR, K. C. (1962): Pacemaker failure in complete heart block. *Circ. Res.*, **10**:295.
13. ALBERT, H. M., GLASS, B. A., LEVY, L. (1965): Therapy of complete atrioventricular block complicating recent myocardial infarction. *Dis. Chest*, **48**:561.
14. ALBERT, H. M., GLASS, B. A., PITTMAN, B., ROBICHAUX, P. (1964): Cardiac stimulation threshold: chronic study. *Ann. N. Y. Acad. Sci.*, **111**:889.
15. ALDINI, G. (1819): *General Views on the Application of Galvanism to Medical Purposes Principally in Cases of Suspended Animation.* London, J. Callow, p. 96.
16. ALDRIDGE, H. E., KAHN, O. (1965): An unusual hazard of fixed-rate cardiac pacemakers. *Canad. Med. Ass. J.*, **93**:95.

17. ALLEN, P., LILLEHEI, C. W. (1957): Use of induced cardiac arrest in open heart surgery. *Minnesota Med.*, **40**:672.
18. ALLEN, P., ROBERTSON, R., TRAPP, W. G. (1964): Indications for treatment of complete atrioventricular dissociation. *Canad. Med. Ass. J.*, **91**:547.
19. ANAGNOSTOPOULOS, C. E., EISENBERG, L., MAURO, A., HOLCOMB, W. G., GLENN, W. W. L. (1965): Slowing of the heart rate and potentiation of myocardial contractility utilizing the standard radiofrequency (RF) pacemaker implant (Abstract). *Circulation*, **32** (Suppl. 2):42.
20. ANGELAKOS, E. T., TORRES, J. C. (1964): The efficiency of electrical pulses for cardiac stimulation. *Cardiologia (Basel)*, **44**:355.
21. AVRAMIDIS, A. V., HSU, I. (1959): Digitalis-induced ventricular fibrillation. *Arch. Intern. Med. (Chicago)*, **104**:277.
22. BAKULEV, A. N., SAVEL'EV, V. S., SAVCHUK, B. D., KONSTENKO, I. G., IGNA-TENKO, S. N. (1964): Indications for a permanent electric stimulation of the heart in atrioventricular blocks. *Grudn. Khir.*, **6**:3.
23. BANG, O., PETERSEN, G., PETERSEN, O. V. C. E. (1917): Two cases of bradycardia in horses: Adams-Stokes disease. Sinus bradycardia. *Heart*, **6**:100.
24. BARR, I. M., YERUSHALMI, S., BLIEDEN, L., NEUFELD, H. N., (1965): Endocardial radio-frequency pacemaking. *Israel J. Med. Sci.*, **1**:1018.
25. BATTYE, C. K. (1960): The synchronizing of electronic and natural cardiac pacemakers. *Medical Electronics* (Proc. 2nd Int. Conference on Medical Electronics, Paris, June 1959) (Ed. by C. N. Smyth). London, p. 250.
26. BAYLEY, T. J., LIGHTWOOD, R. (1966): Double and triple pulse pacemaking in treatment of ventricular tachycardia. *Lancet*, **1**:235.
27. BELLET, S., WASSERMAN, F., BRODY, J. I. (1955): Treatment of cardiac arrest and slow ventricular rates in complete A-V heart block. Use of molar and half molar sodium lactate. *Circulation*, **11**:685.
28. BELLET, S. (1960): Mechanism and treatment of A. V. heart block and Adams-Stokes syndrome. *Progr. Cardiov. Dis.*, **2**:691.
29. BENCHIMOL, A., DIMOND, E. G. (1966): Cardiac functions in man during artificial stimulation of the left ventricle, right ventricle and right atrium (Abstract). *Amer. J. Cardiol.*, **17**:118.
30. BENCHIMOL, A., DUENAS, A., LIGGETT, M. S., DIMOND, E. G. (1965): Contribution of atrial systole to the cardiac function at a fixed and at a variable ventricular rate. *Amer. J. Cardiol.*, **16**:11.
31. BENCHIMOL, A., LI, Y. B., DIMOND, E. G. (1964): Cardiovascular dynamics in complete heart block at various heart rates. Effect of exercise at a fixed heart rate. *Circulation*, **30**:542.
32. BENCHIMOL, A., LUCENA, E. G., DIMOND, E. G. (1965): Stroke volume and peripheral resistance during infusion of isoproterenol at a constant fixed heart rate. *Circulation*, **31**:417.
33. BENCHIMOL, A., PALMERO, H. A., LIGGETT, M. S., DIMOND, E. G. (1965): Influence of digitalization on the contribution of atrial systole to cardiac dynamics at a fixed ventricular rate. *Circulation*, **32**:84.
34. BENCHIMOL, A., LI, Y-B., DIMOND, E. G., VOTH, R. B., ROLAND, A. S. (1963): Effect of heart rate, exercise, and nitroglycerin on the cardiac dynamics in complete heart block. *Circulation*, **28**:510.

35. BENTIVOGLIO, L. G., GOLDBERG, H. (1965): Comparative hemodynamic effects of intravenous isoproterenol and of ventricular pacing matched at the same rates in patients with complete heart block. *Circulation*, 32 (Suppl. 2): 48.

36. BERG, J. W. VAN DEN (1964): Techniek van pacemakers. *Nederl. T. Geneesk.*, 108:2003.

37. BERGH, N. P., ENGEVIK, L., LINDER, E. (1963): Electric stimulation for total heart block and Stokes-Adams syndrome. *Acta Chir. Scand.*, 125:538.

38. BERGLUND, E., BORST, H. G., DUFF, F., SCHREINER, G. L., (1958): The effect of heart rate on cardiac work, myocardial oxygen consumption and coronary blood flow in the dog. *Acta Physiol. Scand.*, 42:185.

39. BERNSTEIN, M. (1938): Auriculoventricular dissociation following scarlet fever. Report of a case. *Amer. Heart J.*, 16:582.

40. BERTHOUD, E., MERCIER, H., SOLMS, H. (1953): Syndrome de Stokes-Adams par intoxication à la prostigmine. *Rev. Méd. Suisse Rom.*, 73:392.

41. BEVEGÅRD, S. (1962): Studies on the regulation of the circulation in man. *Acta Physiol. Scand.*, 57 (Suppl. 200).

42. BEVEGÅRD, S. (1962): Observations on the effect of varying ventricular rate on the circulation at rest and during exercise in two patients with an artificial pacemaker. *Acta Med. Scand.*, 172:615.

43. BEVEGÅRD, S., JONSSON, B., KARLÖF, I., LAGERGREN, H., SOWTON, E. (1967): Effect of changes in ventricular rate on cardiac output and central pressures at rest and during exercise in patients with artificial pacemakers. *Cardiov. Res.*, in press.

44. BIGELOW, W. G., CALLAGHAN, J. C., HOPPS, J. A. (1950): General hypothermia for experimental intracardiac surgery: The use of electrophrenic respirations, an artificial pacemaker for cardiac standstill, and radiofrequency rewarming in general hypothermia. *Ann. Surg.*, 132:531.

45. BINDER, M. J., ROSOVE, L. (1952): Paroxysmal ventricular tachycardia and fibrillation due to quinidine. *Amer. J. Med.*, 12:491.

46. BINET, J. P., LOGEAIS, Y., AIGUEPERSE, J., LANGLOIS, J., DE SAINT-FLORENT, LEMOINE, G., MATHEY, J. (1965): L'entrainement électrosystolique du coeur par pace-maker (P.M.) intracorporel. (Résultats à propos de 221 interventions, de 204 pace-makers implantés chez 161 malades.) *Mem. Acad. Chir. (Paris)*, 91:677.

47. BISHOP, J. (1964): Personal communication.

48. BISS, K. (1965): Stokes-Adams disease of undetermined etiology. A new hemodynamic concept. *Cor Vasa*, 7:85.

49. BJORK, V. O., INTONTI, F., LORKIEWICZ, Z. (1965): Pacemaker treatment in Adams-Stokes syndrome. *Cor Vasa*, 7:93.

50. BLOOMFIELD, D., REDWOOD, D., SOWTON, G. E. (1966): Distinction between the negative inotropic and choronotropic actions of propranalol. *Brit. Heart J.*, in press.

51. BLUESTONE, R., DAVIES, G., HARRIS, A., LEATHAM, A., SIDDONS, H. (1965): Long-term endocardial pacing for heart block. *Lancet*, 2:307.

52. BLUESTONE, R., HARRIS, A. (1965): Treatment of heart block with long-acting isoprenaline. *Lancet*, 1:1299.

53. BLUESTONE, R. H., HARRIS, A. M., DAVIES, G. (1965): Aftercare of artificially paced patients. *Brit. Med. J.*, 1:1589.

54. BONNABEAU, R. C., BILGUTAY, A. M., STERNS, L. P., WINGROVE, R., LILLEHEI, C. W. (1963): Observations on sudden death during pacemaker stimulation in complete atrioventricular block leading to the development of a "P-wave" pacemaker without atrial leads. *Trans. Amer. Soc. Artif. Intern. Organs*, 9:158.

55. BONNABEAU, R. C., FERLIC, R. M., LILLEHEI, C. W., (1965): A new rechargeable epicardial cardiac pacemaker. *J. Thorac. Cardiov. Surg.*, 50:857.

56. BORRIE, J., LICHTER, I. (1964): Artificial pacing for heart block. Experimental and clinical approach. *New Zeal. Med. J.*, 63:31.

57. BORST, H. (1965): In discussion. *Thoraxchirurgie*, 13:277.

58. BOTTI, R. E., YOUNG, F. E. (1959): Myocardial sarcoid, complete heart block and aortic stenosis. *Ann. Intern. Med.*, 51:811.

59. BOURNE, G. (1955): Stokes-Adams attacks in bundle-branch block. *Brit. Med. J.*, 2:1311.

60. BOUVRAIN, Y. (1963): In discussion. *Arch. Mal. Coeur*, 56:428.

61. BOUVRAIN, Y., BINET, J. P., SLAMA, R., GUÉDON, J., AIGUEPERSE, J. (1963): Traitement de la maladie de Stokes-Adams par implantation intracorporelle d'un entraîneur électrosystolique. Expérience portant sur neuf cas. *Presse Med.*, 71:329.

62. BOUVRAIN, Y., SLAMA, R. (1965): Résultats à long terme de l'entraînement électrosystolique par stimulateur intracorporel. Les pannes d'appareil. *Soc. Med. Hôp. Paris*, 116:397.

63. BOUVRAIN, Y., SLAMA, R., MARTINEAUD, J-P., SAUMONT, R., BINET, J. P. (1964): Bilan de l'implantation d'un stimulateur intracorporel chez 50 malades atteints de maladie de Stokes-Adams. *Arch. Mal. Coeur*, 57:241.

64. BOUVRAIN, Y., SLAMA, R., MARTINEAUD, J-P., SAUMONT, R., BOURTHOUMIEUX, A., NEZRY, R. (1964): L'entraînement électrosystolique par sonde endocavitaire. Expérience portant sur 25 cas. *Arch. Mal. Coeur*, 57:1019.

65. BRAUNWALD, E. (1965): Symposium on electrical control of cardiac activity. Buffalo, May, 1965, unpublished.

66. BRAUNWALD, N. S., FRAHM, C. J. (1961): Studies on Starling's law of the heart. IV. Observations on the hemodynamic functions of the left atrium in man. *Circulation*, 24:633.

67. BRAUNWALD, N. S., GAY, W. A., MORROW, A. G., BRAUNWALD, E. (1964): Sustained, paired electrical stimuli. *Amer. J. Cardiol.*, 14:385.

68. BRAUNWALD, N. S., MORROW, A. G. (with the technical assistance of DEBROSKE, J. M. F., HAMILTON, W. D., BORETOS, J. W.) (1965): Accelerated fatigue testing of available pacemaker electrodes and Elgiloy wire coils. *Surgery*, 58:846.

69. BRAUNWALD, E., ROSS, J., FROMMER, P. L., WILLIAMS, J. F., SONNENBLICK, E. H., GAULT, J. H. (1964): Clinical observations on paired electrical stimulation of the heart. *Amer. J. Med.*, 37:700.

70. BRAUNWALD, E., ROSS, J., SONNENBLICK, E. H., FROMMER, P. L., BRAUNWALD, N. S., MORROW, A. G. (1965): Slowing of heart rate, electroaugmentation of ventricular performance, and increase of myocardial oxygen consumption produced by paired electrical stimulation. *Bull. N. Y. Acad. Med.*, 41:481.

226 *Cardiac Pacemakers*

71. BREDIKIS, YuI., KOSTENKO, I. G. (1964): Depression of the automatism of cardiac ventricles in complete atrioventricular block under the effect of rhythmic electrical impulses. *Pat. Fiziol. Eksp. Ter.*, 8:25.
72. BRISTOW, J. D., FERGUSON, R. E., MINTZ, F., RAPAPORT, E. (1963): The influence of heart rate on left ventricular volume in dogs. *J. Clin. Invest.*, 42:649.
73. BROCKMAN, S. K. (1965): Cardiodynamics of complete heart block. *Amer. J. Cardiol.*, 16:72.
74. BROCKMAN, S. K. (1965): Reflex control of the heart in complete A-V block, with special reference to the experimental creation of Adams-Stokes disease. *Amer. J. Cardiol.*, 16:84.
75. BROCKMAN, S. K., WEBB, R. C., BAHNSON, H. T. (1958): Monopolar ventricular stimulation for the control of acute surgically produced heart block. *Surgery*, 44:910.
76. BROOKS, C. McC., GILBERT, J. L., LANGE, G., MAZZELLA, H. M. (1959): Changes in excitability and electrical response in areas of heart muscle made ischemic by coronary artery ligation (Abstract). *Physiologist*, 2:17.
77. BROOKS, C. McC., HOFFMAN, B. F., SUCKLING, E. E., ORIAS, O. (1955): *Excitability of the Heart.* New York, Grune.
78. BROUSTET, P., BERGAUD, A., BLANCHOT, P., BRICAUD, H., LAGARDE, J., CABANIEU, C., GAZEAU, J., DUFOUR, P. (1957): Le traitment des formes graves du syndrome de Stokes-Adams par les perfusions d'adrénaline. *Arch. Mal. Coeur*, 50:541.
79. BRUCE, R. A., BLACKMON, J. R., COBB, L. A., DODGE, H. T. (1965): Treatment of asystole or heart block during acute myocardial infarction with electrode catheter pacing. *Amer. Heart J.*, 69:460.
80. BRÜCK, A. (1965): Gegenwärtiger Stand der Therapie mit elektrischen Schrittmachern. *Z. Kreislaufforsch.*, 34:853.
81. BRUNS, D. L., GARDNER, R. E., RIVKIN, L. M., ROE, B. B. (1963): The problem of complete heart block. *Amer. J. Surg.*, 106:357.
82. BUCHANAN, J. W. (1965): Spontaneous arrhythmias and conduction disturbances in domestic animals. *Ann. N. Y. Acad. Sci.*, 127:224.
83. BÜCHNER, C., BILGER, R., OVERBECK, W., MIKLAW, H., REINDELL, H. (1964): Geburt bei einer Patientin mit künstlichem Schrittmacher des Herzens. *Deutsch. Med. Wschr.*, 89:1932.
84. BURCHELL, H. B. (1961): Hidden hazards of cardiac pacemakers. *Circulation*, 24:161.
85. BURCHELL, H. B., CONNOLLY, D. C., ELLIS, F. H. (1964): Indications for and results of implanting cardiac pacemakers. *Amer. J. Med.*, 37:764.
86. BURKART, F., SOWTON, E. (1965): The effect of atrial asystole at different heart rates. Unpublished data.
87. BURNETT, W. (1827): *Med. Chir. Trans. London*, 13:202. Reported in Mayor, R. H.: *Classic Descriptions of Disease*, 3rd ed. Springfield, Thomas, 1945.
88. BUTLER, S., LEVINE, S. A. (1929): Diphtheria as a cause of late heart-block. *Amer. Heart J.*, 5:592.

89. BUTTERWORTH, J. S., POINDEXTER, C. A. (1942): Short P-R interval associated with a prolonged QRS complex. *Arch. Intern. Med. (Chicago)*, 69:437.

90. BUTTERWORTH, J. S., POINDEXTER, C. A. (1944): Fusion beats and their relation to the syndrome of short P-R interval associated with a long QRS complex. *Amer. Heart J.*, 28:149.

91. BUTTIGLIERO, J. B., COLES, J. C., GERGELY, N. F. (1964): Artificial cardiac pacing. *Canad. Med. Assoc. J.*, 91:331.

92. BYRON, F. X. (1965): In discussion. *J. Thorac. Cardiov. Surg.*, 50:862.

93. CALLAGHAN, J. C., BIGELOW, W. G. (1951): An electrical artificial pacemaker for standstill of the heart. *Ann. Surg.*, 134:8.

94. CAMMILLI, L. (1964): In discussion. *Ann. N. Y. Acad. Sci.*, 111:1044.

95. CAMMILLI, L., POZZI, R., DRAGO, G. (1962): Contrôle du rhythme cardiaque dans le syndrome de Morgagni-Adams-Stokes par stimulation électrique directe du myocarde. Et stimulation à distance par radio-fréquence. *Presse Med.*, 70:813.

96. CAMMILLI, L., POZZI, R., DRAGO, G. (1962): Remote heart stimulation by radio-frequency for permanent rhythm control in Morgagni-Adams-Stokes syndrome. *Surgery,* 52:765.

97. CAMMILLI, L., POZZI, R., DRAGO, G., PIZZICHI, G., DE SAINT-PIERRE, G. (1961): Stimolazione a distanze del cuore nella sindrome de Morgagni-Adams-Stokes mediante transmettitore a radio frequenza e bonina ricevente epicardia (prima applicazione clinica). *Osped. Ital. Chir.*, 5:999.

98. CAMMILLI, L., POZZI, R., PIZZICHI, G., DE SAINT-PIERRE, G. (1964): Radio-frequency pacemaker with receiver coil implanted on the heart. *Ann. N. Y. Acad. Sci.*, 111:1007.

99. CAMPBELL, G. S. (1965): In discussion. *J. Thorac. Cardiov. Surg.*, 50:864.

100. CAMPBELL, M. (1944): Complete heart block. *Brit. Heart J.*, 6:69.

101. CAMPBELL, M., SUZMAN, S. S. (1934): Congenital complete heart-block: account of 8 cases. *Amer. Heart J.*, 9:304.

102. CAMPBELL, M., THORNE, M. G. (1956): Congenital heart block. *Brit. Heart J.*, 18:90.

103. CARLENS, E., JOHANSSON, L., KARLÖF, I., LAGERGREN, H. (1965): New method for atrial-triggered pacemaker treatment without thoracotomy. *J. Thorac. Cardiov. Surg.*, 50:229.

104. CARLETON, R. A., GRAETTINGER, J. S. (1965): Atrial contribution to ventricular performance. *J. Clin. Invest.*, 44:1033.

105. CARLETON, R. A., SESSIONS, R. W., GRAETTINGER, J. S. (1964): Dual-rate pacemaker. *J. Thorac. Cardiov. Surg.*, 48:684.

106. CARLETON, R. A., SESSIONS, W., GRAETTINGER, J. S. (1964): Environmental influence on implantable cardiac pacemakers. *JAMA*, 190:938.

107. CARLETON, R. A., SESSIONS, R. W., GRAETTINGER, J. S. (1966): Cardiac pacemakers: clinical and physiological studies. *Med. Clin. N. Amer.*, 50:325.

108. CARROLL, J. M. (1962): Mathematics of reliability. *Electronics*, 35:54.

109. CASTBERG, T., RASMUSSEN, K. N. (1963): Treatment of recurrent threatening Adams-Strokes attacks by implantation of a pacemaker. *Acta Chir. Scand.*, 125:557.

110. CASTBERG, T., RASMUSSEN, K. N. (1965): Fortsatte erfaringer med pace-makerbehandling af livstruende Adams-Stokes' anfald. *Ugeskr. Laeg.*, **127**:277.

111. CASTELLANOS, A., JOHNSON, D., MAS, I., LEMBERG, L. (1966): Electrical conversion of paroxysmal atrial fibrillation in the Wolff-Parkinson-White (Pre-excitation) syndrome. *Amer. J. Cardiol.*, **17**:91.

112. CASTELLANOS, A., LEMBERG, L., BERKOVITS, B. V. (1966): Repetitive firing during synchronised ventricular stimulation. *Amer. J. Cardiol.*, **17**:119.

113. CASTELLANOS, A., LEMBERG, L., GOSSELIN, A. (1965): Double artificial ventricular parasystole iatrogenic arrhythmia for the study of excitability and conductivity in the human heart. *Cardiologia (Basel)*, **47**:273.

114. CASTLE, C. H., BRIGGS, L. S. (1965): Hazard of ventricular fibrillation from paired pulse stimulation (Abstract). *Circulation*, **32** (Suppl. 2):65.

115. CENTER, S., NATHAN, D. A., (1965): Synchronous pacing of the heart: three years clinical experience (Abstract). *Circulation*, **32** (Suppl. 2):66.

116. CENTER, S., NATHAN, D., WU, C-Y., DUQUE, D. (1964): Two years of clinical experience with the synchronous pacer. *J. Thorac. Cardiov. Surg.*, **48**:513.

117. CENTER, S., NATHAN, D., WU, C-Y., SAMET, P., KELLER, W. (1963): The implantable synchronous pacer in the treatment of complete heart block. *J. Thorac. Cardiov. Surg.*, **46**:744.

118. CERANKE, P., ST. TOMEK (1953): Pilocarpinintoxikation bei Herzblock. *Wien. Med. Wschr.*, **103**:131.

119. CHAFFEE, E. L., LIGHT, R. U. (1934): A method for remote control of electrical stimulation of the nervous system. *Yale J. Biol. Med.*, **7**:83.

120. CHAILLET, J. L., VAN BRUGGEN, H. W., MEESTER, G. T. (1964): Anwendung und Vorteille der Herzstimulation mittels intrakardialer Katheter. *Verh. Deutsch. Ges. Kreislaufforsch.*, **30**:226.

121. CHANDLER, D., CLAPPER, M. I., (1959): Complete atrioventricular block treated with isoproterenol hydrochloride. *Amer. J. Cardiol.*, **3**:336.

122. CHARDACK, W. M. (1964): A myocardial electrode for long-term pacemaking. *Ann. N.Y. Acad. Sci.*, **111**:893.

123. CHARDACK, W. M. (1964): In discussion. *Ann. N.Y. Acad. Sci.*, **111**:962.

124. CHARDACK, W. M. (1964): In discussion. *Ann. N.Y. Acad. Sci.*, **111**:1108.

125. CHARDACK, W. M. (1964): Heart block treated with an implantable pacemaker. Past experience and current developments. *Progr. Cardiov. Dis.*, **6**:507.

126. CHARDACK, W., FEDERICO, A., GAGE, A. (1965): Pacemaker leads routed down jugular. *World Med. J.*, **1**:46.

127. CHARDACK, W. M. (1965): In discussion. *Bull. N.Y. Acad. Med.*, **41**:733.

128. CHARDACK, W. M. (1965): Heart block treated with an implantable pacemaker: past experience and current developments. *Resuscitation & Cardiac Pacing* (Proc. of Conference, Glasgow, March, 1964). London, Cassell, p. 213.

129. CHARDACK, W. M. (1965): Personal communication.

130. CHARDACK, W. M., FEDERICO, A. J., GAGE, A. A., GREATBATCH, W. (1965): Clinical experience with an implanted pacemaker catheter electrode system (Abstract). Circulation, **32** (Suppl. 2):67.

131. CHARDACK, W. M., GAGE, A. A., DEAN, D. C. (1964): Slowing the heart by paired pulse pacemaker. *Amer. J. Cardiol.*, **14**:374.

132. CHARDACK, W. M., GAGE, A. A., DEAN, D. C. (1965): Paired and coupled electrical stimulation of the heart. *Bull. N.Y. Acad. Med.*, **41**:462.

133. CHARDACK, W., GAGE, A. A., FEDERICO, A. J., SCHIMERT, G., GREATBATCH, W. (1964): Clinical experience with an implantable pacemaker. *Ann. N.Y. Acad. Sci.*, **111**:1075.

134. CHARDACK, W. M., GAGE, A. A., FEDERICO, A. J., SCHIMERT, G., GREATBATCH, W. (1965): Five years' clinical experience with an implantable pacemaker: An appraisal. *Surgery*, **58**:915.

135. CHARDACK, W. M., GAGE, A. A., GREATBATCH, W. (1960): A transistorized, self-contained, implantable pacemaker for the long term correction of complete heart block. *Surgery*, **48**:643.

136. CHARDACK, W. M., GAGE, A. A., GREATBATCH, W. (1961): Correction of complete heart block by self contained and subcutaneously implanted pacemaker. *J. Thorac. Cardiov. Surg.*, **42**:814.

137. CHARDACK, W. M., GAGE, A. A., GREATBATCH, W. (1961): Experimental observations and clinical experience with the correction of complete heart block by an implantable, self-contained pacemaker. *Trans. Amer. Soc. Artif. Intern. Organs*, **3**:286.

138. CHARDACK, W. M., GAGE, A. A., GREATBATCH, W. (1962): Treatment of complete heart block with an implantable and self-contained pacemaker. *Bull. Soc. Int. Chir.*, **21**:411.

139. CHARDACK, W. M., GAGE, A. A., SCHIMERT, G., THOMSON, N. B., SANFORD, C. E., GREATBATCH, W. (1963): Two years' clinical experience with the implantable pacemaker for complete heart block. *Dis. Chest*, **43**:225.

140. CITTERS, R. L. V., SMITH, O. A., RUTTENBERG, H. D. (1965): Paroxysmal ventricular tachycardia induced in dogs with chronic complete heart block by hypothalamic stimulation (Abstract). *Circulation*, **32** (Suppl. 2):211.

141. CLARK, N. S. (1948): Complete heart block in children. Report of three cases possibly attributable to measles. *Arch. Dis. Child.*, **23**:156.

142. COHEN, D. B., DOCTOR, L., PICK, A. (1958): The significance of atrioventricular block complicating acute myocardial infarct. *Amer. Heart J.*, **55**:215.

143. COHN, A. E., LEVINE, S. A. (1925): The beneficial effects of barium chlorid on Adams-Stokes disease. *Arch. Intern. Med. (Chicago)*, **36**:1.

144. COLE, D. S., YARROW, S. (1964): Artificial electrical pacing for heart block: A review based on 24 cases treated with implanted pacemakers. *New Zeal. Med. J.*, **63**:126.

145. COOKSON, H. (1942): Fainting and fits in cardiac infarction. *Brit. Heart J.*, **4**:163.

146. COOKSON, H. (1952): Paroxysmal ventricular standstill. *Brit. Heart J.*, **14**:350.

147. COSBY, R. S., CAFFERKY, E. A., LAU, F. Y. K., ROHDE, R. A. (1965): Electrocardiographic and clinical features in the prognosis of complete heart block (Abstract). *Amer. J. Cardiol.*, **15**:128.

148. COSTEAS, F., MASTROYANNIS, H., NICOLAOU, N., KOTSERAS, P. St. (1963): Tachycardia and death due to an artificial pacemaker. *Ann. Intern. Med.*, **63**:308.

149. COURA, J. R. (1966): Contribuição ao estudo da doença de Chagas no estado da guanabara. Unpublished thesis. Faculdade Nacional de Medicina, Universidade do Brasil.
150. COURBIER, R., DEVIN, R., TORRESANI, J., HENRY, E. (1965): Notre expérience de l'implantation des pacemakers. *Cardiologia (Basel)*, 46:275.
151. COURBIER, R., TORRESANI, J., MONTIES, J. R., DEVIN, R., HENRY, E. (1965): Implantation of intra-corporeal electric stimulators (concerning 20 cases). *J. Cardiov. Surg.*, 6:49.
152. COURTER, S. R., MOFFAT, J., FOWLER, N. O. (1963): Advanced atrioventricular block in acute myocardial infarction. *Circulation*, 27:1034.
153. CRANEFIELD, B. F. (1965): Symposium on electrical control of cardiac activity. Buffalo, May, 1965, unpublished.
154. CRANEFIELD, B. F., SCHERLAG, B. J., YEH, B. K., HOFFMAN, B. F. (1964): Treatment of acute cardiac failure by maintained postextrasystolic potentiation. *Bull. N.Y. Acad. Med.*, 40:903.
155. CRASTNOPOL (1964): In discussion. *Ann. N.Y. Acad. Sci.*, 111:958.
156. CRAWFORD, J. H., DI GREGORIO, N. J. (1947): Complete heart block in younger age groups. *Amer. Heart J.*, 34:540.
157. CRAWFORD, T., DEXTER, D., TEARE, R. D. (1961): Coronary-artery pathology in sudden death from myocardial ischemia. *Lancet*, 1:181.
158. CURD, G. W., DENNIS, E. W., JORDAN, J., McNAMARA, D., MONTERO, A. C., PETERSON, P. K., PRUITT, R. D., SCHNUR, S. (1963): Etiology of atrioventricular heart block: a study of its relevance to prognosis and pacemaker therapy. *Cardiov. Res. Cent. Bull.*, 1:63.
159. CURD, G. W., DENNIS, E. W., MONTERO, A. C., PETERSON, P. K., PRUITT, R. D., SCHNUR, S. (1961): Etiology of atrio-ventricular heart block: a study of its relevance to prognosis and pacemaker therapy. *Circulation*, 24:913.
160. DACK, S. (1965): Pacemaker therapy in heart block and Stokes-Adams syndrome. *JAMA*, 191:846.
161. DALESSIO, D. J., BENCHIMOL, A., DIMOND, E. G. (1965): Chronic encephalopathy related to heart block: its correction by permanent cardiac pacemaker. *Neurology (Minneap.)*, 15:499.
162. DASSEN, R. (1933): Atypical typhoid fever. Heart block. Myocarditis posttyphosa (Romberg). Value of atropin test. *Amer. J. Med. Sci.*, 186:499.
163. DAVIES, J. G. (1962): Artificial cardiac pacemakers for the long-term treatment of heart block. *J. Brit. Inst. Radio Engr.*, 24:453.
164. DAVIES, J. G. (1964): Personal communication.
165. DAVIES, J. G., LEATHAM, A., ROBINSON, B. F. (1959): Ventricular stimulation by catheter electrode (Letter). *Lancet*, 1:583.
166. DAVIES, J. G., SIDDONS, H. (1965): Experience with implanted pacemakers: technical considerations. *Thorax*, 20:128.
167. DAVIES, J. G., SOWTON, G. E. (1964): Cardiac pacemakers. *Phys. Med. Biol.*, 9:257.
168. DAVIES, J. G., SOWTON, G. E. (1966): Electrical threshold of the human heart. *Brit. Heart J.*, 28:231.
169. DAVIES, M. J. (1966): Some aspects of the etiology of complete heart block. Cambridge, Associations of Physicians, April, 1966, unpublished.

170. Davis, D., Sprague, H. B. (1929): Ventricular fibrillation; its relation to heart block; report of case in which syncopal attacks and death occurred in course of quinidine therapy. *Amer. Heart J.*, **4**:559.

171. Day, J., Viar, W. N. (1951): A case of heart block treated with I-cyclohexyl-2-methylaminopropane (Benzedrex). *Amer. Heart J.*, **42**:733.

172. Dean, D. C., Gage, A. A., Chardack, W. M. (1965): Paired pulse pacemaking: effects on rate and contractility of the heart (Abstract). *Amer. J. Cardiol.*, **15**:129.

173. De Boer, S. (1952): On the origin and essence of the Morgagni-Adams-Stokes syndrome. *Ann. Intern. Med.*, **37**:48.

174. De Gasperis, A., Donatelli, R., Palminiello, A., Rovelli, F. (1962): Considerazione su 20 casi di malattia di Morgagni-Adams-Stokes trattati con stimolazione ellettrica. *Minerva Med.*, **53**:3457.

175. Dekker, E., Büller, J., Schuilenburg, R. M. (1964): Enkele hulpmiddelen bij de diagnostick van "pacemaker failure." *Nederl. T. Geneesk.*, **108**:2160.

176. Dekker, E., Büller, J., Schuilenburg, R. M. (1965): Aids to electrical diagnosis of pacemaker failure. *Amer. Heart J.*, **70**:730.

177. Delman, A. J., Schwedel, J. B., Escher, D. J. W. (1963): An intracardiac pacemaker in Adams-Stokes attacks in acute myocardial infarction. *JAMA*, **184**:1040.

178. Derom, F., Schoofs, E., Verstraeten, J., Snoeck, J. (1963): Le traitement du syndrome d'Adam-Stokes par pacemaker interne. *Acta. Chir. Belg.* (Suppl. 12):116.

179. De Saint Pierre, G. (1963): Resuscitazione cardiaca. Prolungato arresto cardiaco regredito mediante iniezone intra-cardiaca di Alupent. *Settim. Med.*, **51**:1111.

180. De Saint Pierre, G. (1964): La sindrome post-pericardiotomica. Rivista sintetica e contributo personale a proposito della sua insorgenza dopo implanto di radio-pacemaker. *Cardiol. Prat.*, **15**:538.

181. De Saint Pierre, G., Toscani, G., Pozzi, A., Cammilli, L. (1963): L'azione di un nuovo derivato adrenalinico (Alupent) nei confronti del risveglio dei segnapassi idioventriculari in letargo studiata mediante una nuova tecnica. *Settim. Med.*, **51**:1189.

182. De Sanctis, R. W. (1963): Short term use of intravenous electrode in heart block. *JAMA*, **184**:544.

183. De Vos, P. (1964): Gangmaking met behulp van de intracardiale catheter-methode. *Nederl. T. Geneesk*, **108**:379.

184. Diamond, S., Flaxman, M. (1955): The use of methamphetamine hydrochloride in Stokes-Adams disease. *Amer. Prac. Dig. Treat.*, **6**:1174.

185. Diezel, P. B., Friese, G. (1963): On the subject of prolonged electrical stimulation of the heart. Tissue changes in the area of the myocardial electrode. *Z. Kreislaufforsch.*, **52**:1.

186. Dimond, E. G., Dunn, M., Brosius, F. (1960): Management of arrhythmias in acute myocardial infarction. *Progr. Cardiov. Dis.*, **3**:1.

187. Dittmar, H. A., Friese, G., Holder, E. (1962): Erfahrungen über die langfristige electrische Reizung des menschlichen Herzens. *Z. Kreislaufforsch.*, **51**:66.

188. Dock, W. (1929): Transitory ventricular fibrillation as cause of syncope, and its prevention by quinidine sulphate, with case report and discussion of diagnostic criteria for ventricular fibrillation. *Amer. Heart J.*, 4:707.

189. Donoso, E., Braunwald, E., Jick, S., Grisham, A. (1956): Congenital heart block. *Amer. J. Med.*, 20:869.

190. Donoso, E., Stein, W. G., Schloff, L., Cohn, L. J., Friedberg, C. K. (1965): Effect of digitalis in compensated and decompensated patients with internal cardiac pacemakers (Abstract). *Circulation*, 32 (Suppl. 2):77.

191. Douglas, A. H., Wagner, W. P. (1955): Ventricular control by artificial pacemaker for seven days with recovery. *JAMA*, 157:444.

192. Dragsted, P. J., Møller, P. F. (1958): Behandling af Adams-Stokes' anfald med natriumlactat. *Ugesk. Laeg.*, 120:1458.

193. Dressler, W. (1963): Postcardiotomy syndrome after implantation of a pacemaker. *Amer. Heart J.*, 63:757.

194. Dressler, W. (1964): Observations in patients with implanted pacemakers. III Frequency of ventricular tachycardia as cause of Adams-Stokes attacks and rate of pacing required for its prevention. *Amer. Heart J.*, 68:19.

195. Dressler, W., Jonas, S. (1962): Experimental production of A-V dissociation with ventricular captures by use of an internal pacemaker in patients with 2:1 A-V block. *Amer. J. Cardiol.*, 10:547.

196. Dressler, W., Jonas, S., Kantrowitz, A. (1963): Observations in patients with implanted cardiac pacemaker. 1. Clinical experience. *Amer. Heart J.*, 66:325.

197. Dressler, W., Jonas, S., Rubin, R. (1965): Observations in patients with implanted cardiac pacemaker. IV. Repetitive responses to electrical stimuli. *Amer. J. Cardiol.*, 15:391.

198. Dressler, W., Jonas, S., Schwartz, E. (1965): Supernormal phase of myocardial excitability in man (Abstract). *Circulation*, 32 (Suppl. 2):79.

199. Duchenne, G. B. (1870): Désordres graves de la circulation cardiaque et de la respiration par intoxication diphthéritique. *Un. Med. (Paris)* (3.s.), 9:27.

200. Durrer, D., van der Tweel, L. H. (1954): Spread of activation in the left ventricular wall of the dog. II. Activation conditions at the epicardial surface. *Amer. Heart J.*, 47:192.

201. Edelist, A., Langendorf, R., Pick, A., Katz, L. N. (1963): Physiologic and Pharmacologic studies in Stokes-Adams disease patients during the use of an artificial cardiac pacemaker (Abstract). *Circulation*, 28:715.

202. Effert, S., Greuel, H., Grosse-Brockhoff, F., Sykosch, J. (1962): Die Therapie mit elektrischen Schrittmachern beim Adams-Stokes Syndrom. *Deutsch. Med. Wschr.*, 87:473.

203. Effert, S., Sykosch, H. J., Pulver, K. G. (1964): Langfristige Therapie mit implantierbaren elektrischen Schrittmachern. *Deutsch. Med. Wschr.*, 89:654.

204. Eisenberg, L., Mauro, A., Glenn, W. W. L., Hageman, J. H. (1965): Radio frequency stimulation: a research and clinical tool. *Science*, 147:578.

205. EKESTRÖM, S., JOHANSSON, L., LAGERGREN, H. (1962): Behandling av Adam-Stokes syndrom med intracardiell pacemakerelektrod. *Opuscula Medica*, 7:175.

206. ELLIS, F. H., MANNING, P. C., CONNOLLY, D. C. (1964): Treatment of Stokes-Adams disease. *Mayo Clin. Proc.*, 39:945.

207. ELMQVIST, R., LANDERGREN, J., PETTERSSON, S. O., SENNING, A., WILLIAM-OLSSON, G. (1963): Artificial pacemaker for treatment of Adams-Stokes syndrome and slow heart rate. *Amer. Heart J.*, 65:731.

208. ELMQVIST, R., SENNING, A. (1960): Implantable pacemaker for the heart. *Medical Electronics* (Proc. 2nd Int. Conference on Medical Electronics, Paris, June 1959) (Ed. by C. N. Smyth). London, p. 253.

209. ENGER, C., KENNEDY, J., MICHELL, A. (1966): Tiny pacemaker is powered by heart itself. *World Med.*, 1:11, 8.

210. ENGLE, M. A. (1949): Recovery from complete heart block in diphtheria. *Pediatrics*, 3:222.

211. ERAKLIS, A. J., GREEN, W. T., WATSON, C. G. (1965): Recurrent paroxysms of ventricular tachycardia following mitral valvuloplasty. *Ann. Surg.*, 161.63.

212. ERLANGER, J. (1906): On the physiology of heart-block in mammals, with especial reference to causation of Stokes-Adams disease. *J. Exp. Med.*, 8:8.

213. ERNST, R. W. (1962): Pedicle grafting of the sino-auricular node to the right ventricle for the treatment of complete atrioventricular block. *J. Thorac. Cardiov. Surg.*, 44:681.

214. ERNST, R. W. (1964): Transplant of the sino-auricular node to the right ventricle for the treatment of complete heart block. *Ann. N.Y. Acad. Sci.*, 111:869.

215. ESCHER, D. J. W. (1965): Personal communication.

216. ESCHER, D. J. W., SCHWEDEL, J. B., EISENBERG, R., GITSIOS, C., PERNA, N., JAMSHIDI, A. (1961): Cardiovascular dynamic responses to artificial pacing of patients in heart block (Abstract). *Circulation*, 24:928.

217. ESCHER, D. J. W., SCHWEDEL, J. B., SCHWARTZ, L. S., SOLOMAN, N. (1964): Transvenous electrical stimulation of the heart. *Ann. N.Y. Acad. Sci.*, 111:981.

218. ETTINGER, P. (1965): Synchronization during electrical pacing (Case report). *Amer. Heart J.*, 70:110.

219. FAIVRE, G., CHALNOT, P., GILGENKRANTZ, J. M., FRISCH, R., CHERRIER, F., TENETTE, C., RENAUD, J. (1963): L'entraînement électrosystolique dans le traitement des blocs auriculo-ventriculaires. *Arch. Mal. Coeur*, 56:406.

220. FAIVRE, G., GILGENKRANTZ, J. M., RENAUD, J. (1964): Application au traitement des blocs auriculo-ventriculaires. L'entraînement électrique du Coeur, France. Paris, Masson & Cie.

221. FATZER, G. (1946): Étude de l'électrocardiogramme dans le bloc atrioventriculaire. *Cardiologia (Basel)*, 10:305.

222. FEDERICO, A. J. (1965): Symposium on electrical control of cardiac activity. Buffalo, May, 1965, unpublished.

223. FELDMAN, D. S., KANTROWITZ, A. (1963): Electrical characteristics of human ventricular myocardium stimulated in vivo (Abstract). *Clin. Res.*, 11:22.

224. FERRIS, E. B., CAPPS, R. B., WEISS, S. (1935): Carotid sinus syncope and its bearing on the mechanisms of the unconscious state and convulsions. Study of 32 additional cases. *Medicine*, **14**:377.

225. FINNEY, J. O. (1965): Hemodynamic alterations in left ventricular function consequent to ventricular pacing. *Amer. J. Physiol*, **208**:275.

226. FISCH, C., MARTZ, B. L., PRIEBE, F. H. (1960): Enhancement of potassium-induced atrio-ventricular block by toxic doses of digitalis drugs. *J. Clin. Invest.*, **39**:1885.

227. FISHER, P., SMITH, F. R. (1965): Continuous electrical pacing of a patient with heart block providing 33 months' survival. *Dis. Chest*, **48**:209.

228. FITCH, E. A., BAILEY, C. P. (1959): An electrically conductive cardiac suture. *J. Thorac. Cardiov. Surg.*, **38**:120.

229. FLEMING, G. B., KENNEDY, A. M. (1910): A case of complete heart-block in diphtheria with an account of post-mortem findings. *Heart*, **2**:77.

230. FLEMING, H. A., MIRAMS, J. A. (1963): A clinical trial of a sustained-action preparation of isoprenaline in the treatment of heart-block. *Lancet*, **2**:214.

231. FOLKMAN, J., EDMUNDS, L. H. (1962): Endocrine pacemaker for complete heart block. *Circ. Res.*, **10**:632.

232. FOLKMAN, J., LONG, D. M. (1964): Drug pacemakers in the treatment of heart block. *Ann. N.Y. Acad. Sci.*, **111**:857.

233. FOLKMAN, J., LONG, D. M. (1964): The use of silicone rubber as a carrier for prolonged drug therapy. *J. Surg. Res.*, **4**:139.

234. FOLKMAN, M. J., WATKINS, E. (1957): An artificial conduction system for the management of experimental complete heart block. *Surg. Forum*, **8**:331.

235 FONGI, E. G., BURUCUA, J. E. (1952): Bloqueo sinoauricular con sindrome de Morgagni-Stokes-Adams provocado per la Estreptomicina. *Prensa Med. Argent.*, **39**:1507.

236. FORD, J. M. (1961): In discussion. *J. Thorac. Cardiov. Surg.*, **42**:828.

237. FORSBERG, S. Å., VARNAUSKAS, E. (1963): Medication for heart block. *Acta Chir. Scand.*, **125**:533.

238. FORT, M. L., SHARP, J. T. (1965): Perforation of the right ventricle by pacing catheter electrode. *Amer. J. Cardiol.*, **16**:610.

239. FORTIN, P. (1964): Le traitement du bloc auriculo-ventriculaire du coeur. *Coeur Med. Intern.*, **3**:445.

240. FOWLER, P. B. S. (1962): A syndrome due to transient or changing heart block. *Brit. Med. J.*, **2**:1638.

241. FREUND, H. A., SOKOLOV, R. (1939): Bundle branch block; criteria of classification, diagnosis and prognosis: study of 210 cases, with follow-up data. *Arch. Intern. Med. (Chicago)*, **63**:318.

242. FREY, W. G. (1963): Paroxysmal cardiac arrest. Report of a case with simultaneous atrio-ventricular standstill presumably due to carcinoma of the lung and responding to radiation therapy. *Dis. Chest*, **43**:551.

243. FRIEDBERG, C. K. (1956): *Diseases of the Heart.* London, Saunders, pp. 730 & 837.

244. FRIEDBERG, C. K., DONOSO, E. (1960): Arrhythmias and conduction disturbances due to digitalis. *Progr. Cardiov. Dis.*, **2**:408.

245. FRIEDBERG, C. K., DONOSO, E., STEIN, W. G. (1964): Non-surgical acquired heart block. *Ann. N.Y. Acad. Sci.*, 111:835.

246. FRIEDBERG, C. K., DONOSO, E., STEIN, W. G., KAHN, M., LITWAK, R. (1965): The role of bradycardia in the retention of sodium and water in complete heart block with and without failure in human beings. *Amer. Heart J.*, 69:293.

247. FRIEDBERG, C. K., KAHN, M., SCHEUER, J., BLEITER, S. (1960): Adams-Stokes syndrome associated with chronic heart block. Treatment with corticosteroids. *JAMA*, 172:1146.

248. FRIESE, G., DITTMAR, H. A. (1961): Über die langfristige elektrische Reizung des Herzens. *Verh. Deutsch. Ges. Kreislaufforsch*, 27:326.

249. FROMENT, R., DE GEVIGNEY, D., PERRIN, A., NORMAND, J. (1959): L'angine de poitrine functionelle du bloc A-V. *Arch. Mal. Coeur*, 52:481.

250. FROMMER, P. L. (1965): Studies on coupled pacing technique and some comments on paired electrical stimulation. *Bull. N.Y. Acad. Med.*, 41:670.

251. FROMMER, P. L., ROBINSON, B. F., BRAUNWALD, E. (1965): Suppression of Ouabain-induced ventricular arrhythmias by paired electrical stimulation (Abstract). *Circulation*, 32 (Suppl. 2):91.

252. FURMAN, S. (1965): Cardiac pacing. (Appraisal and reappraisal of cardiac therapy.) *Amer. Heart. J.*, 70:830.

253. FURMAN, S. (1965): In discussion. *J. Thorac. Cardiov. Surg.*, 50:865.

254. FURMAN, S., ESCHER, D. J. W., SCHWEDEL, J. W., SOLOMAN, N., RUBINSTEIN, B. (1964): Motion factors producing breaks in implanted cardiac pacemaker leads. *Surg. Forum*, 15:248.

255. FURMAN, S., ESCHER, D. J. W., SCHWEDEL, J. B., SOLOMAN, N., RUBINSTEIN, B. (1965): Implanted cardiac pacemakers: motion factors producing lead breaks. *Amer. J. Surg.*, 109:743.

256. FURMAN, S., RADDI, W. J., ESCHER, D. J. W., DENIZE, A., SCHWEDEL, J. B., HURWITT, E. S. (1965): Rechargeable pacemaker for direct myocardial implantation. *Arch. Surg.*, 91:796.

257. FURMAN, S., ROBINSON, G. (1958): The use of an intracardiac pacemaker in the correction of total heart block. *Surg. Forum*, 9:245.

258. FURMAN, S., SCHWEDEL, J. B. (1959): An intracardiac pacemaker for Stokes-Adams seizures. *New Eng. J. Med.*, 261:943.

259. FURMAN, S., SCHWEDEL, J. B., ROBINSON, G., HURWITT, E. S. (1961): Use of an intracardiac pacemaker in the control of heart block. *Surgery*, 49:98.

260. GAAL, P. G., GOLDBERG, S. J., MINDE, L. M. (1964): Cardiac output as a function of ventricular rate in a patient with complete heart block. *Circulation*, 30:592.

261. GADBOYS, H. L., WISOFF, B. G., LITWAK, R. S. (1964): Surgical treatment of complete heart block. *JAMA*, 189:97.

262. GASKELL, W. H. (1883): On the innervation of the heart, with special reference to the heart of a tortoise. *J. Physiol.*, 4:43.

263. GAZES, P. C., CULLER, R. M., TABER, E., KELLY, T. E. (1965): Congenital familial cardiac conduction defects. *Circulation*, 32:32.

264. GERBAUX, A. (1965): Sur certains aspects de l'activation cardiaque au cours du bloc auriculo-ventriculaire traité par stimulation électrique. *Cardiologia (Basel)*, 46:268.

265. GERBAUX, A., LENÈGRE, J. (1964): Observations sur les rythmes à double commande (sinusale et par électrostimulation) constatés après implantation d'un stimulateur interne pour maladie d'Adams-Stokes. *Arch. Mal. Coeur,* **57**:286.

266. GERBAUX, A., MOREAU, P., LENÈGRE, J. (1964): Le traitement du bloc auriculo-ventriculaire par stimulateur électrique interne. *Arch. Mal. Coeur,* **57**:273.

267. GERBEZIUS, M. (1719): *Appendix ad Ephemeridum Academiae Carsaro-Leopoldino-Carolinae Naturae Curiosum in Germania.* Nuremberg, 1719, Centuriae vii et viii, p. 23. Reported in Mayor, R. H.: *Classic Descriptions of Disease,* 3rd ed. Springfield, Thomas, 1945.

268. GERBODE, F., KERTH, W., KEEN, W., OGATA, T., POPPER, R. W., OSBORN, J. J. (1963): Surgical heart block. *Arch. Surg.,* **86**:890.

269. GIBSON, J. R. (1838): Case of fits with very slow pulse. *London Med. Gaz.,* **23**:123, 155.

270. GIBSON, T. C., HUGHES, J. P. (1956): Stokes-Adams attacks in acute rheumatic carditis. *Brit. Heart J.,* **18**:427.

271. GILBERT, G., TARDIF, B., LEPAGE, G., DAVID, P. (1963): Évolution d'un bloc auriculo-ventriculaire complet postchirurgical chez une fillette de six ans. *Laval Méd.,* **34**:1198.

272. GILCHRIST, A. R. (1933): Action of atropine in complete heart-block. *Quart. J. Med.,* **2**(n.s.):483.

273. GILCHRIST, A. R. (1958): Clinical aspects of high-grade heart block. *Scot. Med. J.,* **3**:53.

274. GILGENKRANTZ, P. (1964): In discussion. *Arch. Mal. Coeur,* **57**:315.

275. GILMORE, J. P., SARNOFF, S. J., MITCHELL, J. H., LINDEN, R. J. (1963): Synchronicity of ventricular contraction: observations comparing hemodynamic effects of atrial and ventricular pacing. *Brit. Heart J.,* **25**:299.

276. GLASS, H. I. (1965): Problems associated with the design of implantable electronic devices. *Resuscitation & Cardiac Pacing.* (Proc. of Conference, Glasgow, March, 1964). London, Cassell, p. 207.

277. GLASS, H., SHAW, G., SMITH, G. (1963): An implantable cardiac pacemaker allowing rate control. *Lancet,* **1**:684.

278. GLENN, W. W. L., HAGEMAN, J. H., MAURO, A., EISENBERG, L., FLANIGAN, S., HARVARD, M. (1964): Electrical stimulation of excitable tissue by radio frequency transmission. *Ann. Surg.,* **160**:338.

279. GLENN, W. W. L., MAURO, A., LONGO, E., LAVIETES, P. H., MACKAY, F. J. (1959): Remote stimulation of the heart by radio-frequency transmission. Clinical application to a patient with Stokes-Adams syndrome. *New Eng. J. Med.,* **261**:948.

280. GOCHBERG, S. H. (1964): Congenital heart block. *Amer. J. Obstet. Gynec.,* **88**:238.

281. GOETZ, R. H. (1963): Bipolar catheter electrode as temporary pacemaker in Stokes-Adams syndrome. *Surg. Gynec. Obstet.,* **116**:712.

282. GONIN, A. (1938): Le syndrome de Morgagni-Adams-Stokes (vertiges et syncopes dans la dissociation auriculo-ventriculaire). *Arch. Mal. Coeur,* **31**:1172.

283. GORDON, A. J. (1965): Catheter pacing in complete heart block: Techniques and complications. *JAMA,* **193**:1091.

284. GOWANS, J. D. C. (1960): Complete heart block with Stokes-Adams syndrome due to rheumatoid heart disease. *New Eng. J. Med.*, 262:1012.

285. GRASSBERGER, A. (1929): Klinische, elektrokardiographische und histologische Untersuchung eines Falles von Adams-Stokesscher Erkrankung. *Z. Klin. Med.*, 112:389.

286. GRAYBIEL, A., SPRAGUE, H. B. (1933): Bundle branch block; analysis of 395 cases. *Amer. J. Med. Sci.*, 185:395.

287. GRAYBIEL, A., WHITE, P. D. (1936): Complete auriculo-ventricular dissociation. A clinical study. *Amer. J. Med. Sci.*, 192:334.

288. GREATBATCH, W. (1959): Medical cardiac pacemaker. United States Patent Office, 3,057,356. Oct. 9, 1959.

289. GREATBATCH, W. (1966): Electrochemical polarization of physiological electrodes. In press.

290. GREATBATCH, W. (1965): Symposium on electrical control of cardiac activity. Buffalo, May, 1965, unpublished.

291. GREATBATCH, W. (1965): Personal communication.

292. GREENE, J. A., BENNETT, A. W. (1945): Acute rheumatic disease in the aged, with respect of case with Stokes-Adams syndrome treated with paredrine. *Amer. Heart J.*, 30:415.

293. GREINER, T. H., GARB, S. (1950): The influence of drugs on the irritability and automaticity of heart muscle. *J. Pharmacol. Exp. Ther.*, 98:215.

294. GRIFFITH, G. C., ZINN, W. J., VURAL, I. L. (1965): Familial cardiomyopathy. Heart block and Stokes-Adams attacks treated by pacemaker implantation. *Amer. J. Cardiol.*, 16:267.

295. GROEDEL, F. M., KISCH, B. (1942): Morgagni-Adams-Stokes syndrome: what does it represent? *Cardiologia (Basel)*, 6:43.

296. GRONDIN, P., LEPAGE, G., GUIGNARD, J., KARAMEHMET, A. (1964): Evaluation of cardiac drugs in the presence of an electrical pacemaker. *J. Thorac. Cardiov. Surg.*, 48:941.

297. GROSS, L., FRIED, B. M. (1936): Lesions in auriculo-ventricular conduction system occurring in rheumatic fever. *Amer. J. Path.*, 12:31.

298. GUYER, P. B. (1964): Stokes-Adams attacks precipitated by hypokalemia. (Medical memorandum). *Brit. Med. J.*, 2:427.

299. HABER, E., LEATHAM, A. (1965): Splitting of heart sounds from ventricular asynchrony in bundle-branch block, ventricular ectopic beats, and artificial pacing. *Brit. Heart J.*, 27:691.

300. HAGEMAN, J. (1964): In discussion. *J. Thorac. Cardiov. Surg.*, 48:525.

301. HAHN, C. (1965): Stimulateurs électriques. *Cardiologia (Basel)*, 46:246.

302. HALLÉN, A., NORDLAND, S., WARVSTEN, B. (1965): Pacemaker treatment in Adams-Stokes syndrome. *Acta Soc. Med. Upsal.*, 70:17.

303. HAMER, J., SOWTON, E. (1965): Cardiac output after beta-adrenergic blockade in ischemic heart disease. *Brit. Heart J.*, 27:892.

304. HAN, J., GARCIA DE JALON, P., MOE, G. K. (1964): Adrenergic effects on ventricular vulnerability. *Circ. Res.*, 14:516.

305. HARRIS, A., BLUESTONE, R. (1966): Artificial pacing for slow heart rates following acute myocardial infarction. *Brit. Heart J.*, 28:631.

306. HARRIS, A., BLUESTONE, R., BUSBY, E., DAVIES, G., LEATHAM, A., SIDDONS, H., SOWTON, E. (1965): The management of heart block. *Brit. Heart J.*, 27:469.

307. HARRIS, A. M., SLEIGHT, P., DREW, C. E. (1965): The diagnosis and treatment of aortic stenosis complicated by heart block. *Brit. Heart J.*, 27:560.

√308. HARRIS, C. W., HULBURT, J. C., FLOYD, W. L., ORGAIN, E. S. (1965): Percutaneous technic for cardiac pacing with a platinum-tipped electrode catheter. *Amer. J. Cardiol.*, 15:48.

309. HARRIS, R. S., BEEKER, D. J., RODENSKY, P., WOLCOTT, M., DICK, M., WASSERMAN, F. (1963): Symptomatic paroxysmal pacemaker-induced ventricular tachycardia. *Amer. J. Cardiol.*, 11:403.

310. HARRISON, C. V., LENNOX, B. (1948): Heart block in osteitis deformans. *Brit. Heart J.*, 10:167.

311. HAUPT, G. J., MYERS, R. N., DALY, J. W., BIRKHEAD, N. C. (1963): Implanted cardiac pacemakers of variable frequency. *JAMA*, 185:87.

312. HAUPT, G. J., MYERS, R. N., PERRIL, C. V., BIRKHEAD, N. C. (1963): Human tissue response to long term implanted cardiac pacemaker-electrode system. *Surg. Gynec. Obstet.*, 117:484.

313. HAYES, C. (1965): Symposium on electrical control of cardiac activity. Buffalo, May, 1965, unpublished.

314. HAYWOOD, J., WYMAN, M. G. (1965): Effects of isoproterenol, ephedrine, and potassium on artificial pacemaker failure (Abstract). *Circulation*, 32 (Suppl. 2):110.

315. HEINECKER, R. (1963): Zur intravenösen Behandlung des Morgagni-Adams-Stokesschen Syndroms mit Na-Laktat und Alupent. *Thoraxchirurgie*, 11:170.

316. HERBIET, J., DE MAY, D., CLOETENS, W. (1960): Arrêts cardiaques tres prolongés au cours d'un syndrome d'Adams-Stokes. Correction par pacemaker électrique. *Acta Cardiol. (Brux.)*, 15:506.

317. HERNANDEZ-PIERRETI, O., MORALES-ROCHA, J., ACQUATELLA, H., ANDERSON, R., PIMENTEL, R. (1965): Pacemaker implantation in chronic Chagas' heart disease complicated by Adams-Stokes syndrome. *Amer. J. Cardiol.*, 16:115.

318. HERROD, C. E., LEE, R. H., GOGGANS, W. H., McCOMBS, R. K., GERBODE, F. (1952): Control of heart action by repetitive electrical stimuli. *Ann. Surg.*, 136:510.

319. HERSHBERG, P. J., GRÄDEL, F. O., AKUTSU, T., KANTROWITZ, A. (1965): Pathologic effects of recharging Nickel-Cadmium cells through intact skin. A prelim. report. *Trans. Amer. Soc. Artif. Intern. Organs*, 11:143.

320. HILL, P. C. J. (1966): Personal communication from research department, British Broadcasting Corp.

321. HIRSCH, H. H., SCIOR, H., ZIPF, K. E. (1964): Über die Pericardiotomia inferior longitudinalis (Sauerbruch) als Zugang zum Herzen für die Schrittmacherimplantation beim Morgagni-Adams-Stokes-Syndrom. *Bruns Beitr. Klin. Chir.*, 208:446.

322. HIS, W. (1893): *Die Thätigkeit des embryonalen Herzens und deren Bedeutung für die Lehre von der Herzbewegung beim Erwachsenen.* Curschmann (H.) ed. Arbeiten aus der medicinischen Klinik zu Leipzig. Leipzig, Vogel, pp. 14-49.

323. HOFFMAN, B. F. (1965): In discussion. *Bull. N.Y. Acad. Med.*, 41:724.

324. HOFFMAN, B. F. (1965): In discussion. *Bull. N.Y. Acad. Med.*, 41:734.

325. HOFFMAN, B. F., BARTELSTONE, H. J., SCHERLAG, B. J., CRANEFIELD, P. F. (1965): Effects of postextrasystolic potentiation on normal and failing hearts. *Bull. N.Y. Acad. Med.*, **41**:498.

326. HOFFMAN, B. F., BINDLER, E., SUCKLING, E. E. (1956): Postextrasystolic potentiation of contraction in cardiac muscle. *Amer. J. Physiol.*, **185**:95.

327. HOFFMAN, B. F., CRANEFIELD, P. F. (1960): *The Electrophysiology of the Heart.* New York, McGraw.

328. HOFFMAN, B. F., CRANEFIELD, P. F. (1964): The physiological basis of cardiac arrhythmias. *Amer. J. Med.*, **37**:670.

329. HOFFMAN, B. F., GORIN, E. F., WAX, F. S., SIEBENS, A. A., BROOKS, C. McC. (1951): Vulnerability to fibrillation and the ventricular-excitability curve. *Amer. J. Physiol.*, **167**:88.

330. HOFFMANN, B. F., SUCKLING, E. E., BROOKS, C. McC. (1955): Vulnerability of the dog ventricle and effects of defibrillation. *Circ. Res.*, **3**:147.

331. HOFFMAN, F. G., LEIGHT, L. (1965): Complete atrioventricular block associated with rheumatoid disease. *Amer. J. Cardiol.*, **16**:585.

332. HOFMANN, H. (1955): Herzrhythmusstörungen bei Adams-Stokesschem Syndrom und ihre Behandlung. *Z. Ges. Inn. Med.*, **10**:516.

333. HOLBERTON, T. H. (1841): A case of slow pulse with fainting fits. *Med. Chir. Trans.*, **24**:76.

334. HOLCOMB, W. G., ANAGNOSTOPOULOS, C. E., GLENN, W. W. L. (1965): A new method of determining tissue resistance by the reflectometer principle for use with implanted R.F. pacemaker receivers. *Trans. N.Y. Acad. Sci.*, **27**:894.

335. HOLMES, L. B., SPACH, M. S., CANENT, R. V., BROWN, I. W., WHALEN, R. E. (1964): Unusual observations during pacemaker therapy for complete heart block. *Amer. J. Cardiol.*, **13**:828.

336. HOLMGREN, A., JONSSON, B., LEVANDER, M., LINDERHOLM, H., SJÖSTRAND, T., STROM, G. (1957): Low physical working capacity in suspected heart cases due to inadequate adjustment of peripheral blood flow (Vaso regularity asthenia). *Acta Med. Scand.*, **158**:413.

337. HOLMGREN, A., JONSSON, B., SJÖSTRAND, T. (1960): Circulatory data in normal subjects at rest and during exercise in recumbent position, with special reference to the stroke volume at different work intensities. *Acta Physiol. Scand.*, **49**:343.

338. HOLMGREN, A., KARLBERG, P., PERNOW, B. (1959): Circulatory adaptation at rest and during muscular work in patients with complete heart block. *Acta Med. Scand.*, **164**:119.

339. HOLSWADE, G. R., LINARDOS, C. (1961): Induction pacemaker for complete heart block (Abstract). *Circulation*, **24**:958.

340. HOLSWADE, G. R., LINARDOS, C. (1962): Induction pacemaker for control of complete heart block. *J. Thorac. Cardiov. Surg.*, **44**:246.

341. HOPPS, J. A. (1964): Cardiac resuscitation: the present status of defibrillation and stimulation techniques. *Canad. Med. Ass. J.*, **90**:122.

342. HOPPS, J. A., BIGELOW, W. G. (1954): Electrical treatment of cardiac arrest: a cardiac stimulator-defibrillator. *Surgery*, **36**:833.

343. HÖRMANN, J. (1952): Zur Therapie des Adams-Stokesschen Syndroms. *Deutsch. Med. Wschr.*, **77**:1026.

344. Huchard, H. (1899): *Traité clinique du coeur et de l'aorte.* Paris, p. 395, Vol. 1.

345. Hudson, R. E. B. (1965): *Cardiovascular Pathology.* London, Arnold.

346. Hudson, R. E. B. (1963): Personal communication.

347. Hunter, S. W., Roth, N. A., Bernardez, D., Noble, J. L. (1959): A bipolar myocardial electrode for complete heart block. *J. Lancet,* 79:506.

348. Hunter, S. W., Roth, N. A., Bernardez, D., Noble, J. L. (1961): The platform bipolar myocardial electrode for prolonged treatment of total heart block. *J. Lancet,* 81:115.

349. Huo, L.-C., Fang, T-P., Yang, M-H., Yen, H-C., Wu, H-N, Liu, C-Y., Ch'en, H-P. (1964): Experience with two types pacemakers. *Chin. Med. J. (Peking),* 83:307.

350. Hurwitt, E. S. (1960): In discussion. *J. Thorac. Cardiov. Surg.,* 40:296.

351. Hurwitt, E. S. (1964): In discussion. *Ann. Surg.,* 160:363.

352. Hyman, A. S. (1932): Resuscitation of the stopped heart by intracardial therapy. *Arch. Intern. Med. (Chicago),* 50:283.

353. Ide, L. W. (1950): The clinical aspects of complete auriculoventricular heart block: a clinical analysis of 71 cases. *Ann. Intern. Med.,* 32:510.

354. Ikkos, D., Hanson, J. S. (1960): Response to exercise in congenital complete atrioventricular block. *Circulation,* 22:583.

355. Innes, I. R., Nickerson, M. (1965): Drugs acting on postganglionic adrenergic nerve endings and structures innervated by them (sympathomimetic drugs). In Goodman, L. S., and Gilman, A.: *The Pharmacological Basis of Therapeutics,* 3d ed. New York, Macmillan, p. 477.

356. Innes, I. R., Nickerson, M. (1965): Drugs inhibiting the action of acetylcholine on structures innervated by post ganglionic parasympathetic nerves (antimuscarinic or atropinic drugs). In Goodman, L. S., and Gilman, A.: *The Pharmacological Basis of Therapeutics,* 3d ed. New York, Macmillan, p. 521.

357. International Nickel Co. (Mond)Ltd., Development & Research Department. (1965): Platinum tipped catheter from pacemaker. PM/D 1005, Lab. Report. No. 1.

358. Jackson, A., Youmans, R., McCaughey, H., Pickard, C. M., Faw, M. (1959): The cardiac pacemaker: Its use for more than seven months in one patient. *J. Kansas Med. Soc.,* 58:735.

359. James, T. N. (1962): Observations on the cardiovascular involvement, including the cardiac conduction system, in progressive muscular dystrophy. *Amer. Heart J.,* 63:48.

360. James, T. N. (1964): An etiologic concept concerning the obscure myocardiopathies. *Progr. Cardiov. Dis.,* 7:43.

361. James, T. N., Reynolds, E. W. (1963): Pathology of cardiac conduction system in a case of diphtheria associated with atrial arrhythmias and heart block. *Circulation,* 28:263.

362. James, T. N., Rupe, C. E., Monto, R. W. (1965): Pathology of cardiac conduction system in systemic lupus erythematosus. *Ann. Intern. Med.,* 63:402.

363. Jennings, E. R., Hightower, J. A., Addison, B. A. (1963): The percutaneous insertion of an intracardiac electrode in the treatment of complete heart block. *Amer. Surg.,* 29:553.

364. JOHANSSON, B. (1960): A case of Adams-Stokes attacks disappearing after cholecystectomy. *Acta Med. Scand.*, **168**:219.
365. JOHANSSON, B. W. (1961): Adams-Stokes attacks precipitated by swallowing in a patient with bronchial carcinoma. *Amer. J. Cardiol.*, **7**:874.
366. JOHANSSON, B. W. (1961): Adams-Stokes syndrome. A review and follow-up study of forty-two cases. *Amer. J. Cardiol.*, **8**:76.
367. JOHANSSON, B. W., KARNELL, J., MALM, A., SIEVERS, J., SWEDBERG, J. (1963): Electrocardiographic studies on patients with an artificial pacemaker. *Brit. Heart J.*, **25**:514.
368. JOHNSON, A. L., KLASSEN, G. A., McGREGOR, M., DOHELL, A. R. C. (1963): Long-term electrical stimulation of the heart in Stokes-Adams disease. *Canad. Med. Ass. J.*, **89**:683.
369. JUDGE, R. D. (1965): Communication to British Cardiac Society, Nov., 1965, London.
370. JUDGE, R. D. (1965): Personal communication.
371. JUDGE, R. D., PRESTON, T. A., LUCCESI, B. R., BOWERS, D. L. (1966): Myocardial threshold in patients with artificial pacemakers. *Amer. J. Cardiol.*, **18**:83.
372. JUDGE, R. D., WILSON, W. S., SIEGEL, J. H. (1964): Hemodynamic studies in patients with implanted cardiac pacemakers. *New Eng. J. Med.*, **270**:1391.
373. JUE, K. L., RUTTENBERG, H. D., ANDERSON, R. C., ADAMS, P. (1965): Ventricular response to exercise and isoproterenol in atrioventricular dissociation due to congenital or acquired apparent complete and advanced heart block in children (Abstract). *Circulation*, **32** (Suppl. 2): 120.
374. JULIAN, D. G., VALENTINE, P. A., MILLER, G. G. (1964): Disturbances of rate, rhythm and conduction in acute myocardial infarction. *Amer. J. Med.*, **37**:915.
375. JULKUNEN, H., LUOMANMÄKI, K. (1964): Complete heart block in rheumatoid (ankylosing) spondylitis. *Acta Med. Scand.*, **176**:401.
376. KAHN, D. R., STERN, A., SIGMANN, J., SLOAN, H. (1965): An emergency method of handling broken pacemaker wires in children. *Amer. J. Cardiol.*, **15**:404.
377. KAIJSER, L., SOWTON, G. E. (1966): The influence of heart rate on maximum working capacity in patients with artificial pacemakers. In press.
378. KAINDL, F., RUMMELHARDT, K. (1956): Zur Therapie rezidivierender Adams-Stokes-Anfälle. *Wien. Klin. Wschr.*, **68**:583.
379. KAISER, G. C., WILLMAN, V. L., COOPER, T., HANLON, C. R. (1965): Artificial pacemakers in the treatment of heart block: importance of supplemental drug therapy (Abstract). *Circulation*, **32** (Suppl. 2):121.
380. KANTROWITZ, A. (1964): Problems in the clinical use of implantable pacemakers. *J. Cardiov. Surg.*, **5**:668.
381. KANTROWITZ, A. (1964): Implantable cardiac pacemakers. *Ann. N. Y. Acad. Sci.*, **111**:1049.
382. KANTROWITZ, A. (1964): In discussion. *Ann. N. Y. Acad. Sci.*, **111**:1110.
383. KANTROWITZ, A. (1964): In discussion. *J. Thorac. Cardiov. Surg.*, **48**:525.
384. KANTROWITZ, A. (1965): Symposium on electrical control of cardiac activity. Buffalo, May, 1965, unpublished.

385. Kantrowitz, A. (1965): In discussion. *Arch. Surg.*, **91**:815.
386. Kantrowitz, A., Cohen, R., Raillard, H., Schmidt, J., Feldman, D. S. (1962): The treatment of complete heart block with an implanted, controllable pacemaker. *Surg. Gynec. Obstet.*, **115**:415.
387. Karlöf, I. (1965): Symposium on electrical control of cardiac activity. Buffalo, May, 1965, unpublished.
388. Katz, L. N. (1965): Effects of artificially induced paired and coupled beats. *Bull. N. Y. Acad. Med.*, **41**:428.
389. Kay, H. B. (1948): Ventricular complexes in heart block. *Brit. Heart J.*, **10**:177.
390. Keith, A., Flack, M. (1907): The form and nature of muscular connections between the primary divisions of the vertebrate heart. *J. Anat.*, **41**:172.
391. Keller, J. W. (1964): In discussion. *Ann. N. Y. Acad. Sci.*, **111**:1110.
392. Keller, J. W. (1965): Symposium on electrical control of cardiac activity. Buffalo, May, 1965, unpublished.
393. Kempen, R. R., Van Horn, G. (1963): Effects of antiarrhythmic drugs on external fibrillation and defibrillation thresholds. *Cardiov. Res. Cent. Bull.*, **1**:116.
394. Kent, A. F. S. (1893): Researches on the structure and function of the mammalian heart. *J. Physiol.*, **14**:233.
395. Kerr, W. J., Bender, W. L. (1921-1922): Paroxysmal ventricular fibrillation with cardiac recovery in a case of auricular fibrillation and complete heart-block while under quinidine sulphate therapy. *Heart*, **9**:269.
396. Kerth, W. J., Kelly, J. J. (1965): Experience with paired pacing in experimental canine heart failure. *Bull. N. Y. Acad. Med.*, **41**:646.
397. Kieny, R., Sacrez, A., Cuny, A., Fontaine, R. (1964): Le traitement chirurgical du pouls lent par dissociation auriculo-ventriculaire. *Strasbourg Med.*, **15**:777.
398. Kimball, J. T., Killip, T. (1965): A simple bedside method for transvenous intracardiac pacing. *Amer. Heart J.*, **70**:35.
399. Kimball, J. T., Navab, A., LaDue, J. S. (1965): Surgery of the colon in a patient with Adams-Stokes disease. Use of an intracardiac electrode pacer. *JAMA*, **192**:1166.
400. King, B. G. (1934): The effect of electric shock on heart action with special reference to varying susceptibility in different parts of the cardiac cycle. Ph.D. thesis, Columbia University, New York, Aberdeen Press.
401. Kiss, P. (1934): Elektrokardiogramm des während Diphtherie auftretenden Adams-Stokesschen Anfälles. *Z. Ges. Exp. Med.*, **93**:619.
402. Klassen, G. A., Broadhurst, C., Peretz, D. I., Johnson, A. L. (1963): Cardiac resuscitation in 126 medical patients using external cardiac massage. *Lancet*, **1**:1290.
403. Klotz, D. H., Lister, J. W., Jomain, S. L., Hoffman, B. F., Stuckey, J. H. (1963): The most effective site to implant pacemaker wires following right ventriculotomy and heart block. *Trans. Amer. Soc. Artif. Intern. Organs*, **9**:170.
404. Knuckey, L., McDonald, R., Sloman, G. (1965): A method of testing implanted cardiac pacemakers. *Brit. Heart J.*, **27**:483.
405. Kohler, F. P., Mackinney, C. C. (1965): Cardiac pacemakers in electrosurgery. (Letter). *JAMA*, **193**:855.

406. Kornel, L. (1958): A case of calcified ventricular aneurysm with progressive heart block. *Cardiologia (Basel)*, 32:101.
407. Lagergren, H., Johansson, L., Schüller, H., Kugelberg, J., Bojs, G., Alestig, K., Linder, E., Borst, H. G., Schandig, A., Giebel, O., Harms, H., Rodewald, G., Scheppokat, K. D. (1966): 305 cases of permanent intravenous pacemaker treatment for Adams-Stokes syndrome. *Surgery*, 59:494.
408. Lagergren, H. (1965): Personal communication.
409. Lagergren, H., Johansson, L. (1963): Intracardiac stimulation for complete heart block. *Acta Chir. Scand.*, 125:562.
410. Lagergren, H., Johansson, L., Landegren, J., Edhag, O. (1965): One hundred cases of treatment for Adams-Stokes syndrome with permanent intravenous pacemaker. *J. Thorac. Cardiovas. Surg.*, 50:710.
411. Lancaster, J. F., Leonard, J. J., Leon, D. F., Kroetz, F. W., Shaver, J. A. (1965): The experimental production of coronary sinus rhythm in man. *Amer. Heart J.*, 70:89.
412. Landegren, J. (1964): In discussion. *Ann. N. Y. Acad. Sci.*, 111:1043.
413. Landergren, J., Djurck, G. (1963): The clinical assessment and treatment of complete heart block and Adams-Stokes attacks. *Medicine*, 42:171.
414. Lands, A. M., Howard, J. W. (1952): Comparative study of effects of l-arterenol, epinephrine, and isopropylarterenol on heart. *J. Pharmacol. Exp. Ther.*, 106:65.
415. Langedorf, R., Pick, A. (1965). Observations on the clinical use of paired stimulation of the heart. *Bull. N. Y. Acad. Med.*, 41:535.
416. Laranja, F. S., Dias, E., Nobrega, G., Mianda, A. (1956): Chagas' disease: a clinical, epidemiologic and pathologic study. *Circulation*, 14:1035.
417. Laslett, E. E. (1909): Syncopal attacks, associated with prolonged arrest of the whole heart. *Quart. J. Med.*, 2:347.
418. Lasry, J. E., Benchimol, A., Baronofsky, I. D., Carvalho, F. R. (1963): Cardiovascular hemodynamics and the internally placed cardiac pacemaker. *Amer. J. Cardiol.*, 11:399.
419. Lau, F. Y. K., Cosby, R. S., Cafferky, E., Bilitch, M. (1965): Factors affecting survival in 100 paced patients with complete heart block (Abstract). *Circulation*, 32 (Suppl. 2):132.
420. Laurent, D., Bolene-Williams, C., Williams, F. L., Katz, L. N. (1956): Effects of heart rate on coronary flow and cardiac oxygen consumption. *Amer. J. Physiol.*, 185:355.
421. Law, R. (1840): Diseases of the brain dependent on diseases of the heart. *Dublin J.*, 17:201.
422. Lawrence, G. H. (1964): Complete heart block: experience with a totally implantable pacemaker. *Amer. Surg.*, 30:840.
423. Lawrence, G. H., King, R. L., Paine, R. M., Spencer, M. P., Hughes, M. L. (1964): Complete heart block. Patient selection and response to implantation of electronic pacemakers. *JAMA*, 190:1093.
424. Lawrence, G. H., Paine, R. M., Hughes, M. L. (1965): Management of complications associated with the use of implantable electronic cardiac pacemakers for the relief of complete heart block. *Amer. J. Surg.*, 110:177.

425. LEAGUS, C. J., PEMBERTON, A. H., NARODICK, B. G. (1966): Lobectomy in a patient with an internal cardiac pacemaker. *J. Thorac. Cardiov. Surg.*, **51**:268.
426. LEATHAM, A., COOK, P., DAVIES, J. G. (1956): External electric stimulator for treatment of ventricular standstill. *Lancet*, **2**:1185.
427. LEE, J. K., LEWIS, J. A. (1962): Myxoedema with complete A-V block and Adams-Stokes disease abolished with thyroid medication. *Brit. Heart J.*, **24**:253.
428. LEGROS, J., NASSHEUER, R. (1949): Syndrome d'Adams-Stokes après un coqueluche chez une enfant de 12 ans. Étude électrocardiographique. *Acta Paediat. Belg.*, **3**:238.
429. LEMBERG, L., CASTELLANOS, A., BERKOVITS, B. V. (1965): Pacemaking on demand in A. V. block. *JAMA*, **191**:12.
430. LENÈGRE, J. (1962): Les blocs auriculoventriculaires complets chroniques. Étude des causes et des lesions à propos de 37 cas. *Mal. Cardiov.*, **3**:311.
431. LENÈGRE, J. (1964): Etiology and pathology of bilateral bundle branch block in relation to complete heart block. *Progr. Cardiov. Dis.*, **6**:409.
432. LENÈGRE, J. (1964): Traitements actuels du bloc auriculo-ventriculaire complet. *Rev. Prat.*, **14**:2037.
433. LENÈRGE, J. (1965): Les lesions du système de His-Tawara dans les blocs auriculo-ventriculaires d'un haut degrè. *Cardiologia (Basel)*, **46**:261.
434. LENÈGRE, J., MOREAU, P. (1963): Le bloc auriculo-ventriculaire chronique. Étude anatomique, clinique et histologique. *Arch. Mal. Coeur*, **56**:867.
435. LEON-SOTOMAYER, L., MYERS, W. S., HYATT, K. H., HYMAN, A. L. (1962): Digitalis-induced ventricular asystole treated by an intracardiac pacemaker. *Amer. J. Cardiol.*, **10**:298.
436. LEV, M. (1960): The conduction system. In Gould, S. E. (ed.): *Pathology of the Heart*, 2nd ed., Springfield, Thomas.
437. LEV, M. (1964): Anatomic basis for atrioventricular block. *Amer. J. Med.*, **37**:742.
438. LEV, M. (1964): The pathology of complete atrioventricular block. *Progr. Cardiov. Dis.*, **6**:317.
439. LEVITSKY, S., GLENN, W. W. L., MAURO, A., EISENBERG, L., SMITH, P. W. (1962): Long-term stimulation of the heart with radio-frequency transmission. *Surgery*, **52**:64.
440. LEVOWITZ, B. S., FORD, W. B., SMITH, J. W. (1960): The use of direct stimulating myocardial electrodes in complete atrioventricular block. *J. Thorac. Cardiov. Surg.*, **40**:283.
441. LEVY, L., ALBERT, H. M. (1964): Therapy of complete heart block complicating recent myocardial infarction. *JAMA*, **187**:617.
442. LEWIS, D. H., WARNER, H. F., ALLAN, M. B. (1961): Direct measurement of human cardiac excitability (Abstract). *J. Clin. Invest.*, **40**:1058.
443. LEWIS, J. K. (1958): Stokes Adams disease. *Arch. Intern. Med. (Chicago)*, **101**:130.
444. LEWIS, T., ROTHSCHILD, M. A. (1915): The spread of the excitatory process in the vertebrate heart. (Part III. Dog's ventricle). *Phil. Trans. Roy. Soc. London*, **207**:247.

445. Leys, D. G. (1945): Heart block following diphtheria. *Brit. Heart J.*, 7:57.
446. Lichter, I., Borrie, J., Miller, W. M. (1965): Radio-frequency hazards with cardiac pacemakers. *Brit. Med. J.*, 1:1513.
447. Lillehei, C. W. (1964): In discussion. *Ann. N. Y. Acad. Sci.*, 111:951.
448. Lillehei, C. W. (1964): In discussion. *Ann. N. Y. Acad. Sci.*, 111:959.
449. Lillehei, C. W. (1966): Personal communication.
450. Lillehei, C. W., Bilgutay, A. M., Varco, R. L., Long, D. M., Bakken, E. E., Sellers, R. D. (1962): The implantable cardiac pacemaker: present status in the treatment of complete heart block with Adams-Stokes syndrome. *J. Lancet*, 82:68.
451. Lillehei, C. W., Cruz, A. B., Johnstude, I., Sellers, R. D. (1965): A new method of assessing the state of charge of implanted cardiac pacemaker batteries. *Amer. J. Cardiol.*, 16:717.
452. Lillehei, C. W., Gott, V. L., Hodges, P. C., Long, D. M., Bakken, E. E. (1960): Transistor pacemaker for treatment of complete atrioventricular dissociation. *JAMA*, 172:2006.
453. Lillehei, C. W., Levy, M. J., Bonnabeau, R. C., Long, D. M., Sellers, R. D. (1964): The use of a myocardial electrode and pacemaker in the management of acute postoperative and postinfarction complete heart block. *Surgery*, 56:463.
454. Lillehei, C. W., Levy, M. J., Bonnabeau, R. C., Long, D. M., Sellers, R. D. (1964): Direct wire electrical stimulation for acute post-surgical and post-infarction complete heart block. *Ann. N. Y. Acad. Sci.*, 111:938.
455. Lillehei, C. W., Sellers, R. D., Bonnabeau, R. C., Eliot, R. S. (1963): Chronic post-surgical complete heart block. *J. Thorac. Cardiov. Surg.*, 46:436.
456. Lilly, J. C., Hughes, J. R., Alword, E. C., Galki, T. W. (1955): Brief, non-injurious electric waveform for stimulation of the brain. *Science*, 121:468.
457. Lind, J., Wegelius, C., Lichtenstein, H. (1954): The dynamics of the heart in complete A-V block. An angiocardiographic study. *Circulation*, 10:195.
458. Linde, L. M., Goldberg, S. J., Seigel, S. (1964): The natural history of arrhythmias following septal defect repair. *J. Thorac. Cardiov. Surg.*, 48:303.
459. Linden, R. J., Mitchell, J. H. (1960): Relation between left ventricular diastolic pressure and myocardial segment length and observations on the contribution of atrial systole. *Circ. Res.*, 8:1092.
460. Linder, E., Landtman, B., Tauteri, L., Hjelt, L. (1965): Congenital complete heart block. II Histology of the conduction system. *Ann. Paediat. Fenn.*, 11:11.
461. Linenthal, A. J., Zoll, P. M., (1963): Prevention of ventricular tachycardia and fibrillation by intravenous isoproterenol and epinephrine. *Circulation*, 27:5.
462. Linenthal, A. J., Zoll, P. M. (1965): Ventricular fusion beats during electric stimulation in man. Application to conduction velocity and anomalous AV excitation. *Circulation*, 31: 651.

463. LINENTHAL, A. J., ZOLL, P. M. (1965): Theory of atrioventricular block: explanation of supernormal conduction and varying block (Abstract). *Circulation*, **32** (Suppl. 2):138.

464. LINENTHAL, A. J., ZOLL, P. M., GARABEDIAN, G. H., HUBERT, K. (1960): Ventricular slowing and standstill after spontaneous or electrically stimulated runs of rapid ventricular beats in atrioventricular block (Abstract). *Circulation*, **22**:781.

465. LINENTHAL, A. J., ZOLL, P. M., GARABEDIAN, G. H., HUBERT, K. (1962): Retrograde conduction to the atria from electric stimulation of the ventricles in man (Abstract). *Circulation*, **26**:752.

466. LINHART, J. W., BRAUNWALD, E., ROSS, J. (1965): Determinants of the duration of the refractory period of the atrioventricular nodal system in man. *J. Clin. Invest.*, **44**:883.

467. LISTER, J. (1858): Preliminary account of an inquiry into the functions of the visceral nerves, with special ref. to the so-called "Inhibitory system." *Proc. Roy. Soc.*, **9**:367.

468. LISTER, J. W., KLOTZ, D. H., JOMAIN, S. L., STUCKEY, J. H., HOFFMAN, B. F. (1964): Effect of pacemaker site on cardiac output and ventricular activation in dogs with complete heart block. *Amer. J. Cardiol.*, **14**:494.

469. LISTER, J. W., STEIN, E., KOSOWSKY, B. D., LAU, S. H., DAMATO, A. N. (1965): Atrioventricular conduction in man. Effect of rate, exercise, isoproterenol and atropine on the P. R. interval. *Amer. J. Cardiol.*, **16**:516.

470. LISTER, J. W., STEIN, E., LAU, S. H., KOSOWSKY, B. D., DAMATO, A. N. (1965): Control of the heart rate by paired electrical stimulation of the atria (Abstract). *Circulation*, **32** (Suppl. 2):139.

471. LISTER, J. W., STEIN, E., LAU, S. H., KOSOWSKY, B. D., STAM, R. F., DAMATO, A. N. (1965): Postextrasystolic potentiation in the acute and chronic dog, and a report of one case at open-heart surgery in man. *Bull. N. Y. Acad. Med.*, **41**:688.

472. LOCKHART, A., CHARPENTIER, A., BOURDARIAS, J. P., BEN ISMAIL, M., OURBAK, P., SCEBAT, L. (1966): Right ventricular involvement in obstructive cardiomyopathies: hemodynamic studies in 13 cases. *Brit. Heart J.*, **28**:122.

473. LOGUE, R. B., HANSON, J. F. (1945): Complete heart block in German measles. *Amer. Heart J.*, **30**:205.

474. LONG, F. M. (1962): Biological energy as a power source for a physiological telemetering system. *Inst. Radio-Engineers, Convention Record*, Part 9, p. 68.

475. LONGCOPE, W. F., FREIMAN, D. G. (1952): A study of sarcoidosis. *Medicine*, **31**:1.

476. LOPEZ, J. F.. EDELIST, A., KATZ, L. N. (1963): Slowing the heart rate by artificial electrical stimulation with pulses of long duration in the dog (Abstract). *Circulation*, **28**:759.

477. LOPEZ, J. F., EDELIST, A., KATZ, L. N. (1964): Reducing heart rate of the dog by electrical stimulation. *Circ. Res.*, **15**:414.

478. LORD, P. H. (1965): An operation for facilitating external pacing of the heart in the long-term treatment of heart block. *Lancet*, **2**:527.

479. LOUCKS, R. B. (1933): Preliminary report of a technique for stimulation or destruction of tissue beneath the integument and the establishing of conditioned reactions with faradization of the cerebral cortex. *J. Comp. Psychol.*, **16**:439.

480. LOUVROS, N., COSTEAS, F. (1965): Retrograde activation of atria in auriculoventricular block. An electrocardiographic demonstration *Arch. Intern. Med. (Chicago)*, **116**:778.

481. LOWN, B., ARONS, W. L., GANONG, W. F., VAZIFDAR, J. P., LEVINE, S. A. (1955): Adrenal steroids and auriculoventricular conduction. *Amer. Heart J.*, **50**:760.

482. LUAN-CH'IANG, H., TSUO-P'ING, F., MING-HSÜN, Y., HO-CH'ANG, Y., HSIEN-NING, W., CHUNG-YÜ, L., HSIUNG-PIN, C. (1964): Experience with two types of pacemakers. A preliminary report on experimental studies and clinical application. *Chin. Med. J. (Peking)*, **83**:307.

483. LUMB, G., SHACKLETT, R. S. (1960): Human cardiac conduction tissue lesions. *Amer. J. Path.*, **36**:411.

484. LUPPRIAN, K. G., CHURCHILL-DAVIDSON, H. C. (1960): Effect of Suxamethonium on cardiac rhythm. *Brit. Med. J.*, **2**:1774.

485. McGOON, D. C., ONGLEY, P. A., KIRKLIN, J. W. (1964): Surgical heart block. *Amer. J. Med.*, **37**:749.

486. McGOON, D. C., ONGLEY, P. A., KIRKLIN, J. W. (1964): Surgically induced heart block. *Ann. N. Y. Acad. Sci.*, **111**:830.

487. McGREGOR, M., KLASSEN, G. A., (1964): Observations on the effect of heart rate on cardiac output in patients with complete heart block at rest and during exercise. *Circ. Res.* (Suppl. 2), **14-15**:215.

488. MacLEAN, L. D., PHIBBS, C. M. (1960): Relative effect of chronic ischemia and a myocardial revascularization procedure on the ventricular fibrillation threshold. *Circ. Res.*, **8**:473.

489. McLEMORE, G. A., LEVINE, S. A. (1955): Possible therapeutic value of cholecystectomy in Adams-Stokes disease. *Amer. J. Med. Sci.*, **229**:386.

490. MAHAIM, I. (1931): *Les Maladies Organique du Faisceau de His-Tawara.* Paris, Masson.

491. MAHAIM, I. (1945): *Les Tumeurs et les Polypes du Coeur.* Lausanne, Masson.

492. MAHAIM, C. H. (1963): De la réduction d'un bloc A-V par la correction chirurgicale d'une sténose aortique. *Cardiologia (Basel)*, **42**:141.

493. MAJOR, R. H. (1923): Stokes-Adams' disease due to gumma of the heart. *Arch. Intern. Med. (Chicago)*, **31**:857.

494. MANSFIELD, P. B., COLE, A. D. (1963): The design and analysis of myocardial electrodes. *Proc. 16th Annual Conference on Engineering in Medicine and Biology.* Baltimore, Nov., 1963.

495. MANSFIELD, P. B., McDONALD, R. H. (1965): Some metabolic aspects of paired pacing of the heart. *Bull. N. Y. Acad. Med.*, **41**:700.

496. MARION, P. (1964): Intracorporeal cardiac stimulators for Morgagni-Adams-Stokes disease (144 patients operated on by 9 French teams). *J. Cardiov. Surg.*, **5**:657.

497. MARSHALL, R. J. (1964): Hemodynamic effects of endocardial pacemaking in patients with complete heart block. *J. Clin. Invest.*, **43**:1304.

498. MARTIN, R. H., COBB, L. A., LAU, S. H., SAMSON, W. E. (1964): Reduction in cardiac output caused by asynchronous ventricular pacing in man (Abstract). *Circulation,* 30 (Suppl. 3):122.

499. MARVIN, H. M. (1925): The effect of diphtheria on the cardiovascular system. I. The heart in faucial diphtheria. *Amer. J. Dis. Child.,* 29:433.

500. MASSEY, F. C., WALKER, W. J. (1948): Complete atrioventricular block in diphtheritic myocarditis. *Arch. Intern. Med. (Chicago),* 81:9.

501. MASSUMI, R. A., NUTTER, D. O. (1965): Studies on the mechanism of cardiac arrhythmias in Cheyne-Stokes respiration (Abstract). *Circulation,* 32 (Suppl. 2):146.

502. MATTHEWS, R. J. (1965): Prevention of ventricular tachycardia and Stokes-Adams seizures in complete heart block: treatment with large doses of intravenous isoproterenol. *Arch. Intern. Med. (Chicago),* 116:120.

503. MAURO, A.. EISENBERG, L., GLENN, W. W. L. (1964): A review of techniques for stimulation of excitable tissue within the body by electromagnetic induction. *Ann. N. Y. Acad. Sci.,* 118:103.

504. MAYO, H. (1838): Some cases of slowness of pulse. *London Med. Gaz.,* 22:232.

505. MEDTRONIC INC.: (1964) *Procedure Suggested for use with the Implantable Pacemaker Model 5860 Supplied by Medtronic Inc. with Medtronic Pacemakers.*

506. MEIJLER, F. L., DURRER, D. (1965): Physiological and clinical aspects of paired stimulation. *Bull. N. Y. Acad. Med.,* 41:575.

507. MEIJLER, F. L., WIEBERDINK, J., DURRER, D. (1962): L'mportance de la position des électrodes stimulatrices au cours du traitement d'un bloc auriculo-ventriculaire postopératif total. *Arch. Mal. Coeur,* 55:690.

508. MENON, T. B.. RAO, C. K. P. (1945): Tuberculosis of myocardium causing complete heart block. *Amer. J. Path.,* 21:1193.

509. MERKLEN, P. (1908): *Leçons sur les Troubles Functionnels du Coeur.* Paris, Masson.

510. MEYER, P., KIENY, R. (1964): Les effets hémodynamiques de l'implantation d'un pacemaker dans les blocs atrio-ventriculaires. *Strasbourg Med.,* 15:792.

511. MICHAËLSSON, M. (1965): Communication to European Society of Pediatric cardiologists; St. Andrews, unpublished.

512. MICHAËLSSON, M., PETERSSON, P. O. (1964): Pacemaker treatment for total, congenital (?) AV-block. *Acta. Pediat. Scand.* (Suppl. 159):88.

513. MICHEL, D., ZIMMERMAN, W., SCHAUDIG. A., GOLDEL, L., RIECKER, G., BORST, H. (1964): Zur Anwendung intrakardialer Schrittmachersonden. *Verh. Deutsch. Ges. Kreislaufforsch.,* 30:230.

514. MILLER, H., NATHANSON, M. H., GRIFFITHS, G. C. (1952): The action of procaine amide in complete heart block. *Amer. Heart J.,* 44:432.

515. MILLER, D. E., GLEASON, W. L., WHALEN, R. E., MORRIS, J. J., McINTOSH, H. D. (1962): Effect of ventricular rate on the cardiac output in the dog with chronic heart block. *Circ. Res.,* 10:658.

516. MINTZ, S. S., KATZ, L. N. (1947): Recent myocardial infarction: analysis of 572 cases. *Arch. Intern. Med. (Chicago),* 80:205.

517. MITCHELL, J. H., GUPTA, D. N., PAYNE, R. M. (1964): Influence of atrial asystole on effective ventricular stroke volume. *Fed. Proc.,* 23:464.

518. MITCHELL, J. H., GUPTA, D. N., PAYNE, R. M. (1965): Influence of atrial systole on effective ventricular stroke volume. *Circ. Res.*, 17:11.
519. MOBERG, A., TILLGREN, C. (1958): Hjärtarytmi vid lymfogranulomatosis benigna (Schaumanns sjukdom) (Cardiac arrhythmia in benign lymphogranulomatosis). *Opuscul. Med.*, 3:197.
520. MOBITZ, W. (1924): Ueber die unvollständige Störung der Erregungsüberleitung zwischen Vorhof und Kammer des menschlichen Herzens. *Z. Exp. Med. (Berlin)*, 41:180.
521. MOBITZ, W. (1928): Über den partiellen Herzblock. *Z. Klin. Med.*, 107:449.
522. MOE, G. K., ABILDSKOV, J. A. (1965): Antiarrhythmic drugs. In Goodman, L. S., and Gilman, A.: *The Pharmacological Basis of Therapeutics*, 3rd ed. New York, Macmillan, p. 699.
523. MOFFIT, G. R. (1965): Complete atrioventricular dissociation with Stokes-Adams attacks due to disseminated lupus erythematosus: report of a case. *Ann. Intern. Med.*, 63:508.
524. MOLTKE, E. (1955): Adams-Stokes syndrome following acute haemorrhage in an eight year old girl. *Acta Pediat.*, 44:73.
525. MONOPOULOS, S., KEHAYOGLOU, K. STAMATELOPOULOS, S., SIDERIS, D. (1964): Ventricular fibrillation during interim pacing of the heart by a bipolar endocardial electrode. *New Eng. J. Med.*, 271:895.
526. MONTGOMERY, L. H. (1960): An artificial His bundle and ventricular stimulator. *Proc. 3rd Int. Conf. Medical Electronics.* London, p. 233.
527. MOREAU, P. H., GERBAUX, A., LENÈGRE, J. (1963): L'étiologie des blocs A-V. *Arch. Mal. Coeur*, 56:609.
528. MORETTI, G. F., STAEFFEN, J., BERTRAND, E., BRONSTET, A. (1964): Bloc auriculo-ventriculaire complet dans le syndrome de Marfan. *Presse Med.*, 72:605.
529. MORGAGNI, J. B. (1761): *De Sedibus et Causis Morborum per Anatomen Indigatis Diloni Quinque ex Typographia Remondiniana.* Letter 9, art. 7; letter 24, art. 33; letter 44 case 5.
530. MORRIS, J. D., JUDGE, R. D., LEININGER, B. J., VONTZ, F. (1965): Clinical experience and problems encountered with an implantable pacemaker. *J. Thorac. Cardiov. Surg.*, 50:849.
531. MORROW, A. G. (1964): Electrical stimulation of the heart. Technics and instruments for the management of complete heart block. *Amer. J. Med.*, 37:754.
532. MOUQUIN, M., MACREZ, C. (1947): Les troubles du ventriculogramme au cours du pouls lent permanent par dissociation auriculo-ventriculaire. *Arch. Mal. Coeur*, 40:8.
533. MOUQUIN, M., MACREZ, C., SAUVAN, R., GÉLIN, J. (1957): Traitement du pouls lent permanent ou paroxystique et des troubles de conduction auriculo-ventriculaire par le lactate de sodium. *Bull. Soc. Med. Hôp. Paris*, 73:737.
534. MOUQUIN, W., VAYSSE, J., DURAND, M., LAURENT, D., SPROVIERI, L. (1962): Implantation d'un stimulateur interne pour correction d'un bloc auriculo-ventriculaire chirurgical chez un enfant de 7 ans. *Arch. Mal. Coeur*, 55:241.
535. MOWRY, F. M., JUDGE, R. D., PRESTON, T. A., MORRIS, J. D. (1965): Identification and management of exit block in patients with implanted pacemakers. *Circulation*, 32 (Suppl. 2):157.

536. MÜLLER, O. F., BELLET, S. (1961): Treatment of intractable heart failure in the presence of complete atrioventricular heart block by the use of the internal cardiac pacemaker. *New Eng. J. Med.*, 265:768.

537. MURRAY, J. F., BOYER, S. H. (1957): Ventricular arrhythmias after intravenous sodium lactate in heart block. *Circulation*, 15:547.

538. MYERS, G. H., PARSONNET, V., ZUCKER, I. R., LOTMAN, H. A., ASA, M. M. (1963): Biologically-energized cardiac pacemaker. *I.E.E.E. Trans. Biomed. Electronics*, 10:83.

539. NADAS, A. S., ALIMURUNG, M. M., LINENTHAL, A. J. (1951): Persistent ventricular pacemaker following basal skull fracture. *Amer. Heart J.*, 42:888.

540. NAJMI, M., SEGAL, B. L., LIKOFF, W., DREIFUSS, L. S. (1965): Atrial-pacemaker block, a new electrocardiographic syndrome associated with implanted synchronous pacemakers. *Dis. Chest*, 48:1.

541. NAKAMURA, F. F., NADAS, A. S. (1964): Complete heart block in infants and children. *New Eng. J. Med.*, 270:1261.

542. NASH, D. T. (1964): Problems associated with cardiac pacemakers. *Med. Times*, 92:581.

543. NATHAN, D. A. (1965): Symposium on electrical control of cardiac activity. Buffalo, May, 1965, unpublished.

544. NATHAN, D. A., CENTER, S., PINA, R. E., MEDOW, A., KELLER, W. (1966): Perforation during indwelling catheter pacing. *Circulation*, 33:128.

545. NATHAN, D. A., CENTER, S., SAMET, P., WU, C-Y., KELLER, J. W. (1964): The application of an implantable synchronous pacer for the correction of Stokes-Adams attacks. *Ann. N.Y. Acad. Sci.*, 111:1093.

546. NATHAN, D., SAMET, P., CENTER, S., WU, C-Y. (1964): Long-term correction of complete heart block. *Progr. Cardiov. Dis.*, 6:538.

547. NATHAN, D. A., CENTER, S., WU, C-Y., KELLER, W. (1963): An implantable, synchronous pacemaker for the long-term correction of complete heart block. *Circulation*, 27:682.

548. NATHAN, D. A., CENTER, S., WU, C-Y., KELLER, W. (1963): An implantable synchronous pacemaker for the long-term correction of complete heart block. *Amer. J. Cardiol.*, 11:362.

549. NATHAN, D. A., MEDOW, A., PINA, P. (1965): Ectopic cardiac response to electrical stimulation (Abstract). *Circulation*, 32 (Suppl. 2):159.

550. NATHANSON, M. H. (1939): The action of P-hydroxyphenylisopropylamine (paredrine) on the heart: a clinical study of a new epinephrine-like compound. *Ann. Intern. Med.*, 12:1855.

551. NATHANSON, M. H., MILLER, H. (1952): Action of norepinephrine, epinephrine, and isopropyl norepinephrine on rhythmic function of the heart. *Circulation*, 6:238.

552. NEUBAUER, C. (1943): Heart-block in diphtheria. *Brit. J. Child. Dis.*, 40:93.

553. NEUFELD, H. H., GOOR, D., NATHAN, D., LEIBINSOHN, S., FREI, E. (1965): Transvenous pacing of the heart (Abstract). *Circulation*, 32 (Suppl. 2):161.

554. NICHOLSON, M. J., EVERSOLE, U. H., ORR, R. B., CREHAN, J. P. (1959): Cardiac arrest: use of a cardiac monitor-pacemaker in diagnosis and management. *Lahey Clin. Bull.*, 11:179.

555. NICKEL, G. (1965): Oscilloscopic method for the bloodless analysis of conduction disturbances in implanted electric pacemakers (Abstract). *Circulation*, **32**:658; from original (1964): Z. *Kreislaufforsch.* **53**:1149.

556. NICKS, R., STENING, G. F. H., HULME, E. C. (1962): Some observations on the surgical treatment of heart block in degenerative heart disease. *Med. J. Aust.*, **49**(2):857.

557. NISSEN, N. I., THOMSEN, A. C. (1965): Oral treatment of A-V block and other bradycardias with sustained action isoprenaline. *Brit. Heart J.*, **27**:926.

558. NOORDIJK, J. A., OEY, F. T. I., TEBRA, W. (1961): Myocardial electrodes and the danger of ventricular fibrillation. *Lancet*, **1**:975.

559. NORMAN, J. C. (1964): In discussion. *Ann. N.Y. Acad. Sci.*, **111**:1044.

560. NORMAN, J. C. (1965): In discussion. *J. Thorac. Cardiov. Surg.*, **50**:866.

561. NORMAN, J. C., HAYS, C. V., JUDGE, R. D., WILSON, W. S., SLOAN, H. (1964): Experimental observations on the improbability of totally implantable pacemaker-induced ventricular fibrillation. *Trans. Amer. Soc. Artif. Int. Organs*, **10**:378.

562. NORMAN, J. C., LIGHTWOOD, R., ABRAMS, L. D. (1964): Surgical treatment of Adams-Stokes syndrome using long term inductive coupled coil pacemaking. *Ann. Surg.*, **159**:344.

563. NUNEZ-DAY, D., ZALTER, R., EISENBERG, H. (1962): Artificially induced parasystole in man due to surgically implanted myocardial pacemaker. *Amer. J. Cardiol.*, **10**:535.

564. OLMSTED, F., KOLFF, W. J., EFFLEN, D. B. (1958): Electronic cardiac pacemaker after open-heart operation. *Cleveland Clin. Quart.*, **25**:84.

565. PALICKI, B. (1839): De musculari cordis structure. Breslau, dissertation.

566. PALMER, D. G. (1962): Interruption of T waves by premature QRS complexes and the relationship of this phenomenon to ventricular fibrillation. *Amer. Heart J.*, **63**:367.

567. PAPADOPOULOS, G., TSIGOU, C., CHRISOCHOOU, G. (1965): Étude expérimentale d'un traitement chirurgical de la maladie de Stokes-Adams. *Presse. Med.*, **73**:1423.

568. PAPP, C. (1952): Acute cardiac infarction without pain. *Brit. Heart J.*, **14**:250.

569. PARADE, G. W., VOIT, K. (1929): Zur Adrenalin-und Ephetoninbehandling der Adams-Stokesschen Krankheit. *Deutsch. Med. Wschr.*, **55**:179.

570. PARKER, B. M., SHINE, L. C., BURFORD, T., WILLIAMS, K. R. (1963): Indwelling electronic cardiac pacemakers. *JAMA*, **186**:754.

571. PARKINSON, J., PAPP, C., EVANS, W. (1941): The electrocardiogram of Stokes-Adams attack. *Brit. Heart J.*, **3**:171.

572. PARSONNET, V. (1964): In discussion. *Ann. N.Y. Acad. Sci.*, **111**:952-953.

573. PARSONNET, V. (1964): In discussion. *Ann. N.Y. Acad. Sci.*, **111**:958.

574. PARSONNET, V. (1965): In discussion. *J. Thorac. Cardiov. Surg.*, **50**:865.

575. PARSONNET, V., GILBERT, L., ZUCKER, I. R., ASA, M. M. (1963): A plan for the treatment of complete heart block and Stokes-Adams syndrome with an intracardiac dipolar electrode and a permanent implantable pacemaker. *Angiology*, **14**:343.

576. PARSONNET, V., GILBERT, L., ZUCKER, I. R., ASSEFI, I. (1965): Subcostal transdiaphragmatic insertion of a cardiac pacemaker. *J. Thorac. Cardiov. Surg.*, **49**:739.

577. PARSONNET, V., GILBERT, L., ZUCKER, R., MAXIM, M. (1963): Complications of the implanted pacemaker: a scheme for determining the cause of the defect and methods for correction. *J. Thorac. Cardiov. Surg.*, **45**:801.

578. PARSONNET, V., MYERS, G., ZUCKER, I. R., LOTMAN, H. (1964): The potentiality of the use of biologic energy as a power source for implantable pacemakers. *Ann. N.Y. Acad. Sci.*, **111**:915.

579. PARSONNET, V., MYERS, G. H., ZUCKER, I. R., LOTMAN, H., ASA, M. M. (1963): A cardiac pacemaker using biologic energy sources. *Trans. Amer. Soc. Artif. Intern. Organs*, **9**:174.

580. PARSONNET, V., ZUCKER, I. R., GILBERT, L., ASA, M. M. (1962): An intracardiac bipolar electrode for interim treatment of complete heart block. *Amer. J. Cardiol.*, **10**:261.

581. PARSONNET, V., ZUCKER, I. R., GILBERT, L., ASA, M. M. (1962): The development of an intracardiac dipolar catheter electrode for the treatment of complete heart block. *Surg. Forum*, **13**:179.

582. PARSONNET, V., ZUCKER, I. R., GILBERT, L., MYERS, G. H. (1964): A review of intracardiac pacing with specific reference to the use of a dipolar electrode. *Progr. Cardiov. Dis.*, **6**:472.

583. PAUL, M. H., RUDOLF, A. M., NADAS, A. S. (1958): Congenital complete atrioventricular block: problems of clinical assessment. *Circulation*, **18**:183.

584. PAUL, W. D., RHOMBERG, C., COLE, J. (1946): Transitory A-V block occurring during scarlet fever. *Amer. Heart J.*, **31**:138.

585. PAULIN, C., RUBIN, I. L. (1956): Complete heart block with perforated interventricular septum following contusion of the chest. *Amer. Heart J.*, **52**:940.

586. PAULK, E. A., HURST, J. W. (1965): Evaluation of the intracardiac bipolar catheter pacemaker in the management of complete heart block developing as a complication of acute myocardial infarction (Abstract). *Circulation*, **32** (Suppl. 2):169.

587. PAY, P. W., WAVERLEY, VISC. (1961): Adrenocortical steroids in intermittent heart-block. *Brit. Med. J.*, **2**:139.

588. PEARSON, R. S. B. (1945): Sinus bradycardia with cardiac asystole. *Brit. Heart J.*, **7**:85.

589. PENTON, G. B., MILLER, H., LEVINE, S. A. (1956): Some clinical features of complete heart block. *Circulation*, **13**:801.

590. PERASALO, O., HALONEN, P., KYLLONEN, K. E. J. (1963): Experience with an implantable pacemaker in the treatment of total atrioventricular block with Stokes-Adams syndrome. *Acta Chir. Scand.*, **125**:577.

591. PERROTIN, M. (1964): Étude critique des séquelles cardiaques imputables à la diphtérie. *Presse Med.*, **72**:915.

592. PETIT, D. W. (1945): Hemochromatosis with complete heart block with a discussion of the cardiac complications. *Amer. Heart J.*, **29**:253.

593. PHINNEY, A. O. (1961): Sarcoid of the myocardial septum with complete heart block. Report of two cases. *Amer. Heart J.*, **62**:270.

594. PICK, A., LICHTMAN, A. (1957): Effects of isuprel in advanced A-V block (Abstract). *Circulation*, **16**:925.

595. PIEMME, T. E., ZITNIK, R. S., REED, D. P., HAYNES, F. W., DEXTER, L. (1963): Circulatory dynamics of artificial pacing in complete heart block in man. *Circulation*, **28**:785.

596. PONTIUS, R. G. (1963): In discussion. *J. Thorac. Cardiov. Surg.*, **46**:455.

597. POPE, A. (1837): Remarkable slowness of pulse in the horse. *London Med. Gaz.*, **20**:254.

598. PORTAL, R. W., DAVIES, J. G., LEATHAM, A., SIDDONS, A. H. M. (1962): Artificial pacing for the heart. *Lancet*, **2**:1369.

599. PORTHEINE, H., MENGES, G. (1965): Beitrag zur Technik der temporären Elektro-stimulation des Herzens. *Med. Klin.*, **60**:98.

600. POTTER, E. C. (1961): *Electro-chemistry*. New York, Macmillan.

601. POZZI, R., CAMMILLI, L., DE SAINT PIERRE, G., DRAGO, G. (1963): Controllo del ritmo cardiaco nella sindrome di Morgagni-Adams-Stokes mediante pacemaker a radio-frequenza. *Atti del 23 Congresso della Societa Italiana di Cardiologia*. Venezia, 1-3 guigno, 1962.

602. PRESTON, T. A., JUDGE, R. D., BOWERS, D. L., MORRIS, J. D. (1966): Measurement of pacemaker performance. *Amer. Heart J.*, **71**:92.

603. PRIMO, G., VEROFT, R., DELBROUCK, F., WELCH, W. (1964): Le traitement du bloc auriculoventriculaire par implantation d'un pacemaker interne. *Acta. Chir. Belg.*, **63**:400.

604. PRINZMETAL, M., KENNAMER, R. (1954): Emergency treatment of cardiac arrhythmias. *JAMA*, **154**:1049.

605. RACE, D., STIRLING, G. R., EMERY, P., BREMNER, J. (1963): Electrical stimulation of the heart. *Ann. Surg.*, **158**:100.

606. RAILLARD, H. (1962): An implantable cardiac pacemaker. *World Med. Electronics*, **1**:41.

607. RAINER, W. G., DOSCH, E. L. (1964): An improved method for connecting implantable pacemaker electrode wires. *J. Thorac. Cardiov. Surg.*, **48**:132.

608. RAMEY, E. R., GOLDSTEIN, M. S., LEVINE, R. (1951): Action of norepinephrine and adrenal cortical steroids on blood pressure and work performance of adrenalectomized dogs. *Amer. J. Physiol.*, **165**:450.

609. RANTZ, L. A., SPINK, W. W., BOISVERT, P. J. (1946): Abnormalities in the electrocardiogram following hemolytic streptococcus sore throat. *Arch. Intern. Med. (Chicago)*, **77**:66.

610. RAWKINS, M. D., KONSTAM, G. L. S. (1949): Complete heart-block associated with amoebic hepatitis. *Lancet*, **2**:152.

611. REGELSON, W., HOFFMEISTER, F. S. (1958): Antifibrillatory effect of central sedation in acute coronary occlusion (Abstract). *Circulation*, **18**:769.

612. REID, W. D. (1930): Permanent bradycardia following diphtheria. Case report. *Amer. Heart J.*, **5**:524.

613. REID, W. D. (1932): Causation and propagation of heart beat. *New Eng. J. Med.*, **206**:1254.

614. RESNEKOV, L., SOWTON, E., LORD, P., NORMAN, J. (1966): Haemodynamic and clinical effects of paired stimulation of the heart. *Brit. Heart J.*, **28**:622.

615. REULING, R., RAZINSKY, L. (1941): Metastatic bronchiogenic carcinoma of the heart. *Amer. Heart J.*, **21**:470.

616. RICHARDSON, J. W., SCHWARTZ, S. I. (1962): Prevention of thrombosis with the use of a negative electric current. *Surgery*, **52**:636.
617. RICORDEAU, G., PIWNICA, A., CACHERA, J-P., GUILMET, D., MARCILLAC, J-P., LEPOIX, J. (1964): Stimulateurs internes et maladie de Stokes-Adams (A propos 100 interventions). *Presse Med.*, **72**:2907.
618. ROBBIN, S. R., GOLDFEIN, S., SCHWARTZ, M. J., DACK, S. (1955): Adams-Stokes syndrome. *Amer. J. Med.*, **18**:577.
619. ROBERTSON, E. S., MATHEWS, E. S. (1952): Paroxysmal ventricular fibrillation producing Adams-Stokes syndrome. Report of case with review of literature. *Arch. Intern. Med. (Chicago)*, **90**:320.
620. ROBINSON, D. S., FALSETTI, H. L., WHEELER, D. H., MILLER, D. B., AMIDON, E. L. (1965): Ventricular fibrillation associated with two functioning implanted cardiac pacemakers. *Amer. J. Cardiol.*, **15**:397.
621. ROBINSON, J. S., SLOMAN, G., HOGAN, J., McCONCHIE, I. H. (1965): Ventricular tachycardia and fibrillation with implanted electrical pacemakers. *Brit. Heart J.*, **27**:937.
622. RODEWALD, G. (1965): In discussion. *Thoraxchirurgie*, **13**:281.
623. RODEWALD, G., GIEBEL, O., HARMS, H., SCHEPPAKAT, K. T. (1964): Intravenös-intrakardiale Applikation von vorhofgesteuerten elektrischen Schrittmachern. *Kreislaufforsch.*, **53**:860.
624. ROE, B. B. (1965): Intractable Stokes-Adams disease. *Amer. Heart J.*, **69**:470.
625. ROE, B. B., KATZ, H. J. (1965): Complete heart block with intractable asystole and recurrent ventricular fibrillation with survival. *Amer J. Cardiol.*, **15**:401.
626. ROGEL, S., STEIN, H. (1965): The duration of post-pacing asystole in dogs with atrioventricular block. *J. Thorac. Cardiov. Surg.*, **50**:438.
627. ROSE, L. B., WARTONICK, W. (1955): Treatment of a case of Stokes-Adams disease by external electric stimulation. *JAMA*, **159**:1015.
628. ROSENBAUM, H. D. (1965): Roentgen demonstration of broken cardiac pacemaker wires. *Radiology*, **84**:933.
629. ROSENBAUM, M. B., ALVAREZ, A. J. (1955): Electrocardiogram in chronic Chagasic myocarditis. *Amer. Heart J.*, **50**:492.
630. ROSENBERG, D. H. (1945): Electrocardiographic changes in epidemic parotitis (mumps). *Proc. Soc. Exp. Biol. Med.*, **58**:9.
631. ROSS, J., LINHART, J. W., BRAUNWALD, E. (1965): Effects of changing heart rate in man by electrical stimulation of the right atrium. Studies at rest, during exercise and with isoprotorenol. *Circulation*, **32**:549.
632. ROSS, J., HARKINS, G. A. (1959): Percutaneous introduction of cardiac pacemaker electrode. *Lancet*, **2**:1109.
633. ROSS, J., LINHART, J. W., BRAUNWALD, E. (1965): Effects of changing heart rate in man by electrical stimulation of the right atrium. Studies at rest, during exercise and with isoproterenol. *Circulation*, **32**:549.
634. ROSS, J., SONNENBLIK, E. H., KAISER, G. A., FROMMER, P. L., BRAUNWALD, E. (1965): Electroaugmentation of ventricular performance and oxygen consumption by repetitive application of paired electrical stimuli. *Circ. Res.*, **16**:332.

635. Ross, S. M., Hoffman, B. F. (1961): A bipolar pacemaker for immediate treatment of cardiac arrest. In Frommer, P. L. (ed.). *Digest of the 1961 International Conference on Medical Electronics, New York, 1961.* Princeton, N.J., p. 183.

636. Rossi, L. (1961): Histologic study of the pathogenesis of A-V block in 10 cases and observations on the A-V system in 5 hearts with congenital malformations. *Minerva Cardioangiol.*, 9:1.

637. Rossi, L. (1965): Case of cardiac lymphangitis with atrioventricular block. *Brit. Med. J.*, 2:32.

638. Rotem, C. E., Hultgren, H. N. (1965): Corrected transposition of the great vessels without associated defects. *Amer. Heart J.*, 70:305.

639. Rothfeld, E. L., Zucker, I. R., Parsonnet, V., Lotti, L. (1965): Effect of quinidine on competitive cardiac pacing (Abstract). *Circulation*, 32 (Suppl. 2):182.

640. Rowe, J. C., White, P. D. (1958): Complete heart block: A follow-up study. *Ann. Intern. Med.*, 49:260.

641. Rowley, B. A. (1963): Electrolysis—a factor in cardiac pacemaker electrode failure. *I.E.E.E. Trans. Biomed. Electronics*, 10:176.

642. Rubin, R., Dressler, W. (1965): Observations in patients with implanted pacemakers. An electrocardiographic sign of broken electrode wires mimicking interference by alternating current. *Amer. J. Cardiol.*, 15:395.

643. Rylant, P. (1927): Contribution à l'étude de l'automatisme et la conduction dans le cœur. Ablation et gresse intracardiaque du nœud de Keith-Flack (sinus) chez la chèvre, le mouton, le chat et le lapin. Gresses hétérogène du nœud de Keith-Flack chez le chien, la chevre et le mouton. *Bull. Acad. Méd. Belg.*, 7:161.

644. Rytand, D. A. (1946): An auricular diastolic murmur with heart block in elderly patients. *Amer. Heart J.*, 32:579.

645. Rytand, D. A., Lipsitch, L. S. (1946): Clinical aspects of calcification of the mitral annulus fibrosus. *Arch. Intern. Med. (Chicago)*, 78:544.

646. Sacre, J. (1962): Syndrome d'Adams-Stokes et stimulation cardiaque par Pacemaker. *Acta Chir. Belg.*, 61:946.

647. Salvesen, H. A. (1932): Complete heartblock in the course of acute rheumatic infection. *Acta Med. Scand.*, 78:189.

648. Samet, P., Bernstein, W. H., Medow, A., Nathan, D. A. (1964): Effect of alterations in ventricular rate on cardiac output in complete heart block. *Amer. J. Cardiol.*, 14:477.

649. Samet, P., Bernstein, W. H., Nathan, D. A., Lopez, A. (1965): Atrial contribution to cardiac output in complete heart block. *Amer. J. Cardiol.*, 16:1.

650. Samet, P., Jacobs, W., Bernstein, W. H., Shane, R. (1963): Hemodynamic sequelae of idioventricular pacemaking in complete heart block. *Amer. J. Cardiol.*, 11:594.

651. Sarnoff, S. J., Gilmore, J. P., Daggett, W. M., Mansfield, P. B., Weisfeldt, M. L., McDonald, R. H. (1965): Effect of coupled pacing (continuing postextrasystolic potentiation) on the hemodynamics. O_2 consumption and K^+ balance of the heart (Abstract). *Amer. J. Cardiol.*, 15:143.

652. SATINSKY, V., DREIFUS, L., RACINE, P., MASSIE, H., REYNOLDS, L. (1965): Cardiac pacing by means of electrical energy derived directly from the heart. *Circulation,* **32** (Suppl. 2):187.

653. SAYED, H. M. (1965): Complete heart block following open heart surgery. *J. Cardiov. Surg.,* **6**:426.

654. SCHAEFER, J. A., RUDOLPH, L. A. (1957): Corrected transposition of the great vessels. *Amer. Heart J.,* **54**:610.

655. SCHAUB, F. (1965): Die medikamentöse Therapie des Av-Blockes. *Cardiologia (Basel),* **46**:226.

656. SCHAUB, F., HOLZMANN, M., WYSS, S. (1957): Zur Behandlung von Adams-Stokesschen Anfällen und Uberleitungs-störungen des Herzens mit Isopropylnoradrenaline. *Schweiz. Med. Wschr.,* **87**:938.

657. SCHAUB, F., SENNING, A. (1963): Long-term therapy of Adams-Stokes syndrome with a long-term electric miniature pacemaker. *Cardiologia (Basel),* **42**:152.

658. SCHERF, B. (1958): Therapy of arrhythmias in myocardial infarction. *Amer. J. Cardiol.,* **1**:242.

659. SCHERF, D., SCHOTT, A. (1939): The supernormal phase of recovery in man. *Amer. Heart J.,* **17**:357.

660. SCHILD, W., WEISE, H. (1952): Beitrag zur Therapie des sinu-auriculären Blocks. *Klin. Wschr.,* **30**:419.

661. SCHNEIDER, H. (1964): Physical principles of artificial stimulation of the heart. Stimulation of canine heart in situ. *Amer. Heart J.,* **67**:628.

662. SCHNUR, S. (1948): Newer concepts of Stokes-Adams syndrome. *Amer. Heart J.,* **35**:298.

663. SCHUDER, J. C., STOECKLE, H. (1962): A micromodule pacemaker receiver for direct attachment to the ventricle. *Trans. Amer. Soc. Artif. Intern. Organs,* **8**:344.

664. SCHUDER, J. C., STOECKLE, H. (1964): The silicon diode as a receiver for electrical stimulation of body organs. *Trans. Amer. Soc. Artif. Intern. Organs,* **10**:366.

665. SCHÜLLER (1965): In discussion. *Thoraxchirurgie,* **13**:280.

666. SCHWARTZ, L. S., SCHWARTZ, S. P. (1963): The Adams-Stokes syndrome during normal sinus rhythm and transient heart block: the effects of altered posture. *Amer. J. Cardiol.,* **12**:505.

667. SCHWARTZ, S. P. (1936): Auriculoventricular dissociation and Adams-Stokes syndrome in acute coronary vessel closure. *Amer. Heart J.,* **11**:554.

668. SCHWARTZ, S. P., HAUSWIRTH, L. (1934): Studies on transient ventricular fibrillation; observations on alterations in rhythm of heart preceding syncopal seizures in woman with transient auriculoventricular dissociation. *Amer. J. Med. Sci.,* **187**:478.

669. SCHWARTZ, S. P., HELLINGER, L., IMPERIALLI, A. (1952): Transient ventricular fibrillation; effects of procaine amide on patients with transient ventricular fibrillation during established auriculoventricular dissociation. *Circulation,* **6**:193.

670. SCHWARTZ, S. P., SCHWARTZ, L. S. (1960): The Adams-Stokes syndrome during normal sinus rhythm and transient heart block. (2) The effects

of digitalis glucosides on patients with the Adams-Stokes syndrome during normal sinus rhythm and transient heart block. *Arch. Intern. Med. (Chicago)*, **106**:388.

671. SCHWARTZ, L. S., SCHWARTZ, S. P. (1964): The effects of digitalis bodies on patients with heart block and congestive heart failure. *Progr. Cardiov. Dis.*, **6**:366.

672. SCHWEDEL, J. B. (1965): Role of the pacemaker. *J. Chronic Dis.*, **18**:891.

673. SCHWEDEL, J. B., ESCHER, D. J. W. (1964): Transvenous electrical stimulation of the heart. *Ann. N.Y. Acad. Sci.*, **111**:972.

674. SCHWEDEL, J. B., FURMAN, S., ESCHER, D. J. W. (1960): Use of an intracardiac pacemaker in the treatment of Stokes-Adams seizures. *Progr. Cardiov. Dis.*, **3**:170.

675. SEGEL, N., HUDSON, W. A., HARRIS, P., BISHOP, J. M. (1964): The circulatory effects of electrically induced changes in ventricular rate at rest and during exercise in complete heart block. *J. Clin. Invest.*, **43**:1541.

676. SEGERS, M., LEQUIME, J., DENOLIN, H. (1947): Synchronization of auricular and ventricular beats during complete heart block. *Amer. Heart J.*, **33**:685.

677. SELBY, D. M., ANDERSON, L. G., MANDRELL, W. L., COLEMAN, W., CAMPBELL, G. S. (1964): Inductive coupling for recharging nickel cadmium batteries in implanted cardiac pacemakers. *Trans. Amer. Soc. Artif. Intern. Organs*, **10**:371.

678. SELLERS, F. J., DONALD, D. E., WOOD, E. H. (1962): Atrial contribution to stroke volume in dogs with chronic cardiac denervation (Abstract). *Physiologist*, **5**:211.

679. SELLERS, R. D., KANJUH, V. I., ELIOT, R. S., BONNABEAU, R. C., EDWARDS, J. E., LILLEHEI, C. W. (1963): Complete heart block following aortic-valve replacement: anatomic basis, prevention and management (Abstract). *Circulation*, **28**:801.

680. SENN, A. (1965). Erfahrungen mit dem Pacemaker. *Cardiologia (Basel)*, **46**:259.

681. SENNING, A. (1959): In discussion. *J. Thorac. Cardiov. Surg.*, **38**:639.

682. SENNING, A. (1964): Problems in the use of pacemakers. *J. Cardiov. Surg.*, **5**:651.

683. SHAFIROFF, B. G. P., LINDER, J. (1957): The effects of external electrical pacemaker stimuli on the human heart. *J. Thorac. Cardiov. Surg.*, **33**:544.

684. SHEELY, R. F. (1954): Adams-Stokes disease in the geriatric patient. *J. Amer. Geriat. Soc.*, **2**:223.

685. SHOU-CHI, T'AO. (1954): Paroxysmal ventricular fibrillation producing Adams-Stokes syndrome. Report of a case on quinidine therapy with spontaneous recovery. *Chin. Med. J. (Peking)*, **72**:342.

686. SHOU-CHI T'AO. (1957): Cardiac manifestations of the toxic action of potassium antimony tartrate in schistosomiasis patients. Paroxysmal ventricular tachycardia and fibrillation. *Chin. Med. J. (Peking)*, **75**:365.

687. SIDDONS, A. H. M. (1963): Long-term artificial cardiac pacing: experience in adults with heart block. *Ann. Roy. Coll. Surg. Eng.*, **32**:22.

688. SIDDONS, A. H. M. (1965): Implantation of cardiac pacemakers. *Operative Surgery. Service Volume.* London, Butterworth's, Part 5, p. 30.

689. SIDDONS, H. (1965): Cardiac pacing: results with three different techniques. *Ann. Roy. Coll. Surg. Eng.*, 37:155.

690. SIDDONS, H. (1965): A propos de l'entraînement cardiaque. Résultats comparés de trois différentes méthodes. *Mem. Acad. Chir. (Paris)*, 91:675.

691. SIDDONS, A. H. M., BLUESTONE, R., DAVIES, J. G., FARRINGTON, G. H., HARRIS, A. M., LEATHAM, A. (1965): Cardiac pacing. *Thoraxchirurgie*, 13:271.

692. SIDDONS, H., DAVIES, J. G. (1963): A new technique for internal cardiac pacing. *Lancet*, 2:1204.

693. SIDDONS, A. H. M., HUMPHRIES, O'N. (1961): Complete heart block with Stokes-Adams attacks treated by indwelling pacemaker. *Proc. Roy. Soc. Med.*, 54:237.

694. SIEBENS, A. A., HOFFMAN, B. F., CRANEFIELD, P. F., BROOKS, C. McC. (1959): Regulation of contractile force during ventricular arrhythmias. *Amer. J. Physiol.*, 197:971.

695. SIEBENS, A. A., HOFFMAN, B. F., ENSOM, Y., FARRELL, J. E., BROOKS, C. McC. (1953): Effects of L-epinephrine and L-nor-epinephrine on cardiac excitability. *Amer. J. Physiol.*, 175:1.

696. SIEGAL, E. F. (1965): Symposium on electrical control of cardiac activity. Buffalo, May, 1965, unpublished.

697. SIGLER, L. H. (1939): Treatment of Stokes-Adams syndrome by hypertonic glucose solution given intravenously. *Ann. Intern. Med.*, 13:101.

698. SIGUIER, F., BINET, J. P., GODEAU, P., LEVY, R., HAMIDA, B. (1962): Dermatomyosite compliquée de bloc auriculo-ventriculaire complet avec syndrome Adams-Stokes. Implantation d'un stimulateur interne. *Bull. Soc. Med. Hôp. Paris*, 113:1126.

699. SILVER, A. W., ROOT, G., BYRON, F. X., SANDBERG, H. (1965): Externally rechargeable cardiac pacemaker. *Ann. Thorac. Surg.*, 1:380.

700. SILVERMAN, J., ROSENBERG, M. S. (1964): A simplified technique in the use of external cardiac pacemakers. *J. Thorac. Cardiov. Surg.*, 47:109.

701. SIMPSON, J. A., GIBSON, P., STANFORD, R. W., McLERNON, D. (1962): Prolonged cardiac pacemaking in Stokes-Adams disease. *Lancet*, 2:226.

702. SINGER, D. H., GALST, G., WAGNER, M. L. (1965): Effects of sustained paired stimulation of the heart in normal dogs and in dogs following coronary artery ligation. *Bull. N.Y. Acad. Med.*, 41:652.

703. SKINNER, N. S., MITCHELL, J. H., WALLACE, A. G., SARNOFF, S. J. (1963): Hemodynamic effects of altering the timing of atrial systole. *Amer. J. Physiol.*, 205:499.

704. SLAMA, R., GUEDON, J., DORRA, M. (1963): Particularités electrocardiographiques après pose d'un stimulateur interne pour maladie de Stokes-Adams. *Arch. Mal. Coeur*, 56:915.

705. SLOAN, H. E. (1950): The vagus nerve in cardiac arrest. The effect of hypercapnia, hypoxia and asphyxia on reflex inhibition of the heart. *Surg. Gynec. Obstet.*, 91:257.

706. SMALL, J. M., STEPHENSON, S. C. F., CAMPKIN, T. V., DAVISON, P. H., McILVEEN, D. J. S. (1966): Elective circulatory arrest by artificial pacemaker. *Lancet*, 1:570.

707. SMITH, K. S. (1965): The influence of disorders of conduction upon some aspects of cardiac arrest. *Resuscitation and Cardiac Pacing* (Proc. of Conference, Glasgow, March, 1964). London, Cassell, p. 177.

708. SNYDER, J., WOOD, E. H. (1962): Effect of heart rate on atrial contribution to cardiac performance in dogs with complete heart block. *Fed. Proc.,* **21**:137.

709. SOLARZ, S. D., BERKSON, D. M., PICK, A. (1958): Asystole complicating acute myocardial infarction. *JAMA,* **168**:2124.

710. SOLOMON, N., ESCHER, D. J. W. (1963): A rapid method of insertion of the pacemaker catheter electrode. *Amer. Heart J.,* **66**:717.

711. SOMERVILLE, J. (1965): Ostium primum defect: factors causing deterioration in the natural history. *Brit. Heart J.,* **27**:413.

712. SOWTON, E. (1964): Haemodynamic studies in patients with artificial pacemakers. *Brit. Heart J.,* **26**:737.

713. SOWTON, E. (1963): Artificial cardiac pacemaking, with particular reference to cardiac physiology. M. D. Thesis, University of Cambridge.

714. SOWTON, E. (1964): Resuscitation of the heart. The use of artificial pacemaking in cardiac resuscitation. *Proc. Roy. Soc. Med.,* **57**:368.

715. SOWTON, G. E. (1965): Artificial pacemakers: medical aspects and haemodynamic problems. *Resuscitation & Cardiac Pacing* (Proc. of Conference, Glasgow, March, 1964) London, Cassell, p. 187.

716. SOWTON, E. (1965): Artificial pacemaking and sinus rhythm. *Brit. Heart J.,* **27**:311.

717. SOWTON, E., DAVIES, J. G. (1964): Investigations of failure of artificial pacing. *Brit. Med. J.,* **1**:1470.

718. SOWTON, E., JONSSON, B., KAIJSER, L. (1965): The relationship between maximal oxygen uptake and heart rate (Abstract). *Brit. Heart J.,* **27**:948.

719. SOWTON, E., LEATHAM, A., CARSON, P. (1964): The suppression of arrhythmias by artificial pacemaking. *Lancet,* **2**:1098.

720. SPACH, M. S., SCARPELLI, E. M. (1962): Circulatory dynamics and the effects of respiration during ventricular asystole in dogs with complete heart block. *Circ. Res.,* **10**:197.

721. SPEAR, H. C., DAUGHTRY, D. C., CHESNEY, J. G., GENTSCH, T. O. (1965): An appraisal of the surgical management of heart block. *J. Thorac. Cardiov. Surg.,* **49**:743.

722. SPENS, T. (1793): Medical commentaries, Edinburgh, 1793, vii, 463. In Major, R. H.: Classic Descriptions of Disease, 3rd ed. Springfield, Thomas, 1945, pp. 331-332.

723. SPRAWLS, P., MILLER, W. B., LOGAN, W. D. (1965): Observation of electromagnetic signals from implantable pacemakers. *J. Thorac. Cardiov. Surg.,* **49**:748.

724. SPRINKLE, J. D., TAKARO, T., SCOTT, S. M. (1963): Phrenic nerve stimulation as a complication of the implantable cardiac pacemaker. *Circulation,* **28**:114.

725. STACK, M. F., RADER, B., SOBOL, B. J., FARBER, S. J., EICHNA, L. W. (1958): Cardiovascular hemodynamic functions in complete heart block and the effect of isopropylnorepinephrine. *Circulation,* **17**:526.

726. STARMER, C. F., WHALEN, R. E., McINTOSH, H. D. (1964): Hazards of electric shock in cardiology. *Amer. J. Cardiol.*, 14:537.

727. STARZL, T. E., GAERTNER, R. A. (1955): Chronic heart block in dogs. A method for producing experimental heart failure. *Circulation*, 12:259.

728. STARZL, T. E., HERMANN, G., AXTELL, H. K., MARCHIORO, T. L., WADDELL, W. R. (1963): Failure of sino-atrial nodal transplantation for the treatment of experimental complete heart block in dogs. *J. Thorac. Cardiov. Surg.*, 46:201.

729. STEIN, E., DAMATO, A. N., KOSOWSKY, B. D., LAU, S. H., LISTER, J. W. (1966): Cardiovascular response to alterations in heart rate above and below the sinus rate. *Amer. J. Cardiol.*, 17:140.

730. STEPHENSON, S. E. (1960): Direct electrical cardiac stimulators. *Progr. Cardiov. Dis.*, 3:162.

731. STEPHENSON, S. E., BROCKMAN, S. K. (1964): P-wave synchrony. *Ann. N. Y. Acad. Sci.*, 111:907.

732. STEPHENSON, S. E., EDWARDS, W. H., JOLLY, P. C., SCOTT, H. W. (1959): Physiologic P-wave cardiac stimulator. *J. Thorac. Cardiov. Surg.*, 38:604.

733. STEPHENSON, S. E., JOLLY, P. C., BAILEY, H. W., EDWARDS, W. H., MONTGOMERY, L. H. (1960): An evaluation of the P-wave external cardiac stimulator. *Surg. Forum*, 10:612.

734. STETCHER, R. M. (1929): Electrocardiographic changes in diphtheria. I. Complete auriculoventricular dissociation. *Amer. Heart J.*, 4:545.

735. STOCK, R. J. (1965): Quoted by Singer, D. H., *et al. Bull. N. Y. Acad. Med.*, 41:652.

736. STOECKLE, H., SCHUDER, J. C. (1963): Experimental experience with a micromodule pacemaker receiver sutured directly to the left ventricle. *Circulation*, 27:676.

737. STOKES, W. (1846): Observations on some cases of permanently slow pulse. *Dublin J.* (n. s.), 2:73.

738. STOKES, W. (1947): Paroxysmal heart block in bundle branch block. *Brit. Heart J.*, 9:267.

739. STORSTEIN, O. (1949): Adams-Stokes attacks caused by ventricular fibrillation in a man with an otherwise normal heart. *Acta. Med. Scand.*, 133:437.

740. STRAUSS, S., MEYER, J. (1928): The treatment of transient ventricular standstill with barium chloride. *Amer. Heart J.*, 3:328.

741. SUGIE, S., AOKI, T., MURAKAMI, T., KUROSHIMA, S., SAWAGUCNI, R. (1965): Experimental and clinical observation on artificial pacemaker. *Digest of the 6th International Conference on Medical and Biological Engineering. Tokyo*, p. 95.

742. SURAN, J. J. (1956): Circuit properties of the PNPN transistor. *Proc. Nat. Conf. Aeronaut. Electronics.* Quoted by Kantrowitz, A. (1964): *Ann. N. Y. Acad. Sci.*, 111:1049.

743. SURAWICZ, B., CHLEBUS, H., REEVES, J. T., GETTES, L. S. (1965): Increase of ventricular excitability threshold by hyperpotassemia. *JAMA*, 191:1049.

744. SWEDBERG, J., JOHANSSON, E. W., KARNELL, J., MALM, A. (1963): Implantation of pacemaker for Adams-Stokes syndrome. *Acta Chir. Scand.,* **125**:547.

745. SWEET, W. H. (1947): Stimulation of the sino-atrial node for cardiac arrest during operation. *Bull. Amer. Coll. Surg.,* **32**:234.

746. SWIFT, E. V., SMITH, H. L., (1937): Complete heart block associated with pneumonia and peritonitis. Review of the literature and report of a case in which a lesion was demonstrated histologically. *JAMA,* **109**:2038.

747. SYKOSCH, J. (1963): Implantierbare Schrittmacher beim Atrioventrikulären Block. *Chirurg,* **34**:11.

748. SYKOSCH, H. J. (1964): Implantierbare Schrittmacher zur permanenten und intermittierenden Stimulierung des Herzens. *Langenbeck. Arch. Klin. Chir.,* **308**:288.

749. SYKOSCH, J., EFFERT, S., PULVER, K. G., ZACOUTO, F. (1963): Zur Therapie mit elektrischen Schrittmachern. Ein implantierbarer induktiv ausschaltbarer elektrischer Schmittmacher. *Elektromedizin,* **8**:139.

750. TABATZNIK, B., MICHELSON, E. J., WILDER, R. J. (1965): Long-term endocardial pacing (Letter). *Lancet,* **2**:588.

751. TABER, R. E., ESTOYE, L. R., GREEN, E. R., GAHAGAN, T. (1964): Treatment of congenital and acquired heart block with an implantable pacemaker. *Circulation,* **29**:182.

752. TABER, R. E., WEBB, D. F. (1965): Lessons from 118 pacemaker implantations. *JAMA,* **194**:1133.

753. TAMURA, K. (1965): The effects of cations to the digitalis induced arrhythmias: experimental trials of the artificial pacemaker to these arrhythmias. II. The effect of calcium. *Jap. Heart J.,* **6**:165.

754. TATOOLES, C. J., BRAUNWALD, N. S. (1965): The comparative hemodynamic effects of paired and single electrical stimulation of the heart: observations in animals with complete heart block and myocardial failure. *Bull. N. Y. Acad. Med.,* **41**:681.

755. TAVEL, M. E., FISCH, C. (1964): Repetitive ventricular arrhythmias resulting from artificial internal pacemaker. *Circulation,* **30**:493.

756. TAWARA, S. (1906): *Das Reizleitungssystem des Saugetierherzens.* Gustav Fischer Jena.

757. THEVENET, A., HODGES, P. C., LILLEHEI, C. W. (1958): The use of a myocardial electrode inserted percutaneously for control of complete atrioventricular block by an artificial pacemaker. *Dis. Chest,* **34**:621.

758. THOMAS, M., SHILLINGFORD, J. (1965): The circulatory response to a standard postural change in ischaemic heart disease. *Brit. Heart J.,* **27**:17.

759. THORNANDER, H. (1965): Personal communication.

760. THORNANDER, H. (1966): Personal communication.

761. TOBIAN, L. (1961): Prevention of Stokes-Adams seizures with chlorothiazide. *New Eng. J. Med.,* **265**:623.

762. TOBIAN, L. (1964): Prevention of Stokes-Adams seizures with chlorothiazide. *Ann. N. Y. Acad. Sci.,* **111**:855.

763. TOLLES, W. E. (1965): Some considerations of recording and stimulating electrodes. *Trans. N. Y. Acad. Sci.,* **27**:909.

764. TOOLE, A. L., LONGO, E., MAURO, A., GLENN, W. W. L. (1960): Prolonged electrical stimulation of the heart. *Surg. Forum*, 11:247.

765. TORRESANI, J., AUBERT, M., AMBROSI, C. *et al.* (1963): Considerations hemodynamiques sur les blocs auriculo-ventriculaires. *Arch. Mal. Coeur*, 11:1189.

766. TOWNSEND, J. F., STOECKLE, H., SCHUDER, J. C. (1965): Tissue and electrode changes in chronic cardiac pacing. An experimental study. *Trans. Amer. Soc. Artif. Intern. Organs*, 11:132.

767. TRIMBLE, A. S. (1965): The implantable cardiac pacemaker: late failures and their management. *J. Thorac. Cardiov. Surg.*, 50:707.

768. TRIMBLE, A. S., HEIMBECKER, R. O., BIGELOW, W. G. (1964): The implantable cardiac pacemaker. *Canad. Med. Ass. J.*, 90:106.

769. TSUBOI, S., EBINA, K. (1960): Studies on the application of rhythmic stimulation for cardiac dysfunction in heart surgery. *Bull. Heart Inst. Japan*, 4:1.

770. TUNA, N., SCOTT, J. W. (1954): Stokes-Adams attacks with simultaneous auricular and ventricular standstill. *Circulation*, 9:853.

771. U. S. ATOMIC ENERGY COMMISSION (1966): Press release. Washington, Feb. 2.

772. VAGNINI, J., GOURIN, J., STUCKEY, J. H. (1966): Ventricular pacemaker site and myocardial contraction (Abstract). *Amer. J. Cardiol.*, 17:141.

773. VAN DAM, R. T., DURRER, D., STRACKEE, J., DER TWEEL, L. H. (1956): The excitability cycle of the dogs left ventricle determined by anodal, cathodal and bipolar stimulation. *Circ. Res.*, 4:196.

774. VANDAM, L. D., McLEMORE, G. A. (1957): Circulatory arrest in patients with complete heart block during anaesthesia and surgery. *Ann. Intern. Med.*, 47:518.

775. VAN DIJK, O. M. (1964): Het hart dat nooit stilstaat. *Nederl. T. Geneesk.* 108:2007.

776. VAN TYN, R. A., MACLEAN, L. D. (1961): Ventricular fibrillation threshold. *Amer. J. Physiol.*, 201:457.

777. VEREL, D., MAZURKIE, S. J., RAHMAN, F. (1963): Prednisone in the treatment of Adams-Stokes attacks. *Brit. Heart J.*, 25:709.

778. VERZEANO, M., WEBB, R. C., KELLY, M. (1958): Radio control of ventricular contraction in experimental heart block (Abstract). *Science*, 128:1003.

779. VOGEL, J. H. K., TABARI, K., AVERILL, K. H., BLOUNT, S. G. (1964): A simple technique for identifying P waves in complicated arrhythmias. *Amer. Heart J.*, 67:158.

780. VOOKLES, J. T., MILNOR, P. (1965): Criteria for use of internal cardiac pacing. *Circulation*, 32 (suppl. 2):212.

781. VOSSSCHULTE, K., VOEGT, H., KNOTHE, W., GERHARD, W. (1964): Spezielle Beobachtungen nach Implantation elektrischer Schrittmacher mit Bemerkungen über eine neue operative Technik. *Med. Klin.*, 59:501.

782. WALKER, W. J., ELKINS, J. T., WOOD, L. W. (1964): Effect of potassium in restoring myocardial response to subthreshold cardiac pacemaker. *New Eng. J. Med.*, 271:597.

783. WALLACE, H. W., WISOFF, B. G., GADBOYS, H. L., LITWAK, R. S. (1965): Management of malfunctioning implanted cardiac pacemakers. *Circulation*, **32** (suppl. 2):214.

784. WALLGREN, A., WINBLAD, S. (1937): Congenital heart block. *Acta Paediat. (Uppsala)*, **20**:175.

785. WALSHE, W. H. (1862): A practical treatise on diseases of the heart and great vessels, 3rd ed. London, Walton & Maberly, p. 188.

786. WARNER, H. F., LEWIS, D. H. (1961): Effect of increased pulse rate on circulatory dynamics in normal resting man. *Fed. Proc.*, **20**:131.

787. WARNER, H. R., TORONTO, A. F. (1960): Regulation of cardiac output through stroke volume. *Circ. Res.*, **8**:549.

788. WATSON, H. (1964) Electrode catheters and the diagnostic application in intracardiac electography in small children. *Circulation*, **29**:284.

789. WEALE, F. E., DEUCHER, D. C., NIGHTINGALE, A. (1960): Electrical excitability of the human ventricular myocardium. *Guy. Hosp. Rep.*, **109**:157.

790. WEDD, A. M., WILSON, D. C. (1930): Standstill of the heart of vagal origin. *Amer. Heart J.*, **5**:493.

791. WEINBERG, S. J. (1947): Electrocardiogram-electroencephalogram relations in cardiac arrhythmias. *Proc. Soc. Exp. Biol. Med.*, **66**:128.

792. WEINBERG, D. I., ARTLEY, J. L., WHALEN, R. E., MCINTOSH, H. D. (1962): Electric shock hazards in cardiac catheterization. *Circ. Res.*, **11**:1004.

793. WEINMAN, J. (1964): Comments on 'Electrolysis'—a factor in cardiac pacemaker electrode failure (Letter to Editor). *I.E.E.E. Trans. Biomed. Electronics*, **11**:114.

794. WEINMAN, J. (1964): The incorporation of a magnetic switch into an implanted pacemaker. *J. Thorac. Cardiov. Surg.*, **48**:690.

795. WEINMAN, J. (1965): Biphasic stimulation and electrical properties of metal electrodes. *J. Appl. Physiol.*, **20**:787.

796. WEIRICH, W. L., GOTT, V. L., LILLEHEI, C. W. (1957): The treatment of complete heart block by the combined use of a myocardial electrode and an artificial pacemaker. *Surg. Forum*, **8**:360.

797. WEIRICH, W. L., ROE, B. B. (1961): The role of pacemakers in the management of surgically induced heart block. *Amer. J. Surg.*, **102**:293.

798. WEISS, S., BAKER, J. P. (1933): The carotid sinus reflex in health and disease; its role in the causation of fainting and convulsions. *Medicine*, **12**:297.

799. WEISS, S., FERRIS, E. B. (1934): Adams-Stokes syndrome with transient complete heart block of vasovagal reflex origin. *Arch. Intern. Med. (Chicago)*, **54**:931.

800. WELTI, H., WELTI, J. J., RETTORI, R., FONTAINE, G. (1964): A propos de l'implantation des pacemakers: problèmes chirurgicaux. *Mem. Acad. Chir. (Paris)*, **90**:480.

801. WELTI, J-J. (1964): In discussion. *Arch. Mal. Coeur*, **57**:313.

802. WELTI, J-J. (1965): In discussion. *Bull. Soc. Med. Hôp. Paris*, **116**:397.

803. WEYN, A. S., TAKAGI, M., CORRIN, K., BELLET, S. (1965): Hemodynamic comparison of isoproterenol and the artificial pacemaker in patients with complete heart block (Abstract). *Circulation*, **32** (Suppl. 2):218.

804. WHALEN, R. E., STARMER, F., McINTOSH, H. D. (1964): Electrical hazards associated with cardiac pacemaking. *Ann. N. Y. Acad. Sci.*, **111**:922.
805. WIDMANN, W. D. (1963): In discussion. *J. Thorac. Cardiov. Surg.*, **46**:455.
806. WIDMANN, W. D. (1964): In discussion. *Ann. N. Y. Acad. Sci.*, **111**:1043.
807. WIDMANN, W. D., GLENN, W. W. L., EISENBERG, L., MAURO, A. (1964): Radio-frequency cardiac pacemakers. *Ann. N. Y. Acad. Sci.*, **111**:992.
808. WIGGERS, C. J. (1924): The muscular reactions of the mammalian ventricles to artificial surface stimuli. *Amer. J. Physiol.*, **73**:346.
809. WIGGERS, C. J., WEGRIA, R. (1940): Ventricular fibrillation due to single, localized induction and condenser shocks applied during the vulnerable phase of ventricular systole. *Amer. J. Physiol.*, **128**:500.
810. WIGGERS, C. J., WEGRIA, R., PINERA, B. (1940): The effects of myocardial ischaemia on the fibrillation threshold—the mechanism of spontaneous ventricular fibrillation following coronary occlusion. *Amer. J. Physiol.*, **131**:309.
811. WILLIAM-OLSSON, G., ANDERSEN, M. N. (1963): The effect of pacemaker electrode site on cardiac output. *J. Thorac. Cardiov. Surg.*, **45**:618.
812. WILLIUS, F. A. (1923): Ventricular fibrillation in man with temporary cardiac recovery. *J. Lab. Clin. Invest.*, **8**:518.
813. WILSON, W. S., JUDGE, R. D., SIEGEL, J. H. (1964): A simple diagnostic sign in ventricular tachycardia. *New Eng. J. Med.*, **270**:446.
814. WILTSHIRE, H. (1923): A case of heart block illustrating the behaviour of the auricle during periods of prolonged ventricular silence. *Heart*, **10**:201.
815. WINDHOLZ, F., GRAYSON, C. E. (1947): Roentgen demonstration of calcifications in interventricular septum in cases of heart block. *Amer. J. Roentgen.*, **58**:411.
816. WINTERS, W. L., TYSON, R. R., SOLOFF, L. A. (1965): Cardiac pacemaking: I. Clinical experience. *Ann. Intern. Med.*, **62**:208.
817. WISOFF, B. G., GABOR, G. E., DONOSO, E. (1965): Pacemaker-induced ventricular tachycardia. *JAMA*, **192**:258.
818. WOOLFOLK, D., MILLAR, K., EICH, R. H., ABILDSKOV, J. A. (1965): Hemodynamic effects of ventricular activation order in experimental Purkinje net block (Abstract). *Circulation*, **32** (Suppl. 2):222.
819. WORTHINGTON, W. C. (1841): Remarkable slowness of pulse. *Lancet*, **2**:336.
820. WRIGHT, J. C., HEJMANCIK, M. R., HERRMANN, G. R., SHIELDS, A. H. (1956): A clinical study of complete heart block. *Amer. Heart J.*, **52**:369.
821. YATER, W. M. (1929): Congenital heart block: review of literature; report of case with incomplete heterotaxy; electrocardiogram in dextrocardia. *Amer. J. Dis. Child*, **38**:112.
822. YATER, W. M., BARRIER, C. W., McNABB, P. E. (1934): Acquired heart block with Stokes-Adams attacks dependent upon a congenital anomaly (persistent ostium primum): report of a case with detailed histopathologic study. *Ann. Intern. Med.*, **7**:1263.
823. YATER, W. M., CORNELL, V. H., CLAYTON, T. (1936): Auriculo-ventricular heart block due to bilateral bundle-branch lesions. *Arch. Intern. Med. (Chicago)*, **57**:132.

824. YUCEOGLA, Y. Z., LUNGER, M., DRESDALE, D. T. (1966): Transvenous electrical pacing of the heart. *Amer. Heart J.*, **71**:5.
825. ZOLL, P. M. (1952): Resuscitation of the heart in ventricular standstill by external electric stimulation. *New Eng. J. Med.*, **247**:768.
826. ZOLL, P. M., FRANK, H. A., LINENTHAL, A. J. (1964): Implantable cardiac pacemakers. *Ann. N. Y. Acad. Sci.*, **111**:1068.
827. ZOLL, P. M., FRANK, H. A., LINENTHAL, A. J. (1964): Four-year experience with an implanted cardiac pacemaker. *Ann. Surg.*, **160**:351.
828. ZOLL, P. M., FRANK, H. A., ZARSKY, R. N., LINENTHAL, A. J., BELGARD, A. II. (1961): Long-term electrical stimulation of the heart for Stokes-Adams disease. *Ann. Surg.*, **154**:330.
829. ZOLL, P. M., LINENTHAL, A. J., (1963): A program for Stokes-Adams disease and cardiac arrest (Signed editorial). *Circulation*, **27**:1.
830. ZOLL, P. M., LINENTHAL, A. J. (1963): External and internal electric cardiac pacemaker. *Circulation*, **28**:455.
831. ZOLL, P. M., LINENTHAL, A. (1964): External electric stimulation of the heart. *Ann. N. Y. Acad. Sci.*, **111**:932.
832. ZOLL, P. M., LINENTHAL, A. J., GIBSON, W., PAUL, M. H., NORMAN, L. R. (1958): Intravenous drug therapy of Stokes-Adams disease. Effects of sympathomimetic amines on ventricular rhythmicity and atrioventricular conduction. *Circulation*, **17**:325.
833. ZOLL, P. M., LINENTHAL, A. J., NORMAN, L. R. (1954): Treatment of Stokes-Adams disease by external electric stimulation of the heart. *Circulation*, **9**:482.
834. ZOLL, P. M., LINENTHAL, A. J., NORMAN, L. R., PAUL, M. E., GIBSON, W. (1955): Use of external electric pacemaker in cardiac arrest. *JAMA*, **159**:1428.
835. ZOLL, P. M., LINENTHAL, A. J., NORMAN, L. R., PAUL, M. E., GIBSON, W. (1955): External electric stimulation of the heart in cardiac arrest. *Arch. Intern. Med. (Chicago)*, **96**:639.
836. ZOLL, P. M., LINENTHAL, A. J., NORMAN, L. R., PAUL, M. H., GIBSON, W. (1956): Treatment of unexpected cardiac arrest by external electric stimulation of the heart. *New Eng. J. Med.*, **254**:541.
837. ZOLL, P. M., LINENTHAL, A. J., ZARSKY, L. R. N. (1960): Ventricular fibrillation—Treatment and prevention by external electric currents. *New Eng. J. Med.*, **262**:105.
838. ZOLL, P. M., PAUL, M. H., LINENTHAL, A. J., NORMAN, L. R., GIBSON, W. (1956): The effects of external electric currents on the heart. *Circulation*, **14**:745.
839. ZOOB, M., SMITH, K. S. (1963): The aetiology of complete heart block. *Brit. Med. J.*, **2**:1149.
840. ZUCKER, I. R., PARSONNET, V., GILBERT, L., ASA, M. M. (1963): Dipolar electrode in heart block. *JAMA*, **184**:549.
841. ZUCKER, I. R., PARSONNET, V., GILBERT, L., BERNSTEIN, A. (1965): Current status of the treatment of complete heart block. *Dis. Chest*, **47**:314.
842. ZUCKER, I. R., PARSONNET, V., MYERS, G. H., LOTMAN, H. A., ASA, M. M. (1963): Self-energized pacemakers: possibilities of using biologic energy sources (Abstract). *Circulation*, **28**:828.

843. ZUCKER, I. R., ROTHFELD, E. L., PARSONNET, V., GILBERT, L., BERNSTEIN, A. (1965): Competitive idiocardiac and extrinsic pacemaker stimuli in heart block. *Amer. Heart J.*, 69:62.
844. VAN DEN BERG, J., VAN DER HEIDE, J. N. H., NIEVEEN, J., BOONSTRA, E., KRAMER, D. (1962): An implantable transistorized pacemaker for the (human) heart with two gears and control of the resistance of the tissues, the electrodes and the pacemaker. *Konikl. Nederl. Akad. Wetenschappen*, 65:407.
845. BOTTI, R. E. (1966): A variant form of angina pectoris with recurrent transient complete heart block. *Amer. J. Cardiol.*, 17:443.
846. BREDIKIS, YU. I., KOSTENKO, I. G. (1964): The auricular rhythm in patients with the Morgagni-Adams-Stokes syndrome, before and after electrical cardiac stimulation. *Bull. Exp. Biol. Med.*, 55:375.
847. CASTELLANOS, A., LEMBERG, L., JUDE, J. R., BERKOVITS, B. V. (1966): Repetitive firing occurring during synchronized electrical stimulation of the heart. *J. Thorac. Cardiov. Surg.*, 51:334.
848. DACK, S. (1966): Complications of pacemaker therapy for heart block. (Consultant's corner). *Amer. J. Cardiol.*, 17:441.
849. DAVIES, J. G. (1965): Threshold measurements in pacemaking. *Resuscitation & Cardiac Pacing* (Proc. of Conference, Glasgow, March, 1964). London, Cassell, p. 197.
850. ERLANGER, J., BLACKMAN, J. R. (1909-1910): Further studies in the physiology of heart-block in mammals. Chronic auriculo-ventricular heart-block in the dog. *Heart*, 1:177.
851. FAULKNER, J. M. (1930): Adams-Stokes' syndrome in rheumatic fever: report of a case. *New Eng. J. Med.*, 202:1252.
852. FURMAN, S. (1966): Complications of pacemaker therapy for heart block (Consultant's corner). *Amer. J. Cardiol.*, 17:439.
853. FURMAN, S., ESCHER, D. J. W., SCHWEDEL, J. B., SOLOMAN, N. (1966): Transvenous pacing: a seven-year review. *Amer. Heart J.*, 71:408.
854. GILGENKRANTZ, J. M., CHERRIER, F., REBEIX, G., PETITIER, H., FAIVRE, G. (1965): L'entraînement électrosystolique externe au cours des blocs auriculo-ventriculaires du stade initial de l'infarctus myocardique. *Ann. Med. Nancy*, 4:459.
855. GLENN, W. W. L. (1966): Personal communication.
856. JENSEN, N. K., SCHMIDT, R., GARAMELLA, J. J., LYNCH, M. F., PETERSON, C. A. (1966): Intracavitary cardiac pacing. *JAMA*, 195:916.
857. McGUIRE, L. B., BECKWITH, J. R., LITTLEFIELD, J. B., MULLER, W. H. (1966): Experiences with implanted cardiac pacemakers (Annotation). *Amer. Heart J.*, 71:283.
858. MÜLLER, O. F., FINKELSTEIN, D. (1966): Adams-Stokes syndrome due to sinoatrial block. *Amer. J. Cardiol.*, 17:433.
859. MUSTARD, W. T. (1962): New developments in congenital cardiovascular surgery. *Bull. Hosp. Sick Child. Toronto*, 11:41.
860. OVERBECK, W., BÜCHNER, C., BILGER, R., GEBHARDT, W., STEIM, H., WIEMERS, K. (1965): Drei Jahre Erfahrung mit der Anwendung künstlicher Schrittmacher des Herzens. *Deutsch. Med. Wschr.*, 90:1701.
861. PARSONNET, V. (1966): Complications of pacemaker therapy for heart block. (Consultant's corner). *Amer. J. Cardiol.*, 17:440.

862. PENIDO, J. R. F., COTTON, B. H., COSBY, R. S. (1965): Indications for pacemakers in the treatment of heart block. *Amer. Surg.*, 31:659.

863. PIWNICA, A., MARCILLAC, J. P., ECOIFFIER, J. (1965): Stimulation électrique du coeur a long terme par sonde endocavitaire et pacemaker implantable. *Presse Med.*, 73:2561.

864. PRESTON, T. A., JUDGE, R. D. (1966): Letter to the editor. *Amer. J. Cardiol.*, 17:447.

865. SCHWARTZ, L. S., SCHWEDEL, J. B., SCHWARTZ, S. P. (1966): Adams-Stokes syndrome during angina pectoris associated with coronary artery disease. *Amer. J. Cardiol.*, 17:426.

866. SHIMAMOTO, T., MAEZAWA, H., YAMAZAKI, H., ATSUMI, T., FUJITA, T., ISHIOKA, T., SUNAGA, T. (1966): Pyridinolcarbamate, a bradykinin antagonist in veins. A preliminary report on pharmacologic and clinical observations. *Amer. Heart J.*, 71:297.

867. SONNENBLICK, E. H., FROMMER, P. L., BRAUNWALD, E. (1965): Electro-augmentation of human and cat papillary muscle produced by paired electrical stimulation. *Bull. N. Y. Acad. Med.*, 41:554.

868. SOWTON, G. E. (1966): Artificial pacing in intensive coronary care. In Shillingford, J. (ed.): *Intensive Coronary Care.* Oxford, Blackwell Scientific Publications.

869. SOWTON, E., DAVIES, J. G. (1963): Cardiac resuscitation with special reference to the apparatus. *Proc. Roy. Soc. Med.*, 56:278.

870. SUMA, M., FUJIMORI, Y., MITSUI, T., HORI, M., ASANO, K., KIMOTO, S., TOGAWA, T., NAGUMO, J. (1965): Direct induction pacemaker. *Digest of the 6th International Conference on Medical Electronic and Biological Engineering.* Tokyo, p. 96.

871. TAMURA, K., OGURO, M., AOKI, Y., KAWABE, A., MASHIMA, T., OGURO, C. (1966): Bilateral bundle branch block due to cardiac metastasis of pulmonary carcinoma. *Jap. Heart J.*, 4:294.

872. WENNEVOLD, A., MELCHIOR, J. C., SANDOE, E. (1965): Adams-Stokes syndrome in children without organic heart disease. *Acta Med. Scand.*, 177:557.

873. KARLSON, K. E., CARRACCI, W., KRASNOW, N., WECHSLER, B. M. (1966): Electrical pacing of the heart with endocardial and implanted pacemakers. *Ann. Surg.*, 163:339.

874. MARTIN, M. V., LIME, A. B., ALMEIDA, C. S., GERETTO, P., DEL NERO, R., MONFORT, J., SANTOS, RUBENS DE G., FELIPOZZI, H. J. (1966): Implantation of Chardack-Greatbatch adjustable rate and current pacemaker in a 4-months-old infant. *Pediatrics*, 37:323.

875. ZOLL, P. M. (1966): Personal communication.

876. HEIMAN, D. E., HELWIG, J. (1966): Suppression of ventricular arrhythmias by transvenous intracardiac pacing. *JAMA*, 195:1150.

877. MANSFIELD, P. B. (1966): On interference signals and pacemakers (Letter). *Amer. J. Med. Electronics*, 5:61.

878. SLAMA, R., BÉNÉVENT, J., MARNEFFE, H. (1966): Implantation d'un stimulateur intracorporel dans un cas de maladie de Stokes-Adams avec conduction auriculo-ventriculaire normale (Bloc sino-auriculaire ou "maladie" du sinus). *Arch. Mal. Coeur*, 59:292.

879. THALEN, H. J. T. (1966): Personal communication.

880. STAEWEN, W. (1966): Letter. *Amer. J. Med. Electronics,* **5**:64.

881. ALBERT, H. M., GLASS, B. A., ROBICHAUX, P., WILLIAMS, D., HALLER, W. (1966): Atrioventricular pedicle grafts in experimental heart block. *Ann. Thorac. Surg.,* **2**:237.

882. BROCKMAN, S. K., COLLINS, H. A., BLOOMFIELD, D. A., SINCLAIR-SMITH, B. C., GOBBEL, W. G. (1966): Physiological studies and clinical experience in patients with synchronous and asynchronous pacemakers. *J. Thorac. Cardiov. Surg.,* **51**:864.

883. DONATO, L., DENOTH, F. (1966): Self-synchronising cardiac pacemaker (Letter). *Lancet,* **2**:233.

884. FAIVRE, G., GILGENKRANTZ, J-M., CHERRIER, F., FRISCH, R. (1966): L'entraînement électrique du coeur au cours des blocs auriculo-ventriculaires. Résultats éloignés. *Arch. Mal. Coeur,* **59**:587.

885. GOETZ, R. H., DORMANDY, J. A., BERKOVITS, B. (1966): Pacing on demand in the treatment of atrioventricular conduction-disturbances of the heart. *Lancet,* **2**:599.

886. GONIN, A., PERRIN, A., DELAHAYE, J-P., POURCHAIRE, J., LOIRE, P. (1966): Indications et accidents précoces des pacemakers. Premier bilan de l'expérience française. *Arch. Mal. Coeur,* **59**:573.

887. HARRIS, A., DAVIES, M. J. (1966): Personal communication.

888. JOHANSSON, B. W. (1966): Complete heart block. A clinical, hemodynamic and pharmacological study in patients with and without an artificial pacemaker. *Acta Med. Scand.,* **180** Suppl.

889. KAISER, G. C., WILLMAN, V. L., HANLON, C. R. (1966): Implantable pacemakers in heart block. *Arch. Surg.,* **92**:600.

890. LAGERGREN, H., DAHLGREN, S., NORDENSTAM, H. (1966): Cardiovascular tissue response to intracardiac pacemaking. *Acta Chir. Scand.* In press.

891. LAGERGREN, H., JOHANSSON, L., KARLÖF, I., THORNANDER, H. (1966): Atrial-triggered pacemaking without thoracotomy: apparatus and results in twenty cases. *Acta Chir. Scand.* In press.

892. NEVILLE, J., MILLAR, K., KELLER, W., ABIDSKOV, J. A. (1966): An implantable demand pacemaker. *Clin. Res.,* **14**:256.

893. PARSONNET, V., GILBERT, L., ZUCKER, I. R. (1966): Permanent pacemaker insertion. A five-year appraisal. *Ann. Thorac. Surg.,* **2**:561.

894. PARSONNET, V., ZUCKER, I. R., GILBERT, L., MYERS, G. H. (1966): Clinical use of an implantable standby pacemaker. *JAMA,* **196**:784.

895. PELAŠKA, B. (1966): Improved method of long-term pacemaking. Presented at International Symposium *Electric Control of the Heart Beat.* Montecatini, Italy, April 1966.

896. PELAŠKA, B., BIČIK, V. (1966): A new conception of a universal implantable pacemaker. *Československa Fysiologie,* **15**:319.

APPENDIX

ADCOLE (MANSFIELD) IMPLANTED PACEMAKER. MODEL 5080B

Country of origin: USA.

Type: Fixed-rate totally implanted unit.

Manufacturer's
  address: Adcole Corporation
                330 Bear Hill Road
                Waltham, Massachusetts 02154
                USA.

Physical
  specification: Size: 4.8 x 4.3 x 1.1 cm
               Weight: 56 gm (2 oz).
               Construction: Potted in epoxy resin and covered with silicone rubber.

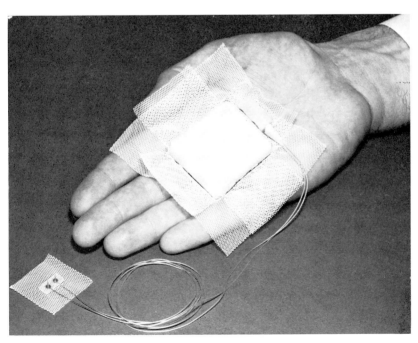

FIGURE 20. Adcole (Mansfield) pacemaker and electrodes.

269

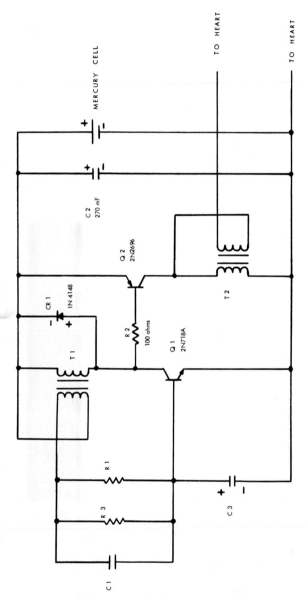

FIGURE 21. Circuit diagram of the Adcole (Mansfield) implantable pacemaker. The output transformer increases the voltage of the single mercury
cell to adequate values for stimulation.

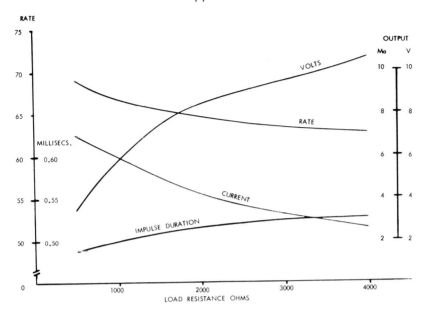

FIGURE 22. Alterations in output current, output voltage, impulse duration and stimulation rate of the Adcole (Mansfield) pacemaker with a resistive load.

Electrical
specification: Circuit: Blocking oscillator driving an amplifier stage which is transformer-coupled to the output. Open circuit 15 v. Internal resistance 1600 ohms.

    Impulse parameters
    Rate: Fixed at preset rate between 50-200/min.
    Impulse duration: 0.5 msec.
    Voltage: 6.5 v (at 5 ma).
    Impulse energy: 18 μJ.
    Impulse wave
    form: Square wave biphasic.
    Batteries: 1 mercury cell.
    Anticipated
    battery life: 3 yr.
    Dependence on
    load: See Fig. 22.

Electrodes: Bipolar. Multistranded stainless steel insulated with silicone rubber and terminating in polished conical stainless steel pins set in an insulating sheet. Electrode resistance is about 1200 ohms.

AIRBORNE INSTRUMENTS (GLENN) CARDIAC PACEMAKER

Country of origin: USA.

Type: Totally implanted receiving unit with bipolar myocardial electrodes. Radio frequency transmission across intact skin from external transmitter.

Manufacturer's address: Airborne Instruments Laboratory
Division of Cutler-Hammer, Inc.
Deer Park, Long Island, New York 11729
USA.

Physical specification: *Transmitter*

Size:	3.5 x 0.8 x 3.1 in.
Weight:	185 gm (6.2 oz).
Case material:	Molded polypropalene.
Operating temperature range:	0-50 C.
Antenna coil:	
Size:	5 x 5 in sq.
Weight:	42 gm (1.4 oz).
Connecting lead:	48 in long.

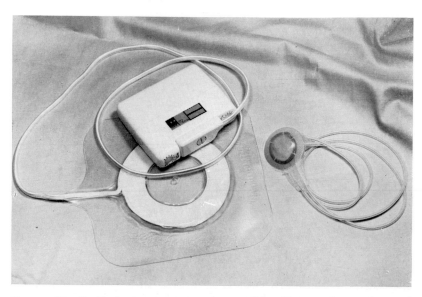

FIGURE 23. Radio frequency pacemaker used by Glenn and manufactured by Airborne Instruments Inc.

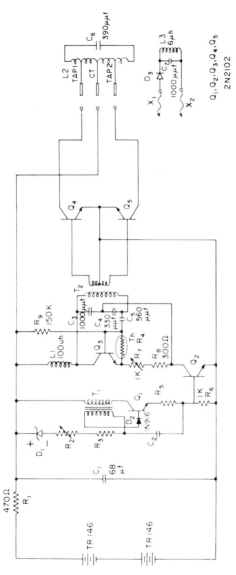

FIGURE 24. Circuit diagram of the Airborne Instruments (Glenn) radio frequency transmitter and implanted pacemaker. Reproduced by permission from *Ann. N.Y. Acad. Sci.*, 111:994-995.

Implanted receiver capsule

Size:	1.5 in diameter, 0.5 in thick.
Weight:	15 gm (0.5 oz).
Material:	Silicone rubber.
Electrodes:	Bipolar, multistrand helical-coil leads. Platinum iridium electrode to mediastinum and Elgiloy electrode to myocardium.

Electrical
specification:

	Rate adjustment:	45/120 beats/min.
	Amplitude adjustment:	3/18 v across electrodes (when heart impedance is 200 ohm).
	Pulse duration:	1 msec.
	Pulse type:	2-megacycle half-wave rectified pulse train.
	Battery life:	In excess of 10,000 hr (14 mo) at nominal pacemaker setting of 60 bpm and 6 v. Higher rates or levels decrease battery life proportionally. Replacement every 6 mo is suggested.
	Battery exhaustion:	Indicated by gradual decrease in pacing rate, giving several days notice.
	Battery replacement:	Pacemaker continues to function for 10 to 20 sec after removal of battery, allowing replacement of battery without interruption of pacing.

CORDIS "ATRICOR" ATRIAL-TRIGGERED PACEMAKER. MODEL 102

Country of origin: USA.
Type: Totally implanted atrial-triggered unit.
Manufacturer's
    address: Cordis Corporation
                             125 N.E. 40th Street
                             Miami, Florida 33137
                             USA.

Physical
specification:

	Size:	2¼ in (5.7 cm) diameter by 15/16 in (2.4 cm) thick.
	Weight:	5 oz (140 gm).
	Construction:	Potted in epoxy resin with stainless-steel indifferent electrode plate.

Electrical
specification:

	Circuit:	1-shot complementary multivibrator with buffer output. Constant current type (8-10 ma short-circuit).
	Atrial amplifier:	Single ended with 2 transistor stages powered by 3 mercury cells.

Lowest P wave: 1 mv. Input impedance 10,000 ohm. Frequency band width 10-250 cps. Voltage gain 300.

A-V delay circuit: 2 transistor 1-shot multivibrator actuated by a positive or negative signal of 0.3 v from the atrial amplifier; powered by 2 mercury cells.

Refractory circuit and self-pacer circuit: 2 transistor stage: free running multivibrator circuit oscillating at 60 cps if atrial input signal is of insufficient amplitude for triggering. Triggered by a negative pulse from the A-V delay circuit, powered by all 5 mercury cells. Free-running multivibrator circuit oscillating at 60 cps if atrial input signal is of insufficient amplitude for triggering. Triggered by a negative pulse from the A-V delay circuit, powered by all 5 mercury cells.

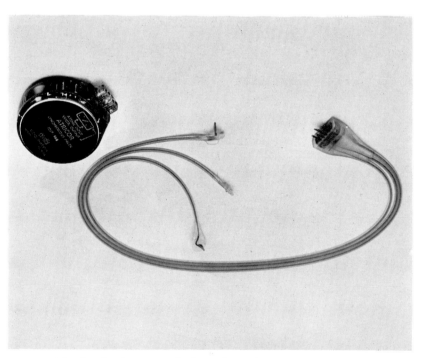

FIGURE 25. Cordis Atricor and electrodes. The atrial pick-up electrode is shown between two ventricular electrodes, only one of which is used: The other is a spare which can be brought into use by rotating the connecting plug through 180°.

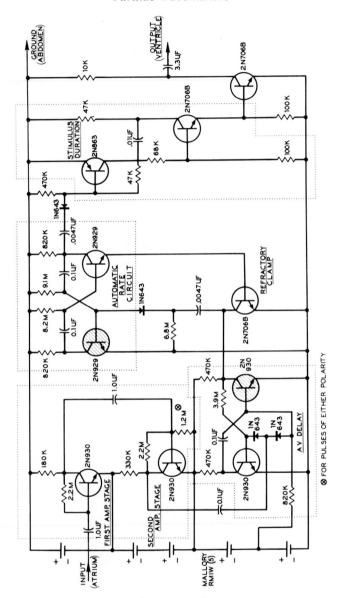

FIGURE 26. Cordis Atricor. Circuit diagram of the Cordis Atricor pace-maker. Reproduced by permission from Nathan *et al.: Progress in Cardio-vascular Diseases 1963/4.* Vol. 6., pp. 538-565.[546]

Output circuit: 2 transistor 1-shot multivibrator.

Output parameters

Rate: Maximum synchronous rate 125/min: If the
                   atrial rate exceeds 125/min a 2:1 atrial ven-
                   tricular block is introduced which changes to
                   3:1 if the atrial rate exceeds 250/min.

Batteries: 5 mercury cells. About 1 mo before batteries
                   are exhausted atrial-triggered pacing ceases
                   and fixed-rate pacing occurs.

Anticipated
battery life: 2 yr (at approximately 70 impulses/min).
Voltage: 6.5 v (open-circuit).
Impulse duration: 2 msec.
Impulse wave   Condenser discharge, initially negative with
form: late slow positive component.
Impulse energy: 50 μJ.

Electrodes: Two ventricular stimulating electrodes and one atrial pickup
                   electrode are attached to the unit with gold-plated pins and in-
                   sulated with a silicone rubber boot. Unipolar stimulation is
                   used, the second ventricular electrode being brought into use
                   when the connecting plug is rotated by 180°. The indifferent
                   electrode is a 5.6 cm diameter stainless steel plate on the pace-
                   maker. Ventricular electrodes (20 in long) are spiral Elgiloy in-
                   sulated with silicone rubber; the terminal 4.5 mm coil penetrates
                   the myocardium. The atrial electrode (20 in long) is spiral
                   Elgiloy insulated in silicone rubber except for the terminal 6.4
                   mm which is half exposed and can be sutured to the surface of
                   the atrium.

Alternative models with higher input sensitivity and/or higher maximum synchronous rates are also available.

CORDIS "VENTRICOR," FIXED-RATE, IMPLANTABLE PACEMAKER. MODEL 111

Country of origin: USA.

Type: Totally implanted fixed-rate unit.

Manufacturer's
address: Cordis Corporation
                   125 NE 40th Street
                   Miami, Florida 33137
                   USA.

Physical
specification: Size: 2¼ in diameter (5.7 cm) times 15/16 in
                                  thick (2.4 cm)
                   Weight: 5 oz (140 gm)
                   Construction: Potted in epoxy resin with stainless steel in-
                                  different electrode plate incorporated.

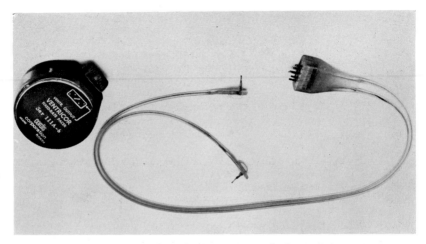

Figure 27. Cordis Ventricor and electrodes.

Electrical
  specification: Circuit: Free-running complementary multivibrator with buffer output, providing a constant current (8-10 ma short-circuit).

                Batteries: 5 mercury cells.
                Anticipated
                  battery life: 3 yr.

                Output parameters
                  Rate: Fixed at 70/min.
                  Impulse wave
                    form: Condenser discharge.
                  Impulse
                    duration: 2 msec.
                  Voltage: 6.5 v (open-circuit).
                  Energy: 50 μJ.

Electrodes: Unipolar spiral "Elgiloy" (nickel-cobalt alloy, Elgin Watch Co.) insulated in silicone rubber tubing and turning to enter myocardium. Stainless steel indifferent plate on pacemaker.

COTELEC IMPLANTABLE PACEMAKER. MODEL GES 999

Country of origin: France.

Type: Fixed-rate totally implanted unit.

Manufacturer's
  address: Cotelec
              Société Francaise d'Etudes et de
              Contructions Electroniques

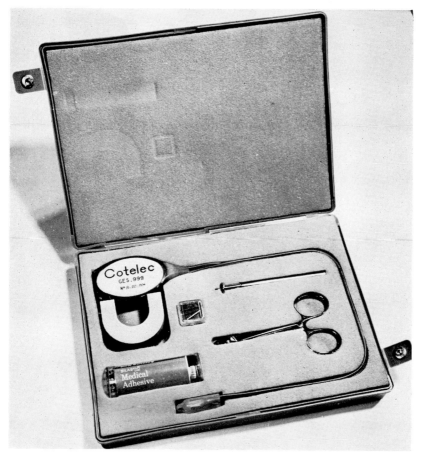

FIGURE 28a. Cotelec pacemaker with integral electrodes and magnet for actuating internal on-off switch.

	64 Rue du Chateau	
	Boulogne (Seine)	
	France.	
Physical specification:	Size:	Flat egg-shaped container, volume 60 cc.
	Weight:	140 gm (5 oz)
	Construction:	Potted in epoxy resin and covered with silicone rubber.
Electrical specification:	Circuit:	Blocking oscillator. On-off magnetic switch can be activated before or after implantation.

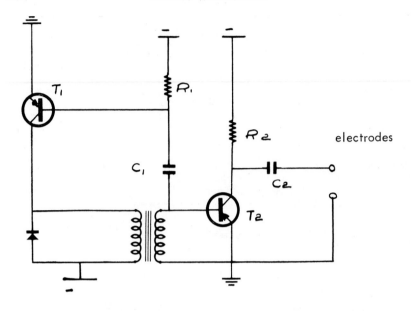

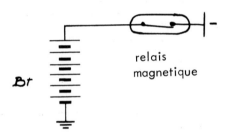

FIGURE 28b. Circuit diagram of the Cotelec pacemaker G.E.S. 999.

Batteries:	5 mercury cells.
Anticipated battery life:	2 yr. Stimulation frequency increases over several weeks as batteries near exhaustion. Batteries can be conserved during storage by use of on-off switch.

Output parameters

Rate:	Fixed at 60/min.
Voltage:	6.5 v leading edge, 5.5 v trailing edge.
Impulse duration:	2 msec

	Impulse wave
form:	Fast rising upstroke with exponential decay.
Impulse energy:	Approximately 170 μJ into 300 ohm.

Electrodes:	Helical platinum-iridium wire insulated with silicone rubber which is hermetically sealed to the coating of the pacemaker.

DEVICES (ST. GEORGE'S HOSPITAL) IMPLANTABLE PACEMAKER (ABDOMINAL TYPE)

Country of origin: England.

Type: Totally implanted fixed-rate unit.

Manufacturer's
address: Devices Implants Ltd.
13-15 Broadwater Road
Welwyn Garden City Hertfordshire
England.

Distributed by: P.J. Reynolds Ltd.
22 Waverly Road
Enfield, Middlesex
England.

Physical
specification:

Size:	5.5 x 4.0 x 2.0 cm.
Weight:	100 gm (3½ oz).
Construction:	Potted in epoxy resin and covered with silicone rubber.

Electrical
specification:

Circuit:	Blocking oscillator with transformer output. See Fig. 30.
Batteries:	4 mercury cells.
Anticipated battery life:	3 yr. Stimulation frequency decreases as batteries near exhaustion.

Output parameters

Rate:	Fixed at 70/min or as required within the range 40-120/min.
Impulse wave form:	Initially square wave but capacitor differentiated to prevent polarization.
Impulse duration:	0.8-1.0 msec.
Voltage:	5.0 v minimum open-circuit. 2.5 v minimum into 47 ohm load.
Energy:	Approximately 60 μJ into 300 ohm load.
Dependence on load:	Impulse duration, stimulation rate and output voltage essentially unchanged with loads between 100-1000 ohm. Impulse energy is load-dependent. See Fig. 31.

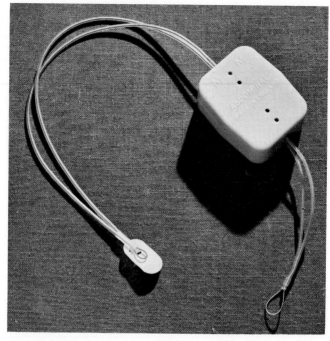

FIGURE 29. Devices (St. George's Hospital) abdominal-type pacemaker and electrodes. The shorter electrode is the platinum indifferent.

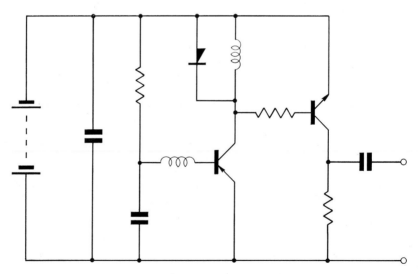

FIGURE 30. Devices. Circuit of Devices (St. George's Hospital) pacemakers.

LOAD TEST ON ABDOMINAL TYPE PACEMAKER

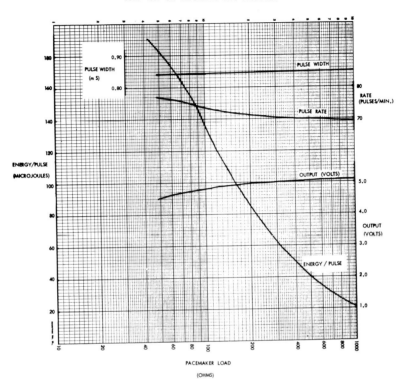

FIGURE 31. Devices abdominal. Relation between pacemaker load and impulse parameters for Devices abdominal-type pacemaker.

Electrodes: Unipolar. A continuous coil of stainless steel, insulated in silicone rubber, runs from the pacemaker to the heart and returns to the pacemaker. A 10 mm length is free of insulation and is sutured onto the epicardium. The two ends of this coil must be attached in the sockets marked "M" (myocardial) which are negative during the impulse. Indifferent electrode is coiled platinum wire partially insulated in silicone rubber.

DEVICES (ST. GEORGE'S HOSPITAL) IMPLANTABLE PACEMAKER (AXILLARY TYPE A)

Country of origin: England.

Type: Fixed-rate totally implanted unit.

Manufacturer's
address: Devices Implants Ltd.
13-15 Broadwater Road

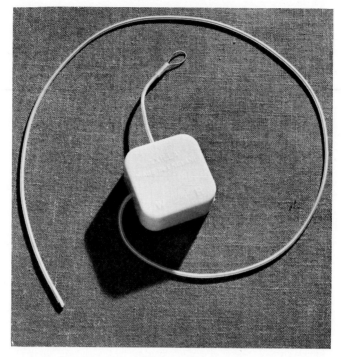

FIGURE 32. Devices (St. George's Hospital) axillary Type A pacemaker. An endocardial and a short platinum indifferent electrode are also shown.

	Welwyn Garden City, Hertfordshire England.	
Distributed by:	P.J. Reynolds Ltd. 22 Waverly Road Enfield, Middlesex England.	
Physical specification:	Size:	4.3 x 4.3 x 2.2 cm.
	Weight:	80 gm (2¾ oz).
	Construction:	Potted in epoxy resin and covered with silicone rubber.
Electrical specification:	Circuit:	Blocking oscillator with transformer output. See Fig. 30.
	Batteries:	3 mercury cells.
	Anticipated battery life:	3 yr. Stimulation frequency decreases as batteries near exhaustion.

LOAD TEST ON AXILLA TYPE PACEMAKER

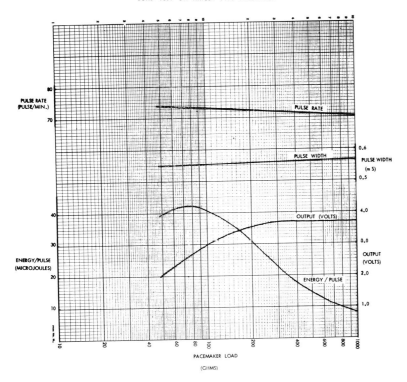

FIGURE 33. Devices axillary. Relation between pacemaker load and impulse parameters for Devices axillary pacemaker.

Output parameters

Rate:	Fixed at 70/min or as required within the range 40-120/min.
Impulse wave form:	Initially square wave but capacitor differentiated to prevent polarization.
Impulse duration:	0.5-0.8 msec.
Voltage:	3.5 v minimum open-circuit.
	2.5 v minimum into 150 ohm load.
Energy:	Approximately 25 μJ into 300 ohm load.
Dependence on load:	Impulse duration, stimulation rate and output voltage essentially unchanged with loads between 200 and 1000 ohm. Impulse energy load-dependent.

Electrodes: Any transvenous catheter electrode with small area terminal contacts. One suitable unipolar electrode must be connected to the socket marked "C" (catheter) which is negative during the impulse. The indifferent electrode is a platinum helical spring insulated in silicone rubber and terminating in a loop which makes tissue contact.

ELA STIMULATEUR CARDIAQUE INTRACORPOREL. MODEL SC1-4 (ALSO KNOWN AS HELLIGE-FRANCE PACEMAKER MODEL SIC4)

Country of origin: France.

Type: Totally implanted unit with preset rate and amplitude.

Manufacturer's address:

L'Electronique Appliquée
Services Commerciaux
96-100 Rue Maurice Arnoux
Montrouge (Seine)
France.

Distributed by:

Hellige-France
88 Route de Bischwiller
Strasbourg-Schiltigheim
France.

Physical specification:

Size: 6.1 x 5.6 x 2.1 cm.
Weight: 154 gm (5½ oz).
Construction: Potted in epoxy resin. Countersunk, screwdriver actuated controls for on/off, stimulation rate and amplitude for use before implantation.

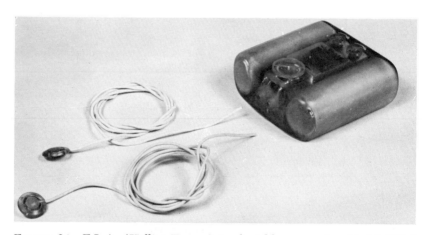

FIGURE 34. E.L.A. (Hellige-France) implantable pacemaker Model SCI-4 and epicardial electrodes.

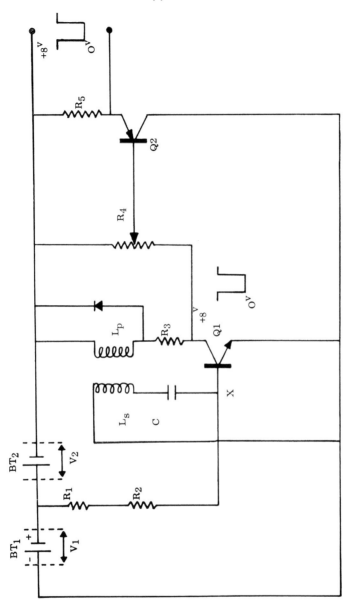

FIGURE 35. E.L.A. Circuit of E.L.A. (Hellige-France) pacemaker.

Electrical
specification:

Circuit: Blocking oscillator with constant output impedance.

Batteries: 6 mercury cells arranged in 2 groups of 3.

Anticipated
battery life: 2 yr. Stimulation frequency increases as batteries near exhaustion.

Impulse parameters

Rate: Can be preset to any value between 40-110/min before implantation. Normally set at 70/min.

Voltage: Can be preset to any value up to 8 v before implantation; normally set at 6.5 v. On/off switch can be used to prevent battery drain during storage.

Impulse duration: 2 msec.

Impulse wave
form: Square wave.

Impulse energy: Dependent upon load impedance.

Electrodes: Silver-plated steel wires attached to platinum discs which are sutured to the epicardium.

Note: When the pacemaker is viewed end-on with the set-screws uppermost, the right-hand electrode socket is negative during the impulse; the right-hand control adjusts the rate and the left-hand control the amplitude.

ELECTRODYNE IMPLANTABLE PACEMAKER. MODEL TR-14

Country of origin: USA.

Type: Totally implanted fixed-rate unit.

Manufacturer's
address:
Electrodyne Company Inc.
15 Southwest Park
Westwood, Massachusetts 02091
USA.

Physical
specification:

Size: 6.5 x 5.0 x 2.0 cm.

Weight: 176 gm (4½ oz).

Construction: Two independent complete inner coatings with epoxy resin and an outer coating of a different epoxy resin which is well tolerated by human tissue. The whole instrument is enclosed in a Teflon® mesh bag so that tissue growth will anchor the pacemaker.

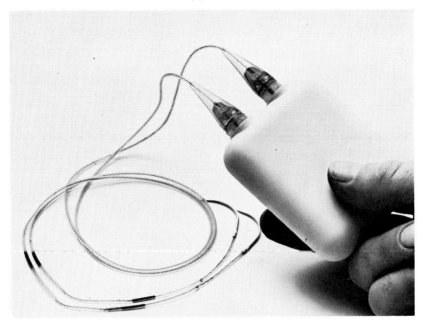

FIGURE 36. Electrodyne pacemaker Model TR 14 and electrodes.

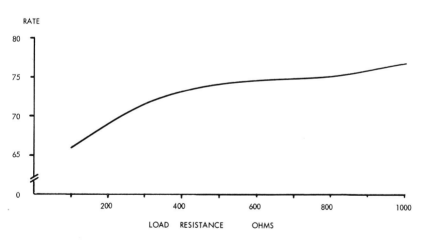

FIGURE 37. Electrodyne. Relation between pacemaker load and stimulation rate for Electrodyne Model TR 14. Drawn from data published by Zoll: *Ann. N.Y. Acad. Sci.*, 111:1072.

Electrical
specification: Circuit: Blocking oscillator. 15 ma constant current
                                            output.
                      Batteries: 6 mercury cells.
                      Anticipated
                        battery life: 3-5 yr. Stimulation frequency decreases by
                                            about 5% as batteries near exhaustion.

                      Output parameters
                        Rate: Fixed at 70/min.
                        Impulse wave
                          form: Sharp rising, rounded with a late positive
                                            wave so that total net charge transfer is zero.
                        Impulse duration: 2 msec.
                        Voltage: 7.5 v.
                        Energy: 190 μJ into 500 ohms.
                        Dependence on
                          load: Stimulation rate increases with increasing
                                            load. See Fig. 37.

Electrodes: Bipolar coiled stainless steel wires, plated with gold and sited
                      in the ventricular wall.

ELEMA-SCHÖNANDER PACEMAKER. MODEL EM 138

Country of origin: Sweden.

Type: External adjustable unit for long-term direct myocardial stimula-
                      tion.

Manufacturer's
  address: Elema-Schönander AB
                      Industrivägen 23
                      Stockholm-Solna
                      Sweden.

Physical
specification: Size: 10.5 x 7.5 x 3.2 cm.
                      Weight: 400 gm (14 oz).
                      Construction: Enclosed in white plastic case and carried in
                                            a shoulder sling beneath the patient's clothes.

Electrical
specification: Circuit: High stability multivibrator with comple-
                                            mentary transistors.
                      Batteries: 9 mercury cells.
                      Anticipated
                        battery life: Over 9 mo, batteries easily replaceable.

                      Output parameters
                        Rate: Selected by 6-position switch.
                                            Position   1. 25-30/min
                                                        2. 45-50/min
                                                        3. 70-75/min

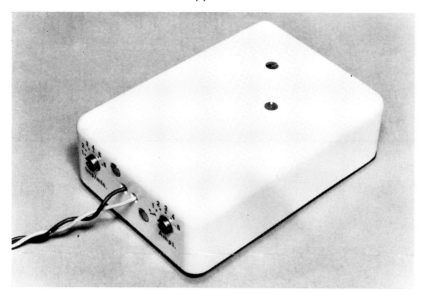

FIGURE 38.   Elema 138. Elema-Schönander pacemaker Model EM 138. The
unit is carried externally in a sling and connected to a transvenous catheter.

	4. 85-90/min
	5. 100-110/min
	6. 140-150/min
Impulse wave form:	Differentiated biphasic.
Impulse duration:	2-2.5 msec.
Voltage:	Selected by 5-position switch with on/off position.
	Position 1. 2 v (leading edge)
	2. 5 v
	3. 6 v
	4. 8.5 v
	5. 11 v
Electrodes:	As for implantable pacemakers Models EM 139 and EM 141. The red lead is negative during the stimulus with respect to the yellow lead.

ELEMA-SCHÖNANDER IMPLANTABLE PACEMAKER. MODEL EM 139

Country of origin:	Sweden.
Type:	Fixed-rate totally implanted unit.
Manufacturer's address:	Elema-Schönander AB Industrivägen 23

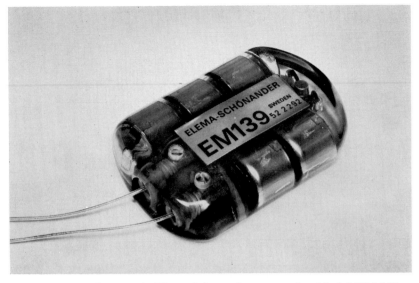

FIGURE 39. Elema 139. Elema-Schönander pacemaker Model EM 139.

Stockholm-Solna
Sweden.

Physical
specification:

Size: Approximately 30 sq cm by 2.2 cm thick.
Weight: 130 gm (4½ oz).
Construction: Potted in epoxy resin.

Electrical
specification:

Circuit: High stability multivibrator with complementary transistors.
Batteries: 5 mercury cells.
Anticipated
battery life: 2 yr. Stimulation frequency increases by 1-2% when batteries near exhaustion. Complete failure of one cell increases frequency by 2%.

Output parameters

Rate: Fixed at 70/min or at any rate between 50-90/min to special order.
Impulse wave
form: Differentiated biphasic.
Impulse duration: 2-2.5 msec.
Voltage: Over 6 v (leading edge).
Impulse energy: Approximately 100 μJ into 300 ohm load.
Dependence on
load: Stimulation frequency and impulse duration are dependent on load.

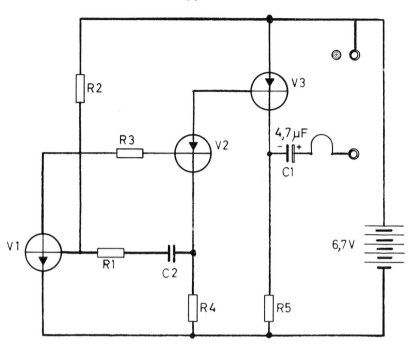

FIGURE 40. Elema 139. Circuit of Elema-Schönander pacemaker Model
EM 139.

Electrodes: Myocardial electrode Type EMT 567: 9 mm diameter platinum
               disc to be sutured to epicardium; attached to 600 mm long mul-
               tistrand, stainless steel tape coiled and insulated with polythene.
               The attachment to the platinum disc is protected with epoxy
               resin.

               Endocardial catheters Types EMT 570 and EMT 588: uni-
               polar. Platinum tip 6 mm long and 2.5 mm (EMT 588) or 3
               mm (EMT 570) diameter attached to similar wire as used for
               myocardial electrodes but with an additional outer insulation of
               silicone rubber.

               Indifferent electrode EMT 564, 2 cm diameter flat stainless steel
               disc attached to similar wire.

ELEMA-SCHÖNANDER IMPLANTABLE PACEMAKER. MODEL EM 141

Country of origin: Sweden.

Type: Totally implanted atrial-triggered unit.

Manufacturer's
address: Elema-Schönander AB
Industrivägen 23
Stockholm-Solna

Physical Sweden.
specification: Size: 6.5 x 6.0 x 2.2 cm.
Weight: 125 gm.
Construction: Potted in epoxy resin.

Electrical
specification: Circuit: P wave amplifier is a common emitter grounded 2-stage amplifier. PQ-delay circuit is a 1-shot multivibrator. Blocking circuit is a 1-transistor stage. Fixed-rate generator is a multivibrator with complementary transistors. Output stage is a 1-transistor amplifier. Lowest P wave amplitude 0.9 mv. PQ-delay time 100-120 msec.

Output parameters

Rate: Highest synchronous rate 140-150/min. When atrial rate exceeds 150/min, intermittent ventricular stimuli are dropped so that

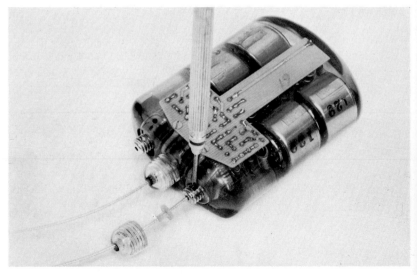

FIGURE 41. Elema 141. Elema-Schönander atrial-triggered pacemaker Model EM 141 (laboratory model).

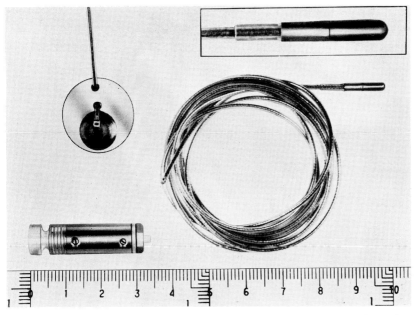

FIGURE 42. Elema 141. Elema-Schönander endocardial catheter electrode, indifferent electrode and external connector.

as the atrial rate increases to 10% over the synchronous limit a 2:1 block is slowly introduced. Fixed minimum rate 50/min.

Impulse wave form:	Capacitor discharge.
Duration:	2-2.5 msec.
Voltage:	Over 5 v (leading edge).
Energy:	Approximately 35 μJ into 300 ohm load.
Electrodes:	As for fixed-rate type EM 139. Atrial potential pick-up electrode is a unipolar catheter, Type EMT 588, positioned outside the atrium against the posterior wall, with a mediastinoscope.

IMPLANTABLE PACEMAKER. MODEL EKS 2

Country of origin:	USSR.
Type:	Fixed-rate totally implanted unit.
Manufacturer's address:	VO Medexport Moscow G-200 USSR.

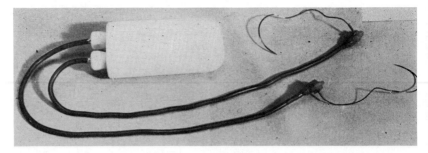

FIGURE 43. Russian EKS-2 stimulator and myocardial electrodes.

Physical
  specification: Construction: Flat container with rounded corners.
                     Weight: 125 gm (4½ oz).
                     Anticipated
                     battery life: 2.5-3 yr.

                     Output parameters
                      Rate: Fixed at 60/min.
                     Impulse duration: 1.8 msec.

Electrodes: Platinum-iridium spirals covered with silicone rubber and at-
                     tached to the pacemaker by a boot.

FLORENCE UNIVERSITY (CAMMILLI-GRASSI) RADIO FREQUENCY
PACEMAKER

Country of origin: Italy.

Type: External radio frequency transmitter with internal receiving unit
                     attached directly to the heart.

Manufacturer's
  address: Developed at
                     Arcispedale di Santa Maria Nuova
                     (Professor Dott. Leonardo Cammilli)
                     (Surgical Service)
                     Florence
                     Italy.

Physical
  specification: *External Unit*
                     Size: 10 cm x 2 cm thick.
                     Weight: 75 gm (2½ oz) plus batteries.
                     Construction: Plastic case with removable covers held by
                                      screws. An aluminium battery container (9
                                      x 7 x 4 cm) is connected by flexible cable.

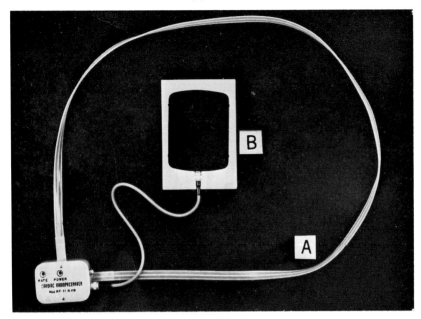

FIGURE 44. Florence University (Cammilli-Grassi) radio frequency pacemaker. Antenna A is attached to the skin overlying the implanted receiving unit. The transmitter is powered by a separate battery pack B.

	Internal Unit	
	Size:	3.2 cm diameter by 0.5 cm thick.
	Weight:	5.6 gm.
	Construction:	Insulating plate with both surfaces coppered and silver plated, carrying electronic components and covered in silicone rubber.
Electrical specification:	*External Unit*	
	Circuit:	Relaxation oscillator with electronic (transistor) switch regulated by Shokley diode controlling capacitor discharge. Pulses transmitted via oscillator circuit with approximately 20 w RF power dissipated.
	Power supply needed:	36 v, continuous current of 0.6 ma peak current 800 ma.
	Internal Unit:	Inductance composed of 20 concentric turns photoengraved on plated disc, with 80 pF tuning condenser and silicone diode (OA95-TD) for half-wave rectification.

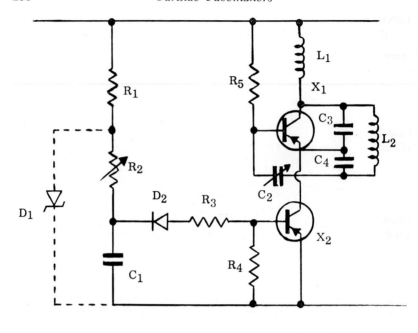

R1	-	10k	C1	-	22ufS 35vw
R2	-	50k	C2	-	150-470 pf
R3	-	33.39	C3	-	850 pf
R4	-	180	C4	-	33 pf
R5	-	2.7k	X1	-	2N1046
L1	-	3uH	X2	-	**ASZ** 18

FIGURE 45. Florence University (Cammilli-Grassi). Transmitter circuit of Cammilli-Grassi radio frequency pacemaker. Reproduced by permission from *Ann. N.Y. Acad. Sci.*, **111**:1009.

Output parameters

Rate: 30-150/min.
Impulse duration: 1-10 msec (Standard is 2 msec).
Voltage: Limited by Zener diode in internal unit to 6.8 v.
Impulse wave
form: Rectilinear biphasic.
Batteries: 4 x 9 v units in series provide power for 5 days continuous pacing. Rate slows as batteries near exhaustion.

Electrodes: Bipolar spike electrodes of 10% platinum-iridium; size: 1 mm diameter, 7 mm long, 1 cm apart and connected by a Zener diode and a capacitor. Integral with internal unit.

GENERAL ELECTRIC COMPANY (USA) IMPLANTABLE PACEMAKERS (DUAL-RATE MODEL A2070AA. BASIC-RATE MODEL A2070AB)

Country of origin: USA.

Type: Fixed-rate totally implantable units.
The dual-rate model has a switch activated by an externally applied magnet. Both models can be controlled via an externally applied induction coil.

Manufacturer's
address: General Electric Company
Pacemaker Division
4855 Electric Avenue
Milwaukee, Wisconsin
USA.

Physical
specification: Construction: 6 x 5 x 2 cm.
Size· 140 gm (5 oz).
Weight: Potted in epoxy resin and covered with silicone rubber.

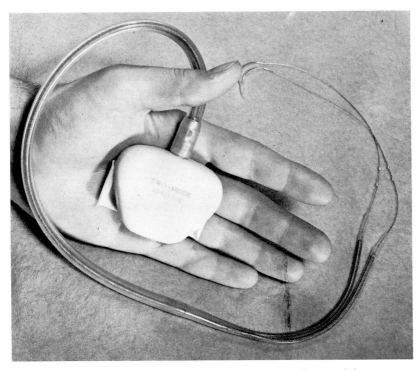

FIGURE 46. General Electric (USA) dual-rate pacemaker Model A2070 AB with electrodes.

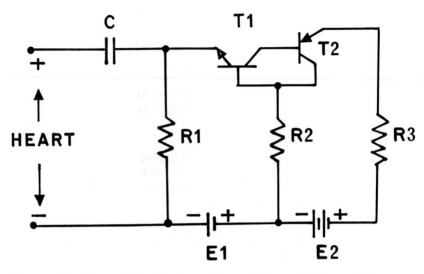

FIGURE 47. General Electric. Basic circuit of General Electric (USA) pacemakers.

Electrical
specification: Circuit: Basic circuit is a complementary multivibrator with capacitor coupled output. A coil is wound round the assembled components and connected at two points. Constant energy output.

                   Batteries: 5 mercury cells.
                   Anticipated
                    battery life: 4 yr. Stimulation frequency decreases as batteries near exhaustion.

Output parameters
                   Rate: Basic rate fixed at 70/min.
                                     Active rate fixed at 85/min.
                                     Rate changed in dual-rate model by temporary application of external magnet. Rate may be temporarily increased up to 120/min by an optional external control (both models).
                   Voltage: 3.8 v (leading edge) into 300 ohm load.
                   Impulse duration: 1.7-2.0 msec effective duration. Approximately 8 msec total duration.
                   Impulse wave
                    form: Biphasic differentiated (capacitor discharge).
                   Impulse energy: Constant at any one rate; 40-68 μJ, at 70/min. Impulse energy is approximately halved if rate is doubled.

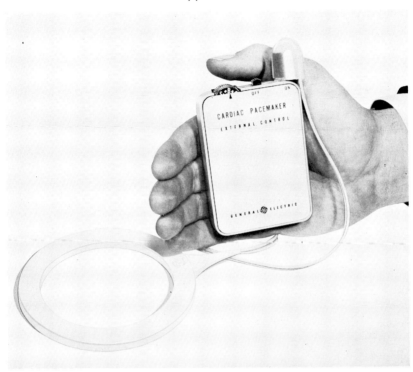

FIGURE 48. General Electric. External control and primary coil for General Electric (USA) pacemakers.

Dependence on
load: Rate increases if load impedance increases; impulse energy falls as rate increases.

External control unit:

Physical
specification: Aluminium case 9 x 6 x 1.5 cm connected by a 38 cm cable to a flat induction coil 8.5 cm diam.

Electrical
specification: Circuit is similar to implanted unit. In use the external induction coil is taped to the patient's skin over the implanted unit.

Electrodes: Bipolar spirally wound coils of 343 filaments of stainless steel bonded with silver and floating in silicone fluid within sealed silicone rubber tubing. Contact is made within the myocardial wall by 1.5 cm of noninsulated wire.

HOKKAIDO IMPLANTABLE PACEMAKER. MODEL MS-21

Country of origin: Japan.

Type: Fixed-rate totally implantable unit.

Manufacturer's
  address: Developed by
                    Research Institute of Applied Electricity
                    and Second Department of Surgery
                    Hokkaido University
                    Sapporo
                    Japan.

Physical
  specification: Size: 6.5 x 7.2 x 2.2 cm.
                    Weight: 180 gm (6½ oz).
                    Construction: Potted in epoxy resin.

Electrical
  specification: Circuit: Blocking oscillator. See Fig. 49.
                    Batteries: 6 mercury cells.

                    Output parameters
                    Rate: Fixed, 65 to 75/min.
                    Voltage: 7.8 v.
                    Impulse duration: 1.75 to 2.0 msec.
                    Impulse wave
                      form: Square wave biphasic.

Electrodes: Stainless steel coil with an internal straight wire.

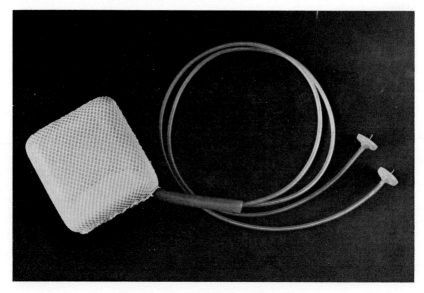

FIGURE 49. Hokkaido pacemaker.

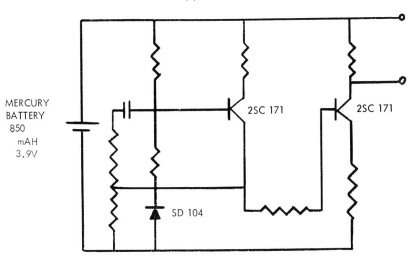

F<small>IGURE</small> 50. Hokkaido. Circuit of Hokkaido implantable pacemaker.

HYCON IMPLANTED RECHARGEABLE PACEMAKER. MODEL AD NOS. 1-10

Country of origin: USA.

Type: Fixed-rate totally implantable unit with rechargeable batteries.

Manufacturer's
address: Hycon Manufacturing Company
700 Royal Oaks Drive
Monrovia, California 91017
USA.

Physical
specification: *Internal unit*

Size:	7 cm diameter x 2.2 cm thick.
Weight:	192 gm (6¾ oz).
Construction:	Potted in epoxy resin.
External unit:	Metal-cased charging equipment connected by cable to a small hand-held electromagnet which can be placed over the pacemaker for recharging.

Electrical
specification: *Internal unit*

Circuit: RC complementary oscillator with additional charging circuitry. Average current drain 25 μa. Internal source impedance 500 ohm.

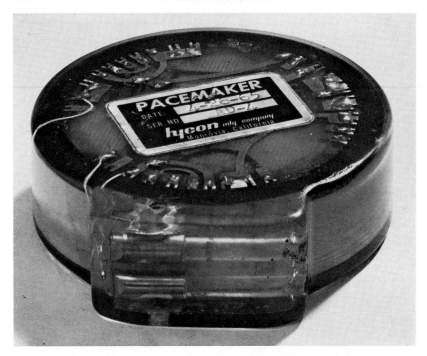

FIGURE 51.   Hycon implantable rechargeable pacemaker.

Batteries:	6 nickel-cadmium cells.
Anticipated battery life:	Approximately 3 mo without recharging. Since frequent recharging prolongs battery life this is recommended every day, thus limiting current drain to less than 1% of total cell capacity. Without recharging, batteries lose 50% of capacity in 150 days at 100 F (38 C).

Impulse parameters

Rate:	Fixed at 72/min or preset at factory to other rates.
Voltage:	3.2 v into 1000 ohm load.
Impulse duration:	2 msec.
Impulse wave form:	Square wave biphasic.
Impulse energy:	20 μJ.

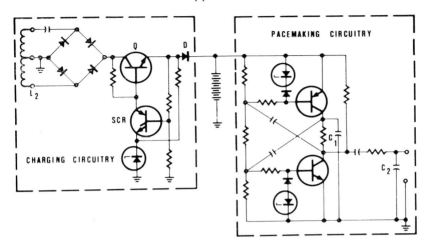

FIGURE 52. Hycon. Circuit of Hycon implantable, rechargeable pacemaker. Reproduced by permission from Silver *et al.* (1965): *Ann. Thorac. Surg.*, 1:380-388.[699]

External (charging) unit:

Circuit:	Phase-shift oscillator (5 kc) and push-pull amplifier driving electromagnet (L1). See Fig. 52.
Power supply:	Main line supply converted to 15 v dc. Total consumption 4 w.
Battery recharging:	Performed for a few minutes each day. The external electromagnet (L1) is held over the pacemaker and an induced current flows in the tuned coil (L2). The additional current flow in L1 associated with this flow in L2 is monitored on a meter (M), which indicates when the batteries are fully charged (or that charging is faulty). The induced current in the pacemaker is fed to the batteries via a transistor (Q) and a diode (D); when the battery voltage reaches a preset level a silicon-controlled rectifier (SCR) fires and prevents transistor (Q) passing current, to prevent overcharging. The cessation of current flow is reflected in the reading of meter (M) in the external unit. When charging is complete current leakage through the charging circuitry is prevented by the diode (D).

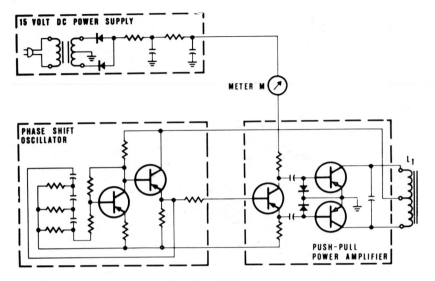

FIGURE 53. Hycon. Circuit of external charging equipment for Hycon pacemaker. Reproduced by permission from *Ann. Thorac. Surg.*, 1:380-388, 1965.

During charging a 5 kc sine wave voltage appears across the pacemaker output, but the amplitude is reduced by capacitors C1 and C2. Maximum ripple voltage during charging is 20 mv RMS.

Electrodes: Medtronic-Chardack coil electrodes used.

LUCAS (ABRAMS-LIGHTWOOD) INDUCTIVELY COUPLED CARDIAC PACEMAKER

Country of origin: England.

Manufacturer's   Joseph Lucas Ltd.
address: Monkspath
                    Shirley
                    Solihull
                    Warwickshire
Physical   England.
specification: Sizes:
                    External
                    electronic unit: 3¾ in (9.4 cm) x 2⅞ in (7.2 cm) x 1⅝ in
                                       (4.1 cm).

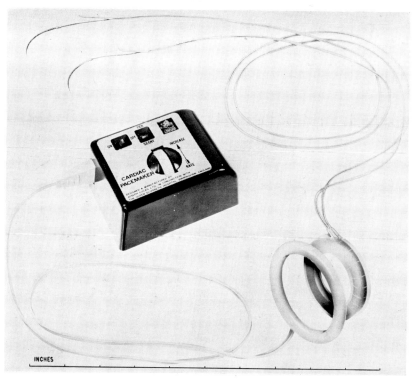

FIGURE 54. Lucas induction pacemaker, with external primary coil, internal secondary coil and bipolar myocardial electrodes.

Implanted coil
(adult size): $2\frac{5}{16}$ in (9.4 cm) outside diameter 1¼ in (3.18 cm) inside diameter $\frac{5}{16}$ in (0.785 cm) thick.
(child size): $1\frac{11}{16}$ in (4.26 cm) outside diameter, ¾ in (1.9 cm) inside diameter, $\frac{5}{16}$ in (0.785 cm) thick.

Weights:
External
electronic unit: 12.9 oz (366 gm)
Implanted coil
and leads
(adult):   1.95 oz (55.4 gm)
Implanted coil
and leads
(child):   1.08 oz (30.7 gm)
Surface material:
Electronic unit: Molded polycarbonate (Makrolon).
Implanted coils: Hot cured silicone rubber.

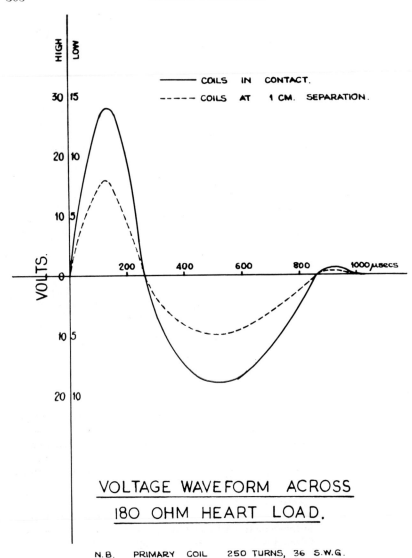

FIGURE 55. Lucas. Impulse wave form produced by Lucas induction pacemaker.

Electrical
  specification: Circuit: Voltage converter circuit charging a capac-
                                       itor whose energy is discharged into the pri-
                                       mary (external) coil via an S.C.R. The stim-

ulating pulse is induced in the secondary (implanted) coil and conducted to the heart by stainless steel electrodes. The pulse rate is varied by adjusting the rate of energy conversion in the voltage converter circuit. The output pulse characteristic is constant and does not vary with battery voltage or pulse rate. The wave form of the pulse appearing across the heart is shown in the diagram, for the two levels of pulse energy (*high* and *low* power) which are available from the electronic unit. The pulse width can be varied, if desired, by changing the design of the primary (external) coil, between 250 ps and 3 ms. The pulse width does not vary with load impedance. If the external coil fractures or is not correctly connected, the pacemaker emits a loud warning noise.

Pulse rate is patient-controlled between 30 and 100 ppm. The rate does not vary with load impedance.

Power source: Single U2 cell (life one month on low power operation, one week on high power). Battery changing easily accomplished by patient. Pulse rate falls slowly as battery is used, but impulse power remains constant: patient restores rate to appropriate value until end of the control is reached, indicating need to replace battery.

Electrodes: Endocardial catheter electrode No. 997.200.01: unipolar. Wound from three strands of 0.008 in diameter stainless steel wire as a helix of internal diameter 0.024 in. Insulated with silicone rubber sleeve of 0.1 in external diameter. Platinum tip welded to wire. Standard length of catheter is 31 in (80 cm), but other lengths available to special order.

A single wire stainless steel stylet is used during manipulation but withdrawn later. The catheter is connected via a push-fit self-sealing adaptor requiring no adhesive, so the stylet can be reinserted for any subsequent manipulation.

MEDTRONIC (GREATBATCH-CHARDACK) IMPLANTABLE CARDIAC PACEMAKERS. MODELS 5860, 5870 AND 5870C

Country of origin: USA.

Type: Fixed-rate totally implanted units.
Models 5870 and 5870C include provision for percutaneous adjustment of rate and amplitude.

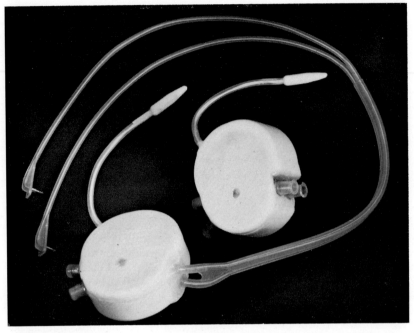

FIGURE 56. Medtronic Chardack-Greatbatch Model 5870 variable rate, variable output implanted pacemaker with Medtronic Chardack Model 5814 myocardial electrodes.

Manufacturer's address:	Medtronic, Inc. 3055 Highway 8 Minneapolis 18, Minnesota USA.	
Physical specification:	Size:	2½ in (6.3 cm) diameter by 1 in (2.5 cm) thick.
	Weight:	5 oz (140 gm).
	Construction:	Potted in epoxy resin and covered with silicone rubber.
Electrical specification:	Circuit:	Blocking oscillator/amplifier, with capacitor discharge output. The units do not provide constant current, voltage or power.
	Batteries:	6 mercury cells in fixed-rate unit, 5 mercury cells in variable rate unit.

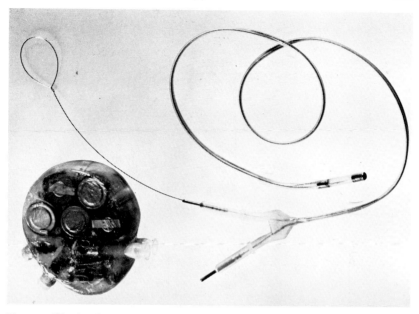

FIGURE 57. Medtronic Chardack-Greatbatch Model 5870C variable rate, variable output implantable pacemaker with Medtronic Chardack Model 5816 endocardial catheter electrode.

Anticipated battery life:	3 yr. Stimulation frequency increases slightly as batteries near exhaustion, but impulse intensity falls so the patient returns to idioventricular rhythm.

Output parameters Model 5860.

Rate:	Fixed at 60/min.
Impulse wave form:	Biphasic, capacitor discharge.
Impulse duration:	1.6 msec.
Voltage:	1.5 v (trailing edge).
Current:	3 ma (trailing edge).
Impulse energy:	Approximately 10 μJ.

Model 5870.

As for model 5860 with variable amplitude (0-5 ma) and rate (40-100/min and off) by means of controls adjusted with needles inserted percutaneously.

Model 5870C.

As for model 5870 with amplitude adjustable

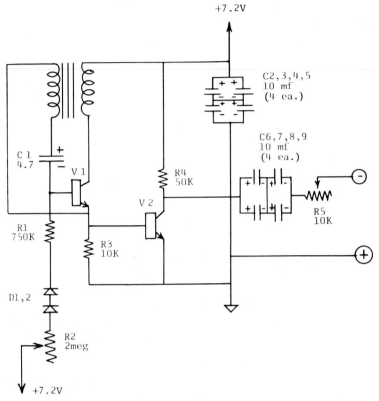

FIGURE 58. Circuit of Medtronic Greatbatch pacemakers. Reproduced by permission from Chardack *et al.* (1964): *Ann. N.Y. Acad. Sci.*, **111**:1075.[133]

up to 5.0 v and rate adjustable as for model 5870.

Electrodes: Medtronic/Chardack Model 5814 Myocardial Electrode: Platinum-iridium alloy wire (diameter 0.01 in) coil spring (diameter 2.044 in) freely movable within an insulating sleeve of silicone rubber tubing. The coil extends in one piece from the pacemaker terminal to an electrode plate where it turns to terminate as the electrode pin, the last three turns of the coil being opened slightly to permit ingrowth of fibrous tissue between the spirals.

Medtronic/Chardack Model 5816 Endocardial Catheter Electrode: Bipolar transvenous electrode of two adjacent stainless steel springs running in silicone rubber insulation and terminating in platinum electrode terminals. Stainless steel stylets can be inserted into the lumen of the coils to aid initial positioning, but should be withdrawn later.

PELAŠKA IMPLANTABLE PACEMAKERS

Country of origin: Czechoslovakia.

Type: Totally implanted fixed-rate units.

Manufacturer's
address: Research Institute for Medical Electronics
                (Director: B. Pelaška, M.D., Sc.D.)
                Prague 4-Krč
                Budejovicka 800
                Czechoslovakia.

Physical
specification: Varies with number of cells.

Size: 2-cell unit: 4.6 x 3.9 x 2.2 cms.
                            7-cell unit: 6.8 x 5.3 x 2.2 cms.

Weight: 2-cell unit: 55 gm.
                            7-cell unit: 150 gm.

Construction: Both potted in special epoxy resin.

Electrical
specification: 6 units are available containing from 2 to 7
cells. The circuit is identical for all models
(see Fig. 60).

Output parameters

Rate: Fixed rate, normally at 76 impulses/min.
Impulse duration: Approx. 1.3 msec.
Voltage: 2.6 v (2 cell model).
                            9.1 v (7 cell model).

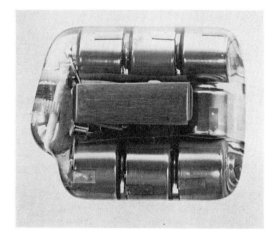

FIGURE 59. Peleška pacemaker (Czechoslovakia).

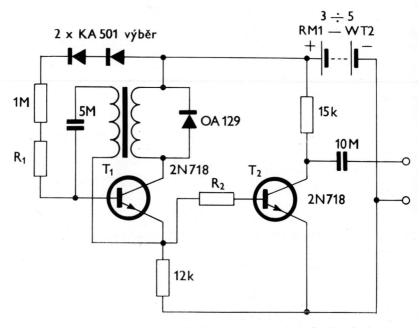

FIGURE 60. Circuit of Peleška pacemaker (Czechoslovakia).

Energy: Varies with model and load. Approx. 30 μJ
                 for 2 cell model and 300 ohm load.
Battery: 2 to 7 mercury cells.

Estimated battery
  life: Varies with model and load from 1.8 years
                 (7 cell model, 300 ohm load) to 5.8 years
                 (2 cell model, 300 ohm load). Rate increases
                 as batteries near exhaustion.

Electrodes: Indifferent (positive) electrode attached to body of pacemaker.
                 Elema catheter electrode (q.v.) used for transvenous pacing.
                 Devices myocardial electrode (q.v.) used for epicardial or in-
                 tramural pacing.

PRESBYTERIAN-ST. LUKE'S HOSPITAL IMPLANTED PACEMAKER

Country of origin: USA.

Type: Totally implanted fixed-rate unit. A dual-rate version provides
                 a choice of two fixed rates.

Manufacturer's
  address: Designed by
                 Robert W. Sessions

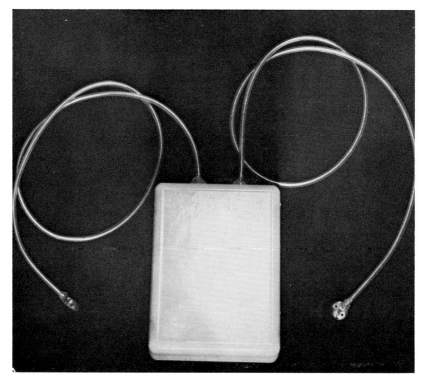

FIGURE 61. Presbyterian-St. Luke's Hospital implantable pacemaker and epicardial electrodes.

Presbyterian-St. Luke's Hospital
Chicago, Illinois
USA.

Physical specification:	Size:	8 x 6 x 2 cm (single and double rate units).
	Weight:	Single rate unit—184 gm.
		Double rate unit—204 gm.
	Construction:	Potted in epoxy resin and covered with medical grade silicone rubber.
Electrical specification:	Circuit:	Blocking oscillator with capacitor output. Constant impulse energy.
	Batteries:	4 or 5 mercury cells.
	Anticipated battery life:	3 yr. Stimulation frequency decreases as batteries near exhaustion. Prophylactic replacement of pacemaker recommended after 2 yr.

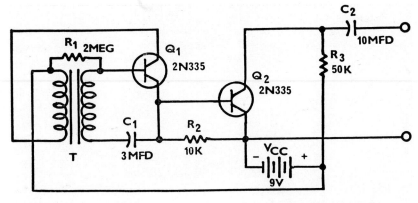

FIGURE 62.   Circuit of Presbyterian-St. Luke's Hospital pacemaker.

Output parameters

Rate: Fixed at 75/min. Dual-rate unit provides fixed rates of 75/min and 100/min selected by a switch operated with an external magnet.

Impulse wave
  form: Square wave biphasic.
Impulse duration: 2 msec.
Voltage: 5.6-7.0 v.
Energy: Approximately 50-60 μJ into 1200 ohm load.
Dependence on
  load: Impulse voltage, but not stimulation rate, is load-dependent.

Electrodes: Stainless steel ribbon coiled on polythene core and insulated in polythene and silicone rubber tubing; termination at 9 mm diameter platinum disc electrode which is sutured onto the epicardium.

PYE IMPLANTABLE PACEMAKER. MODEL EM 1005

Country of origin: England.

Type: Totally implanted fixed-rate unit with optional external rate control.

Manufacturer's
  address: Pye Laboratories Ltd.
                    Pacemaker Division
                    St. Andrews Road
                    Cambridge
                    England.

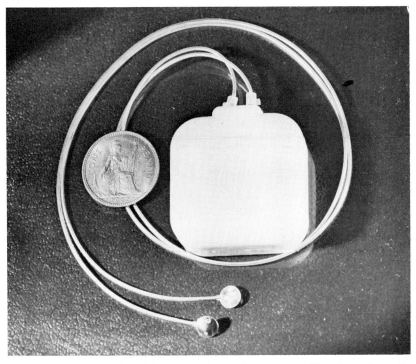

FIGURE 63. Pye implantable pacemaker with screw-in self-sealing electrode attachments.

Physical specification:	Internal unit:	
	Size:	5.0 x 5.0 x 1.8 cm.
	Weight:	100 gm (3½ oz).
	Construction:	Potted in epoxy resin and covered with silicone rubber.
Electrical specification:	Internal unit:	
	Circuit:	A stable RC controlled multivibrator containing no transformer. Substantially constant voltage output.
	Batteries:	5 mercury cells.
	Anticipated battery life:	4 yr. Stimulation frequency increases as batteries near exhaustion.
Output parameters		
	Rate:	Fixed at 66/min or as required to special order. The rate may be temporarily slowed to

Cardiac Pacemakers

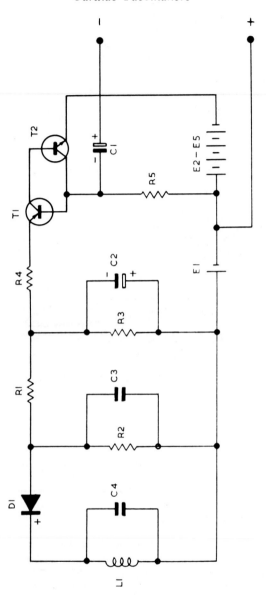

FIGURE 64. Circuit of Pye implantable pacemaker.

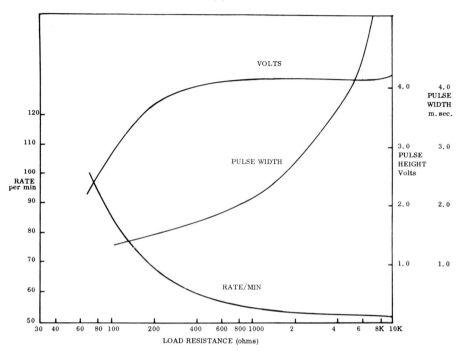

FIGURE 65. Pye. Relation between output parameters and load resistance for Pye pacemakers.

	30/min by the use of an inductively coupled external control.
Impulse wave form:	Differentiated biphasic wave form with a rise time of less than 20 μsec.
Impulse duration:	1.75 msec at 90% amplitude.
Voltage:	5 v peak (leading edge) into 1000 ohm load.
Energy:	Approximately 90 μJ into 300 ohm load.
Dependence on load:	Variations between 300 and 2000 ohms result in changes of less than ±5% in amplitude and rate and less than ±25% in duration and rise time. See Fig. 65.
Electrodes:	Epicardial Disc Type EM 1006: Consists of 4 helical stainless steel tape conductors welded at separate sites to a platinum hemisphere 0.7 cm radius. The covering is medical grade polythene and sealing is with medical grade epoxy resin. Length 50 cm; diameter 1.6 mm.

Intramural Electrode Type EM 1007: Consists of a double spiral of platinum-ruthenium wire 4.0 cm long wound on a terylene suture and replacing the platinum hemisphere of Type EM 1006.

SUMA-TOGAWA INDUCTION PACEMAKER

Country of origin: Japan.

Type: External generator with induction to implanted receiving unit. Both primary (external) and secondary (internal) coils are iron-cored.

Manufacturer's
  address: Developed by Dr. K. Suma and
                   Dr. T. Togawa.
                   Institute for Medical Electronics
                   Faculty of Medicine
                   University of Tokyo
                   Hongo, Tokyo
                   Japan

Commercial
  version available
  from: Medical Electronics Division
                   Nippon Electric Company

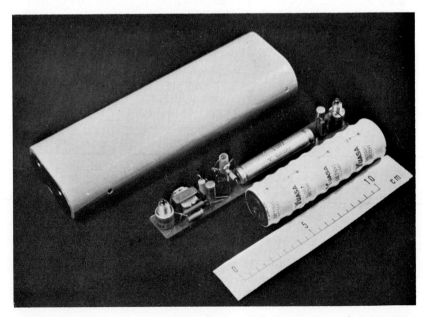

FIGURE 66. Suma-Togawa. External unit of Suma-Togawa induction pacemaker.

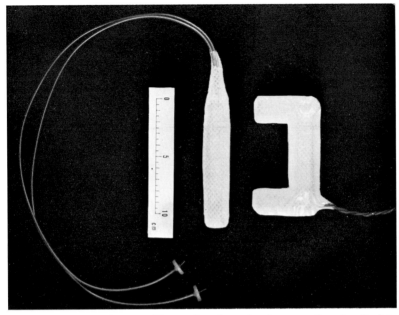

FIGURE 67. Suma-Togawa. External U-shaped primary coil and cylindrical implantable secondary coil attached to bipolar myocardial electrodes. Both coils are iron cored.

		Honjuku, Fuchushi, Tokyo Japan.
Physical specification:	External unit: Size: Internal unit: Size: Construction:	U-shaped primary coil. 9 x 5 cm. Secondary coil wound on iron core. 10 x 1.0 x 0.1 cm. The entire internal unit is covered with silicone rubber.
Electrical specification:	External unit: Circuit: Batteries: Internal unit: Circuit: Impulse wave form:	 Condenser discharge with S.C.R. electronic switch. Primary coil wound with 500 turns of 0.5 copper wire. Nickel-cadmium. Secondary coil wound with 3000 turns of 0.1 polyurethane-coated copper wire. Biphasic modified sine-wave.
Electrodes:	Bipolar. Integral with secondary coil.	

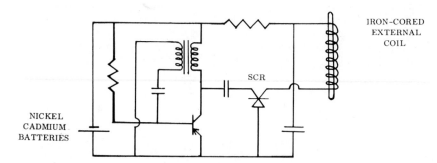

IRON–CORED
EXTERNAL
COIL

SCR

NICKEL
CADMIUM
BATTERIES

FIGURE 68. Suma-Togawa. Circuit of external unit of Suma-Togawa induction pacemaker.

VITATRON IMPLANTABLE PACEMAKERS. MODELS MIP 100 AND MIP 200

Country of origin: Holland.

Type: Totally implanted unit with two fixed rates; switching actuated by an external magnet.

Manufacturer's
address: 1. Vitatron N V

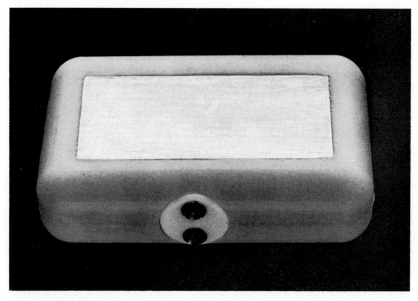

FIGURE 69. Vitatron pacemaker, Model MIP 100, showing the stainless steel plate indifferent electrode and the locking screws for attachment of the myocardial electrode.

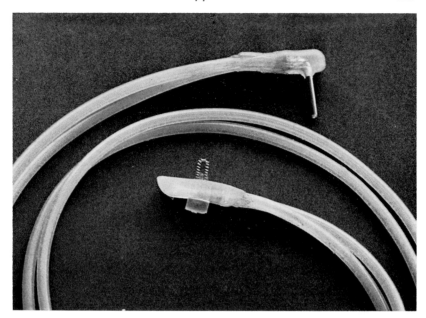

FIGURE 70. Vitatron myocardial electrode MIP 120 with silicone rubber button (to be removed later) to aid implantation in the heart muscle. The pin for connection to the pacemaker is also shown.

		Spoorstraat 23
		Dieren
		Holland.
	2.	Vitatron N V
		Medical Instrument Department
		Lindenstraat 44
		Amsterdam C
		Holland.

Physical specification:	Size:	8.0 x 5.0 x 2.2 cm.
	Weight:	155 gm.
	Construction:	Potted in epoxy resin and covered with medical grade silicone rubber.

Electrical specification:	Circuit:	Multivibrator. Protected against high frequency current during electrocauterization.
	Batteries:	Model MIP 100: 5 mercury cells.
		Model MIP 200: 6 mercury cells.
	Anticipated battery life:	Model MIP 100: 3-5 yr.
		Model MIP 200: 2-3 yr.
		Stimulation frequency decreases slightly as

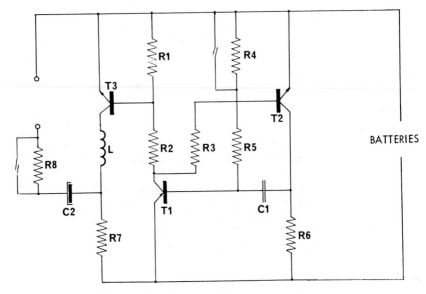

FIGURE 71. Circuit of Vitatron pacemakers.

batteries near exhaustion, with a very rapid increase later. The life of the unit can be temporarily extended by strapping the external magnet to the chest wall over the pacemaker ("prolonged lifetime mode"). A reed switch then short-circuits an internal resistor.

Output parameters

Rate:	Fixed at 70/min or 95/min. Rates are
Impulse wave	switched by means of an external magnet.
form:	Monophasic square wave with late positive component providing area-matching.
Impulse duration:	Model MIP 100: 2 msec.
	Model MIP 200: 3 msec.
Voltage:	Model MIP 100: 6.5 v peak.
	Model MIP 200: 7.8 v peak.
Maximum impulse	
charge:	Model MIP 100: approximately 45 microcoulombs.
	Model MIP 200: approximately 120 microcoulombs.
Impulse energy:	Model MIP 100: 125 μJ.
	Model MIP 200: 325 μJ.

Dependence on
   load: Stimulation rate increases slightly as load resistance increases. Impulse voltage independent of load.

Electrodes: Intramural Type MIP 120: consists of two spirals of platinum: iridium (90%:10%) imbedded in solid silicone rubber. The wire coil runs from the pacemaker connecting pin to the heart and back to the connecting pin.

The pacemaker has sockets for two connecting pins but only one is electrically live (marked "-"). The other socket (marked "R" for reserve) is intended for a spare electrode as an aid to rapid location.

Indifferent electrode: stainless steel plate, size 26 x 58 mm attached to pacemaker. Adaptors are available for connection to other manufacturers' electrodes.

PRELIMINARY REPORTS ON NEW IMPLANTABLE PACEMAKERS

First Author (reference no.)	*Year*	*Pacemaker*
Byron [92]	1965	2-cell rechargeable pacemaker used in dogs.
Bonnabeau [55]	1965	Epicardial pacemaker using 2 nickel-cadmium cells which run down in 50 days unless recharged.
		Size: 2 x 4 x 1 cm, sutured to heart. Used for up to 7 months in dogs.
		Impulse: 2-5 v, 5 ma. 2 msec square wave. Circuit used free running. Complementary multivibrator.
Campbell [99]	1965	Rechargeable pacemaker using nickel-cadmium cells used in dogs. Skin burns produced during recharging.
Furman [253]	1965	Rechargeable pacemaker using nickel-cadmium cells.
		Size: 3.5 cm diameter x 1 cm thick.
		Weight: 30 gm. Sutured to heart with stainless steel electrodes acting as electrodes.
		Rate: 70/min. Impulse: 0.5 msec. Interval between charging 4-5 mo. Used in dogs.
Lillehei [54]	1963	P wave pacemaker detecting atrial potentials via bipolar ventricular electrodes which are also used for stimulation. Not used clinically by 1966.[449]
Luan-Ch'iang [482]	1964	Induction type: external unit uses cold cathode discharge tube (circuit given in reference). Internal unit 3.5 cm diameter, covered with silicone rubber, connected to heart by bipolar electrode wires.
		Impulse wave form: monophasic 2 msec duration.
		Rate: 60-130/min. Used in dogs and clinically.

INDEX